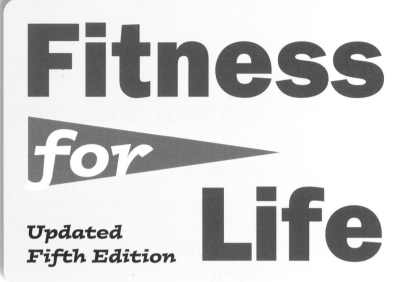

Fitness for Life

Updated Fifth Edition

Authors:

Charles B. Corbin
Arizona State University

Ruth Lindsey
California State University

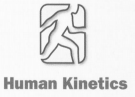

Human Kinetics

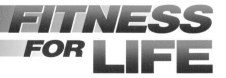

Library of Congress Cataloging-in-Publication Data

Corbin, Charles B.
 Fitness for life / Charles B. Corbin, Ruth Lindsey.-- Updated 5th ed.
   p. cm.
 Includes index.
 ISBN-13: 978-0-7360-6676-1 (soft cover)
 ISBN-10: 0-7360-6676-4 (soft cover)
 1. Physical fitness. I. Lindsey, Ruth, 1926- II. Title.
 RA781.C584 2007
 613.7--dc22

                        2006004028

ISBN-10: 0-7360-6676-4
ISBN-13: 978-0-7360-6676-1

The Web addresses cited in this text were current as of February 2006, unless otherwise noted.

Acquisitions Editor: Scott Wikgren; **Developmental Editor:** Jennifer Clark; **Managing Editor:** Kathleen Bernard; **Assistant Editor:** Derek Campbell; **Copyeditor:** Joanna Hatzopolous Portman; **Proofreader:** Kim Thoren; **Indexer:** Sharon Duffy; **Permission Manager:** Dalene Reeder; **Graphic Designer:** Robert Reuther; **Graphic Artists:** Angela K. Snyder and Denise Lowry; **Photo Manager:** Dan Wendt; **Cover Designer:** Keith Blomberg; **Photographer (cover):** Dan Wendt; **Photographer (interior):** © Human Kinetics unless otherwise noted: © Photodisc—photos on pp. 26, 53(l/r), 60, 80, 124, 153, 175, 176(r), 190 (t/b), 200, 201(t), 211, 233(b), 288, 298, and 313; © DigitalVision—photos on pp. 15(l/r), 37(l/r), 70(r), 93, 97(l/r), 112(r), 126, 127(l/r), 146, 233(t), 270, 277, 278, 292, and 314(l/r); © Eyewire—photos on p. 3, 85(t), 102, 107, 120(l), and 121; © 1994 CMSP All Rights Reserved—photos on p. 44; © Urban Leisure—photo on p. 145; photo on p. 47 courtesy of Sankyo Pharma (l = left; r = right; t = top; b = bottom); **Art Manager:** Kelly Hendren; **Illustrators:** Argosy (medical art) and Mic Greenberg; **Printer:** Custom Color Graphics

Printed in the United States of America   10 9 8 7 6 5 4 3 2

Human Kinetics
Web site: www.HumanKinetics.com

United States: Human Kinetics, P.O. Box 5076, Champaign, IL 61825-5076
800-747-4457
e-mail: humank@hkusa.com

Canada: Human Kinetics, 475 Devonshire Road Unit 100, Windsor, ON N8Y 2L5
800-465-7301 (in Canada only)
e-mail: orders@hkcanada.com

Europe: Human Kinetics, 107 Bradford Road, Stanningley, Leeds LS28 6AT, United Kingdom
+44 (0) 113 255 5665
e-mail: hk@hkeurope.com

Australia: Human Kinetics, 57A Price Avenue, Lower Mitcham, South Australia 5062
08 8277 1555
e-mail: liaw@hkaustralia.com

New Zealand: Human Kinetics, Division of Sports Distributors NZ Ltd., P.O. Box 300 226 Albany, North Shore City, Auckland
0064 9 448 1207
e-mail: info@humankinetics.co.nz

contents

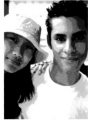
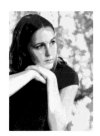
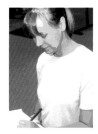

editorial board

Phil Abbadessa, MEd
Physical Education Department Chair
Mountain Pointe High School
Phoenix, Arizona

Rick Amundson
Curriculum, Instruction, and Assessment Specialist
Webster School District
Webster, New York

Marybell Avery, PhD
Curriculum Specialist for Health and
    Physical Education
Lincoln Public Schools
Lincoln, Nebraska

Chris F. Corley
Physical Education Coordinator
Vista Ridge High School
Leander, Texas

Donna L. Cunningham, MS
Boy Scouts of America
Venturing Division
Amarillo, Texas

Doris Dorr
Health Fitness Teacher
Toppenish School District
Toppenish, Washington

Jim Hart, EdD
K-12 Physical Education Specialist
Eugene School District 4J
Eugene, Oregon

Richard C. Hohn
Professor Emeritus
Department of Physical Education
University of South Carolina
Columbia, South Carolina

Martha Hyder
Clinical Instructor
Southern Utah University
Cedar City, Utah

Ray D. Martinez, EdD
Department of Exercise & Sport Science
University of Wisconsin-La Crosse
La Crosse, Wisconsin

Guy C. Le Masurier, PhD
Arizona State University
Mesa, Arizona

Karen E. McConnell, PhD, CHES
Associate Professor
Pacific Lutheran University
Tacoma, Washington

Marilu D. Meredith, EdD
Vice-President, IT
Project Director, *FITNESSGRAM*
The Cooper Institute
Dallas, Texas

Julio Morales, PhD
Department of Health and Kinesiology
Lamar University
Beaumont, TX

Sarajane V. Quinn
Coordinator of Health, Physical Education, and
    Dance
Baltimore County Public Schools
Baltimore County, Maryland

Janet A. Seaman, PED, MBA, CAPE
Executive Director
American Association for Active Lifestyles and Fitness
A national association of AAHPERD
Reston, Virginia

Joan Van Blom
Physical Education Curriculum Leader
Long Beach Unified School District
Long Beach, California

Robert A. Widen
Adjunct Faculty
Prescott College
Prescott, Arizona

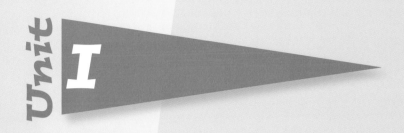

Getting Started

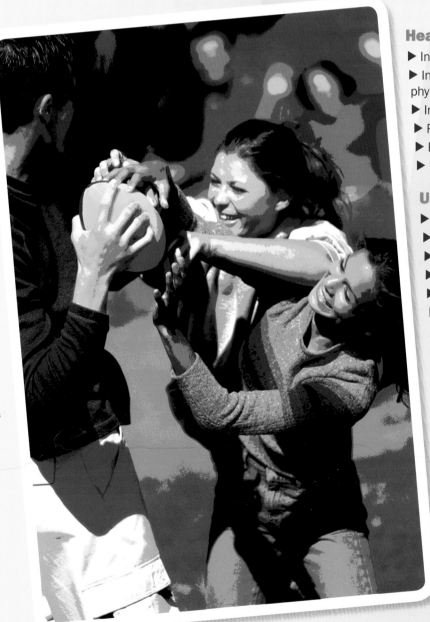

Healthy People 2010 Goals

▶ Increase daily physical activity for all people.
▶ Increase quality of life and fitness through physical activity.
▶ Increase years of healthy life.
▶ Reduce risk of chronic disease.
▶ Reduce back pain.
▶ Reduce incidence of overweight.

Unit Activities

▶ Starter Workout
▶ Health- and Skill-Related Fitness Stunts
▶ Fitness Games
▶ Safe Exercise Circuit
▶ Cooperative Games
▶ Back Exercise Circuit

1

Fitness and Wellness for All

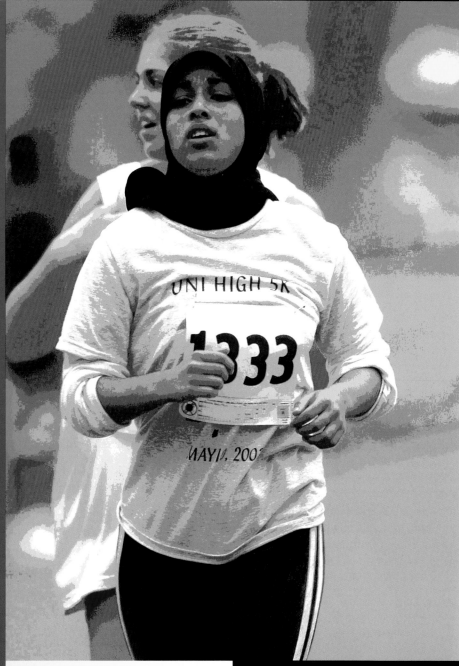

In this chapter...

Activity 1
Starter Workout

Lesson 1.1
Fitness for Life

Self-Assessment
Exercise Basics

Lesson 1.2
Fitness Through Physical Activity

Taking Charge
Learning to Self-Assess

Self-Management Skill
Learning to Self-Assess

Activity 2
Health- and Skill-Related Fitness Stunts

Activity 1

STARTER WORKOUT

This starter workout is designed to help you begin exercising. You will find the instructions for it on the sheet provided by your teacher. The workout can help you prepare for more advanced activities in the book. You probably will not find it to be difficult if you already do regular physical activity, but if you don't exercise regularly, it can be a good workout to get you started.

Lesson 1.1

Fitness For Life

Lesson Objectives

After reading this lesson, you should be able to
1. Define physical fitness, health, and wellness.
2. Describe some of the benefits of fitness, health, and wellness.

Lesson Vocabulary

exercise (p. 4), health (p. 4), physical activity (p. 4), physical fitness (p. 3), wellness (p. 4)

 www.fitnessforlife.org/student/1/1

Physical fitness. What is it? Do you need it? And how can you achieve it? As you read this book, you will find answers to these and many more questions. This book will help you decide which types of physical activities you need. Early in the book you will learn how to prepare for safe, smart physical activity. You will learn about each type of physical fitness and which physical activities are best for developing them. You will learn how physical activity and other healthy lifestyle choices improve your health and wellness as well as your physical fitness. Later in the book you will learn how to plan a personal physical activity program that will help you to improve your current fitness and your fitness throughout life. You will also learn how to use self-management skills to help you stick with your plan. The goal of this book is to help you to become an informed consumer who can make informed and effective decisions about fitness, health, and wellness.

Before you get started on your physical activity plan, you need some basic information about fitness. In this lesson you will learn the definitions of some words you will use throughout this course. You will better understand the meaning of the words fitness, health, and wellness. You will also learn how physical activity provides fitness, health, and wellness benefits.

 www.fitnessforlife.org/student/1/2

What Is Physical Fitness?

Physical fitness is the ability of your body systems to work together efficiently to allow you to be healthy and effectively perform activities of daily living. Being efficient means being able to do daily activities with the least amount of effort. A fit person is able to perform schoolwork as well as responsibilities at home and still have enough energy and vigor to enjoy school sports and other leisure activities. A fit person has the ability to respond to normal life situations such as raking the leaves at home, stocking shelves at a part-time job, or marching in the band at school. A fit person also has the ability to respond to emergency situations such as running to get help or aiding a friend in distress.

As a child you were probably very active and thought little about improving or maintaining your fitness. However, most people become less active as they grow older. Developing a personal plan for regular physical activity can help you keep your activity level high and avoid sedentary living. The activities you choose can be those that you like doing best and those that are best for you. Getting fit and staying fit can be fun when you choose activities that you enjoy.

Look at the picture at the bottom of this page. The biker is doing physical activity that promotes physical fitness. There are many other types of activity, and each has its own benefits. You might wonder what some of those benefits are.

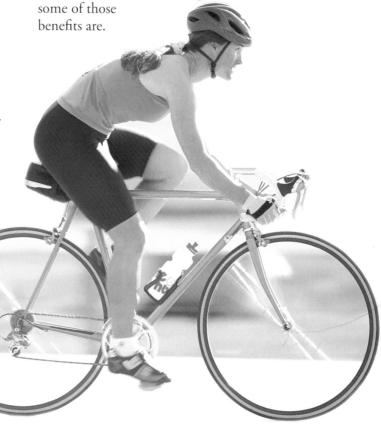

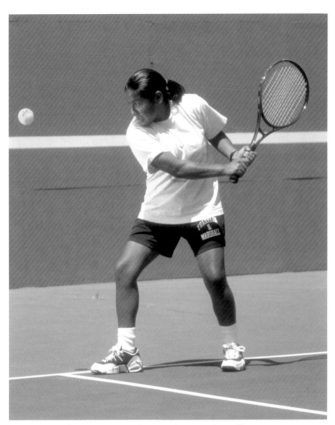
Each type of physical activity has its own benefit.

FI T FACTS

The Surgeon General is a leading medical doctor appointed by the president of the United States. The Surgeon General is the leading spokesperson on matters of public health.

Physical activities not only help you to be physically fit but also they help promote wellness. The *Surgeon General's Report on Physical Activity and Health* indicates that physical inactivity is a major risk factor for many diseases. Increasing physical activity should be a major health goal for people of all ages.

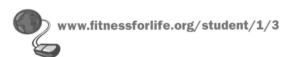
www.fitnessforlife.org/student/1/3

Health and Wellness

So what are some specific benefits of regular physical activity? Understanding the meaning of some basic words may help you answer this question.

Health is a word often associated with good fitness. Early definitions of health focused on illness. The first medical doctors concentrated on helping sick people get well; they treated illnesses. Health was considered as nothing more than absence from

disease (the World Health Organization [WHO] uses this term). But as medical and public health experts received better training, they began to focus on prevention of illness and disease as well as on the treatment of people who were already sick. This new focus led world health experts to define health as more than absence from disease.

In recent years the definition of health has been expanded to include **wellness,** a state of being that enables you to reach your fullest potential. Wellness includes intellectual, social, emotional, physical, and spiritual aspects. It has to do with feeling good about yourself and with having goals and purposes in life. Wellness is more likely to be present in individuals who assume responsibility for their own health. So illness is the negative component of health that we want to treat or prevent, while wellness is the positive component of health that we want to promote.

Physical Activity and Exercise

Good physical fitness, health, and wellness are all states of being that a person possesses. One of the principal ways that you achieve these states of being is by performing regular physical activity. The people in the pictures in this lesson are all engaged in **physical activity**—movement using the large muscles of the body. Physical activity is a general term that includes sports, dance, and activities done at home or work, such as walking, climbing stairs, or mowing the lawn. You may do physical activity to complete a specific job, to enjoy recreation, or to improve your physical fitness. Sometimes you do physical activity with a specific purpose in mind; other times you just do it with no real purpose other than enjoyment.

When people do physical activity especially for the purpose of getting fit, we say they are doing **exercise.** Even though the terms physical activity and exercise have slightly different meanings, they are sometimes used interchangeably. What you should remember is that physical activity and exercise are important to your fitness, health, and wellness.

Fitness, Health, and Wellness Benefits

Performing physical activity has many benefits. Regular exercise leads to improved physical fitness. Both regular physical activity and good fitness provide benefits to health and wellness. As the diagram on page 5 shows, being active provides you a double benefit: The first benefit is improved physical fitness. Good fitness leads to the second benefit—improved health and wellness. Good health and wellness, in turn, make you

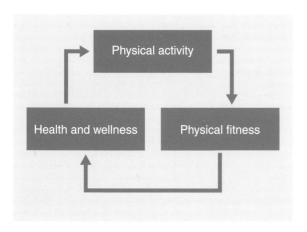

Cycle of Physical Activity Benefits.

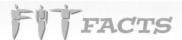

more likely to be physically active. This cycle is called the Cycle of Physical Activity Benefits. A goal of this book is to help you find ways to keep the cycle going throughout your life.

You might not be concerned with the fact that physical activity has been shown to be effective in preventing and treating various illnesses. You might assume that because illness and disease are most common later in life, you don't have to worry about them now. You might even share a common attitude among many teenagers that "I am young and healthy; it can't happen to me." But evidence indicates that the disease process begins early in life. Choosing and adopting healthy life-

styles such as performing regular physical activity early in your life can do much to prevent disease and illness. You will learn more about the benefits of physical activity in preventing illness in chapter 3.

The benefits derived from physical activity not only help you later in life—you can enjoy many benefits now. These benefits include those associated with fitness and wellness such as looking good, feeling good, meeting emergencies, and being physically fit. Making healthy lifestyle choices, including choosing to be physically active and to eat well, is necessary for achieving the benefits described in the following section. As you will learn throughout this book, healthy lifestyle choices have positive consequences that are in your control.

Looking Good

Do you care about how you look? Most people do. In fact, one study showed that 94 percent of all men and 99

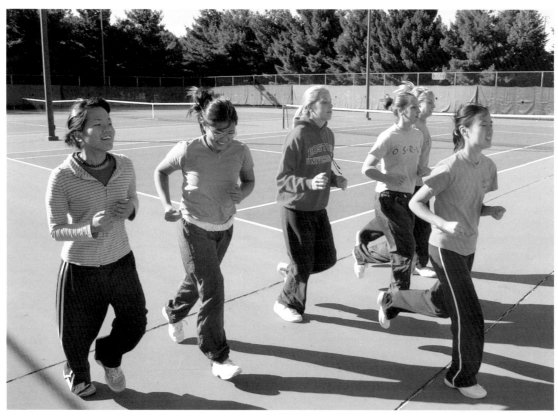

It is important to learn how to warm up before participating in a physical activity.

percent of all women would change some part of their appearance if they could. People are most concerned with weight (weighing too much or too little); the size of their waist or thighs; and their muscles, teeth, and hair. Experts agree that regular physical activity is one healthy lifestyle choice that can help you look your best. Others are proper nutrition, good posture, and good body mechanics.

Feeling Good

Besides looking better, people who do regular physical activity feel better. If you are active and therefore more physically fit, you can resist fatigue, are less likely to be injured, and are capable of working more efficiently. National surveys indicate that active people sleep better, do better in school, and are less depressed than people who are less active.

 www.fitnessforlife.org/student/1/4

Enjoying Life

Like most people, enjoying life is important for your personal wellness. But what if you are too tired on most days to participate in activities you really enjoy? Regular physical activity results in physical fitness, which is the key to being able to do more of the things you want to do.

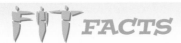 **FACTS**

The national health goals (Healthy People 2010) are established every decade and reviewed every five years. The review in 2005 resulted in changing some goals and eliminating others. The good news is that there has been a decrease in deaths from three of the most deadly diseases (heart disease, cancer, and stroke) since the Healthy People 2010 goals were established. Also, the number of Americans who are totally sedentary (inactive) has decreased in the last few years. While more American adults are doing some activity, most do not get enough physical activity to promote optimal health benefits. Continued effort is necessary if we are to reach our national health goals by the year 2010.

FITNESS Technology

In recent years new technology has been developed to help athletes improve performance and to help nonathletes to become more active. The World Wide Web (Internet) allows the average person to get immediate access to all kinds of health and fitness information. As you will learn later in this book, some of this information is good, but much of it is inaccurate. In each chapter of this book you will find Internet addresses that will lead you to sound information about fitness, health, and wellness. Special Web symbols are included throughout the book. Type in the address by the Web symbol and you will find good, reliable information. At these special Web sites you will also find links to other good sources of fitness and health information.

Meeting Emergencies

Another important health and wellness benefit of physical activity is that it allows you to be fit enough to meet emergencies and day-to-day demanding situations. If you are physically fit and active, you will be able to run for help, change a flat tire, and offer assistance to others when needed.

The Warm-Up and Cool-Down

In addition to your learning in the classroom, you will be participating in many different physical activities. Before you participate in these activities, it is important to learn about warming up and cooling down. It is also important for you to learn how to count your heart rate at rest and immediately after performing physical activity. The self-assessment on the following pages will show you how to perform a simple set of exercises that you can do before and after the physical activities that you will do later in this class. You will also learn to count your heart rate.

Lesson Review
1. What is physical fitness?
2. What are some benefits of being physically active?

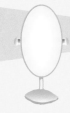

Self-Assessment

Exercise Basics

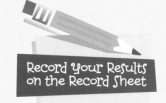

Record Your Results on the Record Sheet

In each chapter of this book, you will find a self-assessment to help you determine your own fitness level. The record sheet that your teacher will provide for each self-assessment will help you record and analyze your assessment results.

This self-assessment will teach you some basics you will need to know to do activities in the following chapters. You will learn how to count your heart rate and how to do a warm-up and cool-down. In chapter 2 you will learn some of the reasons why a warm-up and cool-down are recommended before and after your physical activity sessions. You also will learn how to plan your own personal warm-up and cool-down. However, because you will be doing some physical activities before reading chapter 2, you can use the following general warm-up and cool-down before and after most physical activities.

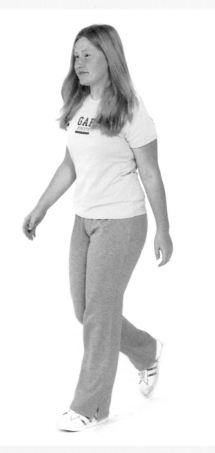

This exercise increases the heart rate and blood circulation.

PART 1: The Warm-Up and Stretch

Try the warm-up activities described here. You can use them to warm up for future activities. Keep these guidelines in mind:

▶ Do the stretching exercises on a soft but firm surface, such as carpeting, a mat, a towel, or grass. Do not do them on a very soft surface, such as a bed.

▶ Do each stretch 1 to 3 times. Hold each stretch for 15 to 30 seconds.

▶ It is best to stretch the muscles while they are warm. That is why you walk or jog several minutes before stretching. A longer and more general warm-up period is even better and is recommended when possible.

Heart Warm-Up

1. Walk slowly for 1 minute, then jog slowly for 1 minute.
2. If you do not have enough room to jog or walk, jog in place for 2 minutes.
3. It is best to complete the heart warm-up before your muscle stretch warm-up.

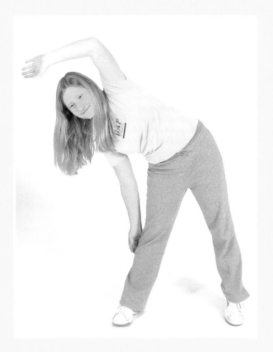

Side Stretch

1. Stand with your feet about shoulder-width apart.
2. Lean to your left.
3. Reach down to your left foot with your left hand. Reach over your head with your right arm. Hold for a count of 15.

 Caution: Do not twist or lean your body forward.

4. Repeat the exercise on your right side.

Safety Tips: Stretch slowly. Try to stretch the muscles slightly, but do not stretch too far. Avoid stretching until you feel pain. Do not bounce or jerk.

This exercise stretches the muscles of the arms and shoulders as well as the side of the body.

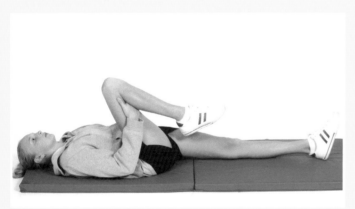

Knee-to-Chest Stretch

1. Lie on your back. Lift one leg off the floor with the knee bent.
2. Reach behind your knee and hug the thigh of the lifted leg with your hands. Pull further with your arms only if you can fully straighten your leg.
3. Try to keep your other leg straight and flat on the floor. Hug the bent leg for 15 seconds.
4. Repeat the exercise with your other leg.

This exercise stretches the muscles of the lower back and buttocks.

This exercise stretches the lower back and buttocks muscles.

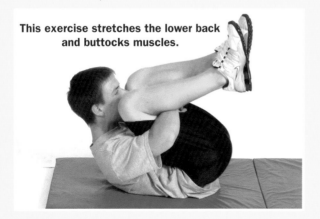

Back and Hip Stretch

1. Lie on your back. Bend your knees and bring them up to your chest.
2. Reach behind your knees and hug your thighs with your arms.
3. Lift your head and shoulders off the floor as you pull your legs to your chest. Hold for 15 seconds.

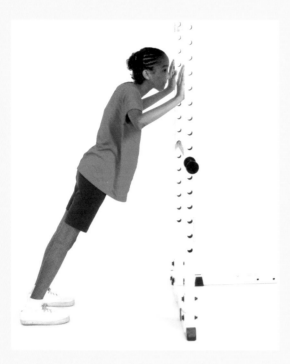

This exercise stretches the calf muscles.

Two-Leg Calf Stretch

1. Face a wall and stand 2 or 3 feet away from it.
2. Reach forward and touch the wall with your hands.
3. Slowly bend your arms and let your body lean forward. Keep your knees straight and your heels on the floor.

 Caution: Do not arch your back.

4. Turn your toes in slightly. Hold for 15 seconds.
Note: The single-leg calf stretch can also be used (see page 172).

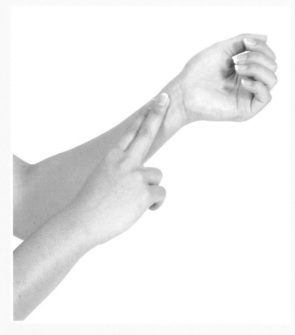

Use the first and second finger to find a pulse at your wrist.

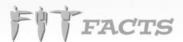

You can determine your one-minute heart rate in other ways. For example, you can count the number of beats in 10 seconds and multiply by 6, or count your pulse for 6 seconds and add a zero.

PART 2: Counting Heart Rate

To perform many of the activities that you will do in future weeks, you will need to be able to determine your one-minute heart rate. These activities will teach you how.

Counting Resting Heart Rate

Your resting heart rate is the number of times your heart beats when you are relatively inactive. Follow these instructions to learn how to determine your resting heart rate:

1. Sit and take your heart rate by using the first and second fingers of your hand to find a pulse at your wrist. Do not use your thumb. This is your radial pulse. Practice so that you can locate the pulse quickly.
2. Count the number of pulses for 1 minute. Record your one-minute heart rate on your record sheet.
3. Take your resting (seated) heart rate again, this time counting the pulse at your neck. This is your carotid pulse. If you use your right hand count your neck pulse on the left side, and if you use your left hand count your pulse on the right side of the neck. Be careful not to press too hard. Record your results.
4. Try taking your pulse using a 15-second count. First, count the heart rate for 15 seconds; then multiply

(continued)

Counting Resting Heart Rate (continued)

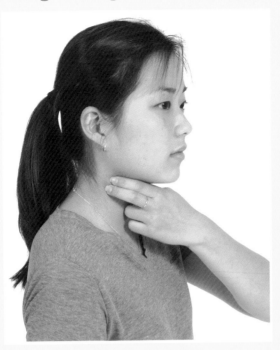

Use the first and second finger to find a pulse at your neck.

the number by 4. This method is considered to be especially good because you can do it quickly and because counting your heart rate for longer periods after exercise is less accurate. This is because your heart rate slows down quickly when you stop exercising, so long counts underestimate your heart rate during exercise. Counting for shorter periods can result in error because a single beat error in counting is multiplied several times. You can use table 1.1 to help you determine your one-minute heart rate from your 15-second count.

5. Now take both your wrist and neck pulse while you are standing. Repeat the pulse (both wrist and neck) count while sitting. Compare your results. Usually your standing pulse is faster than your sitting pulse. Record your results on your worksheet.

6. Take the pulse of a partner while a partner takes your pulse (standing). Compare your self-counted heart rate with your heart rate determined by your partner. You may use different methods of counting, but use the same one as your partner when making comparisons. Record your results.

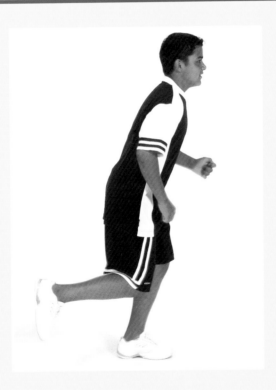

Counting Exercise Heart Rate

Counting your pulse during activities such as jogging can be difficult, but you can get a good estimate of your exercise heart rate during a physical activity by determining your heart rate immediately after exercising. To estimate your heart rate during exercise using your after-exercise pulse count, follow these instructions:

1. Walk at a fast pace for 1 minute.

2. Immediately after the walk, locate your pulse (within 5 seconds) and use one of the methods described to determine your heart rate. You may want to continue to walk slowly while you count your heart rate because slow walking can help you recover faster. If you have trouble counting your heart rate while walking, stand still when you count then begin moving after the count. Your heart rate should be faster than it was at rest. Record your results on your record sheet.

3. Jog or run at a moderate pace for 1 minute. Immediately after the jog, determine your heart rate while you continue to walk slowly or stand still. Your heart rate should be faster than it was at rest. Record your results on your record sheet.

4. Play an active fitness game. Immediately after the game, count your heart rate. If it was a vigorous game, your heart rate will be higher than after the run. Record your results on your record sheet.

Table 1.1

Heart Rate in 15-Second Intervals

15-s rate	1-min rate	15-s rate	1-min rate
15	60	33	132
16	64	34	136
17	68	35	140
18	72	36	144
19	76	37	148
20	80	38	152
21	84	39	156
22	88	40	160
23	92	41	164
24	96	42	168
25	100	43	172
26	104	44	176
27	108	45	180
28	112	46	184
29	116	47	188
30	120	48	192
31	124	49	196
32	128	50	200

Find your 15-second heart rate in a blue column; your one-minute heart rate is in the white column to the right of it.

PART 3: The Cool-Down

A cool-down after activity helps you recover. Until you learn to plan your own cool-down, you can use the same exercises as you used for the warm-up to cool down. Repeat the exercises again to get additional practice in doing them properly.

Fitness Through Physical Activity

Lesson Objectives

After reading this lesson, you should be able to

1. Name and describe the five parts of health-related physical fitness.
2. Name and describe the six parts of skill-related physical fitness.
3. Explain how to use the Stairway to Lifetime Fitness.

Lesson Vocabulary

agility (p. 13), balance (p. 13), body fatness (p. 13), cardiovascular fitness (p. 12), coordination (p. 13), flexibility (p. 13), health-related physical fitness (p. 12), hypokinetic conditions (p. 13), muscular endurance (p. 12), power (p. 13), reaction time (p. 13), skill-related physical fitness (p. 12), speed (p. 13), strength (p. 12)

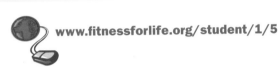

www.fitnessforlife.org/student/1/5

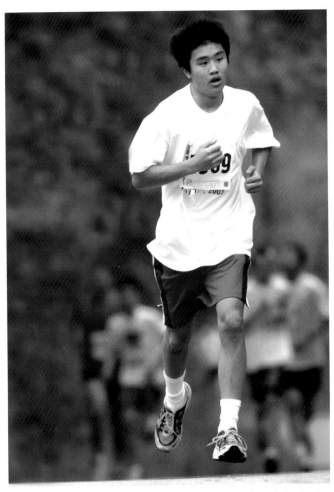

Running is a good way to achieve some health-related physical fitness benefits.

The Parts of Physical Fitness

When you see a person who is good at sports, such as the runner in the photo, do you assume that the person is physically fit? You might be surprised to know that this assumption is not always true. It is true that a person who excels in sports needs a certain degree of physical fitness. However, being good at a specific skill such as running may not be a good indicator of total physical fitness; some sports require only certain parts of physical fitness.

Physical fitness is made up of 11 different parts; 5 parts are health related and 6 parts are skill related. As the terms imply, **health-related physical fitness** helps you to stay healthy, while **skill-related physical fitness** helps you perform well in sports and activities that require certain skills. The activity at the end of this chapter will help you better understand the differences among the 11 parts. Each part of physical fitness is described in more detail later in this chapter.

Health-Related Physical Fitness

Think about the runner again. He probably can run a long distance without tiring. He has good fitness in

at least one area of health-related physical fitness. But does he have good fitness in all five parts? Running is an excellent form of physical activity but it does not guarantee that he will be fit in all areas of health-related physical fitness. Like the runner, you may be more fit in some parts of fitness than in others. As you read about each part of health-related physical fitness next, ask yourself how fit you think you are in each.

▶ **Cardiovascular fitness** is the ability to exercise your entire body for long periods of time without stopping. Cardiovascular fitness requires a strong heart, healthy lungs, and clear blood vessels to supply the cells of your body with the oxygen they need.

▶ **Strength** is the amount of force your muscles can produce. Strength is often measured by how much weight you can lift or how much resistance you can overcome. People with good strength can perform daily tasks efficiently—that is, with the least amount of effort.

▶ **Muscular endurance** is the ability to use your muscles many times without tiring. People with good muscular endurance are likely to have better posture and fewer back problems.

▶ **Flexibility** is the ability to use your joints fully through a wide range of motion. You are flexible when your muscles are long enough and your joints are free enough to allow adequate movement. People with good flexibility have fewer sore and injured muscles.

▶ **Body fatness** is the percentage of body weight that is made up of fat when compared to the other body tissues, such as bone and muscle. For example, a person who weighs 100 pounds, 20 pounds of which is fat, is said to have a body fat level of 20 percent. People who are in a healthy range of body fatness are more likely to avoid illness and even have lower death rates than those outside the healthy range. The extreme ranges are most dangerous. Too little or too much body fat can cause health problems.

How much of each of the five health-related parts of fitness do you think you have? To be healthy, you should have some of each. If you do, you are less likely to develop **hypokinetic conditions**—health problems caused partly by lack of physical activity. Examples include heart disease, high blood pressure, diabetes, osteoporosis, colon cancer, and being over-fat. You will learn more about hypokinetic conditions in chapter 3.

People who are physically fit feel better, look better, and have more energy. You do not have to be a great athlete to have good health and to be physically fit. Regular physical activity can improve anyone's health-related physical fitness.

 www.fitnessforlife.org/student/1/6

Skill-Related Physical Fitness

Just as the runner may not possess a high rating in all parts of health-related physical fitness, she also may not possess the same amount of fitness in all parts of skill-related physical fitness. Different sports require different parts of skill-related physical fitness. Most sports require several parts.

▶ **Agility** is the ability to change the position of your body quickly and to control your body's movements. People with good agility are likely to be good at activities such as wrestling, diving, soccer, and ice skating.

▶ **Balance** is the ability to keep an upright posture while standing still or moving. People with good balance are likely to be good at activities such as gymnastics and ice skating.

▶ **Coordination** is the ability to use your senses together with your body parts or to use two or more body parts together. People with good eye-hand or eye-foot coordination are good at hitting and kicking games such as baseball, softball, tennis, and golf.

▶ **Power** is the ability to use strength quickly. It involves both strength and speed. People with good power might have the ability to put the shot, throw the discus, high jump, play football, and speed swim.

FIT FACTS

Power is sometimes called a "combined part of fitness" because it requires speed (a skill-related part of fitness) and strength (a health-related part of fitness).

▶ **Reaction time** is the amount of time it takes to move once you realize the need to act. People with good reaction time are able to make fast starts in track or swimming or to dodge a fast attack in fencing or karate. Good reaction time is necessary for your own safety while driving or walking.

▶ **Speed** is the ability to perform a movement or cover a distance in a short period of time. People with good leg speed can run fast, while people with good arm speed can throw fast or hit a ball that is thrown fast.

Remember, most sports require different parts of skill-related fitness. For example, a skater might have good agility but may not possess good power. Some people have more natural ability in some areas than in others. No matter how you score on the skill-related parts of physical fitness, you can enjoy some type of physical activity. Keep in mind that good health does not come from being good in skill-related physical fitness; it comes from doing activities designed to improve your health-related physical fitness and can be had by people who consider themselves poor athletes as well as by those who see themselves as great athletes.

The Stairway to Lifetime Fitness

You are probably quite active now; most teens are. But will you be as active as you grow older? Will you do the same kinds of activities you do now? If you answered "no" to either of these questions, you need to begin learning now for lifetime fitness and activity. One way to accomplish this goal is to climb the Stairway to Lifetime Fitness. As you can see in the diagram, when you climb the stairway, you move from a level of dependence to a level of independence, allowing you to make good decisions about lifetime physical activity.

Step 1: Doing Physical Activity

Think about the various physical activities you are involved in. If you are like many people your age, much of your activity results from community or school activities. You also have other opportunities to do physical activity, such as in physical education classes. As you become an adult, school programs will no longer serve as your incentive to exercise, and other opportunities for physical activity will probably decrease. Doing activity planned by others is a good first step, but it is important to keep climbing the stairway.

Step 2: Getting Fit

Because getting fit depends on physical activity and exercise patterns, fitness is something that people often planned for you when you were young. For example, coaches prescribe exercises to get kids fit for sports, and physical education teachers plan activities to get students fit. But when do young people learn to get or keep fit without depending on others? Moving up the stairway means learning to become responsible for your own physical fitness. When you move to the third step in the stairway, you begin to make your own decisions.

Step 3: Self-Assessment

Before you can make good decisions about your own personal fitness and activities, you need to know your own personal fitness level. No doubt you have had your fitness tested before, but probably it was something someone else did for you, rather than something you did for yourself. When you learn to assess your own fitness you will have reached the third step on the Stairway to Lifetime Fitness. You can use the skills of self-assessment all your life to help in self-planning for lifetime activity and fitness. You will find a self-assessment in each chapter of this book.

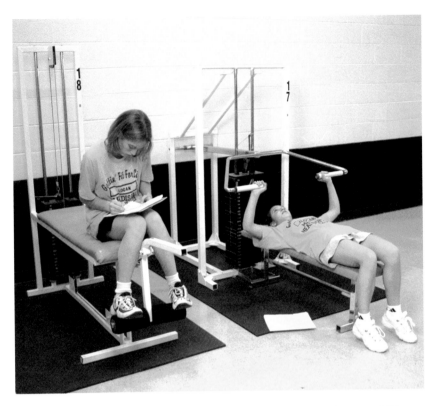

Learning to keep track of your own assessment and fitness is an important life skill.

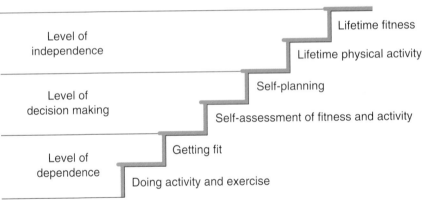

Stairway to Lifetime Fitness.

Step 4: Self-Planning

When you have learned to assess your own fitness, you are ready to progress to self-planning. You use your own fitness results (a personal fitness profile) to help plan your own fitness and activity program. No two people will have identical fitness needs and no two people will have exactly the same program. The information you learn from this book and in this class will help you self-plan.

Taking Charge: Learning to Self-Assess

Testing yourself to see what you can do is referred to as a self-assessment. Many kinds of self-assessments exist. For example, you can assess your physical fitness, your health, your knowledge, and your ability in sports. The self-assessments in this book focus on physical fitness and health.

Julia and Troy are friends who want to know more about their current health-related physical fitness levels. They have taken fitness tests in school in the past, but they learned little about why they were doing the tests or how to test themselves in the future. They wanted to learn how to assess their own fitness.

Julia remembered some of the tests she took in elementary school, such as running a 50-yard dash, seeing how far she could jump, and performing something called a shuttle run. Troy had not taken a fitness test in physical education, but he had been tested for his baseball team to see how many push-ups and jumping jacks he could do.

Julia and Troy thought about doing a self-assessment that included all of the tests Julia had been given in

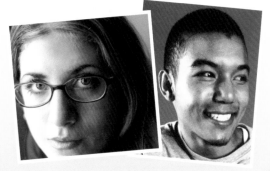

school and all of the tests that Troy had done for his baseball team. But they were not sure how to do the tests the correct way, and they were not sure that these were the best tests. They especially wanted to learn self-assessments for health-related physical fitness.

For Discussion

Discuss a plan of self-assessment that Julia and Troy can follow to determine their current levels of health-related physical fitness. Did the tests Julia performed in elementary school assess health-related physical fitness? Did the tests Troy performed for his baseball team measure health-related physical fitness? What do you think the tests they performed really measured? Fill out the self-assessment questionnaire (provided by your teacher) for this chapter to learn more about self-assessments for health-related physical fitness. Consider the guidelines on page 16. You will get a chance to practice many fitness self-assessments as you do the activities in this book.

Step 5: Lifetime Activity

When you climb to step 5, you will have moved from the level of decision making and problem solving to the level of lifetime activity. This means you have learned *why* activity is important, *what* your fitness needs are, and *how* to plan for a lifetime. You will be a lifetime activity participant. This step is much like step 1 in the stairway, but now you are making your own decisions.

Step 6: Lifetime Fitness

When you reach the top level of the stairway, you will have taken responsibility for your own lifetime fitness. You will have moved from dependence on others to keep you fit. Throughout your life, you will use the skills you learned to reevaluate your fitness needs and to adjust your physical activity program as needed to maintain your fitness.

A major purpose of this book and this class is to help you to achieve lifetime fitness as a result of healthy lifestyle choices, including regular lifetime physical activity. In the chapters that follow, you will learn how to climb the stairway and reach this highest step.

 www.fitnessforlife.org/student/1/7

Lesson Review
1. Name and describe the five parts of health-related physical fitness.
2. Name and describe the six parts of skill-related physical fitness.
3. Use the Stairway to Lifetime Fitness to explain how you can develop a lifetime habit of physical fitness.

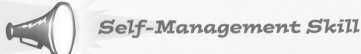

Self-Management Skill

Learning to Self-Assess

Before you go on a trip you use a map to make plans. The map helps you decide where you want to go. Assessing your own fitness is much like using a map. You can assess your current fitness and physical activity levels to help you learn what you need to improve and determine the direction of your future plans.

The following guidelines will be useful as you learn to do personal fitness and activity self-assessments.

1. **Try a wide variety of tests.** There are many different parts of fitness and many types of physical activity. It is important to try a variety of ways to self-assess so that you can get a total picture of your fitness and activity needs. In this class you will get the opportunity to learn various self-assessment techniques.

2. **Choose self-assessments that work best for you.** You will try all the self-assessments you learn in this book, but ultimately you will not need to use them all. You should choose at least one assessment for each type of health-related physical fitness and one assessment to determine your current activity level. After you have tried many self-assessments, you will have the opportunity to select the ones that are best for you.

3. **Practice.** When you first drive a car it is not easy, but the more you practice, the better you get. And the first time you do self-assessments you will make mistakes, but the more you practice, the better you will get. When you decide which assessments you will use on a regular basis, it is essential that you practice using them.

4. **Use self-assessments for personal improvement.** Once you have learned to use self-assessments, repeat them from time to time to monitor your progress. Avoid making assessments too often, but check yourself periodically to see how you are doing.

5. **Use health standards rather than comparisons to others.** Sometimes people are discouraged when they get test results. Often this is because they have set unrealistic standards. Rather than comparing yourself to others, it is wise to compare yourself to health standards and to your own previous performances. This type of comparison helps you stay realistic. You will learn more about health-based standards for fitness in chapter 4. *The standards used in this book are not based on comparisons of one person to another; they are based on the level of fitness needed for good health and wellness.*

16

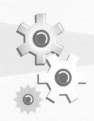

Activity 2

Health- and Skill-Related Fitness Stunts

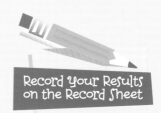

Record Your Results on the Record Sheet

At the end of each chapter of this book, you will find an activity, such as the one that follows, which will help you apply what you learned in the chapter. Your teacher will provide you with a record sheet for each activity where you can record your results. Many of these activities can be used as part of your lifetime fitness plan.

In this activity you will try 11 different stunts. They are called stunts because *they are not meant to be tests of fitness nor are they meant to be exercises that you do to get fit.* The stunts are designed to help you see the differences among the various parts of fitness. It is important that you do not draw conclusions about your fitness based on your performance on these stunts. Later in the book you will learn to make many different self-assessments to determine your fitness level. Trying these stunts is a fun way to get a better understanding of the various parts of physical fitness. Remember to warm up before and cool down after doing the activity.

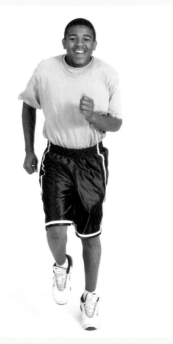

This activity focuses on cardiovascular fitness.

PART 1: Health-Related Physical Fitness Stunts

Run in Place (Cardiovascular Fitness)

1. Determine your one-minute heart rate at rest.
2. Run 120 steps in the same place for 1 minute. A step is every time a foot hits the floor.
3. Rest for 1 minute. Count your heart rate for 30 seconds. People with good cardiovascular fitness recover quickly after exercise. Is your heart rate less than 15 beats above your resting heart rate?

Two-Hand Ankle Grip (Flexibility)

1. With your heels together, bend forward and reach with your hands between your legs and behind your ankles.
2. Clasp your hands in front of your ankles.
3. Interlock your hands for the full length of your fingers. You must keep your feet still.
4. Hold the position for 5 seconds.

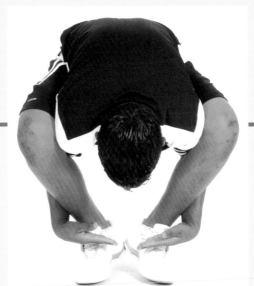

This activity focuses on flexibility.

17

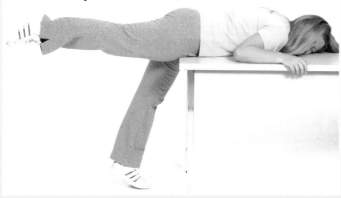

This activity focuses on muscular endurance.

Single-Leg Raise (Muscular Endurance)

1. Position your upper body on a table so that your feet touch the floor. Extend one leg straight out.
2. Complete several leg raises. Performing more than 8 is an indicator of muscular endurance. For this stunt, stop when you reach 25.

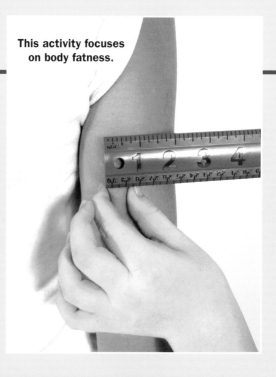

This activity focuses on body fatness.

Arm Pinch (Body Fatness)

1. Let your right arm hang relaxed at your side. Have a partner pinch the skin and fat under the skin on the back of your arm, halfway between your elbow and shoulder.
2. Have your partner use a ruler to measure the skinfold thickness. Thicker skinfolds generally mean greater total body fatness.

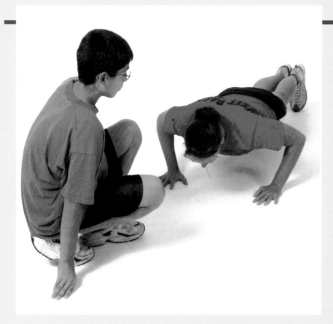

This activity focuses on strength.

90-Degree Push-Up (Strength)

1. Lie facedown on a mat or carpet with your hands under your shoulders, your fingers spread, and your legs straight. Your legs should be slightly apart and your toes should be tucked under.
2. Push up until your arms are straight. Keep your legs and back straight. Your body should form a straight line.
3. Lower your body by bending your elbows until they are each parallel to the floor (at a 90-degree angle), then push up until the arms are fully extended. Do one push-up every 3 seconds. You may want to have a partner say "up-down" every 3 seconds to help you.
4. Stronger people can do more repetitions. Once you are able to do 10 push-ups, this stunt becomes an indicator of muscular endurance.

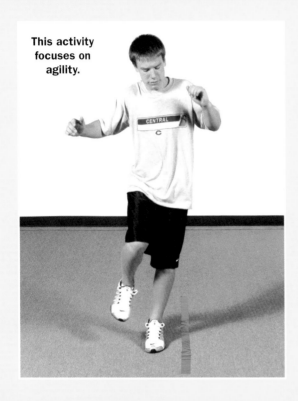

This activity focuses on agility.

PART 2: Skill-Related Physical Fitness Stunts

Line Jump (Agility)

1. Balance on your right foot on a line on the floor.
2. Leap onto the left foot so that it lands to the right of the line.
3. Leap across the line onto the right foot; land to the left of the line.
4. Leap onto the left foot, landing on the line.

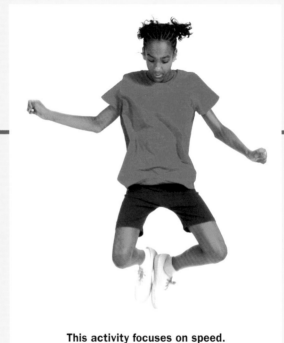

This activity focuses on speed.

Double Heel Click (Speed)

1. Jump into the air and click your heels together twice before you land.
2. Your feet should be at least 3 inches apart when you land.

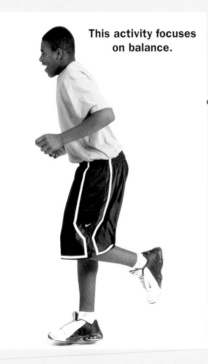

This activity focuses on balance.

Backward Hop (Balance)

1. With your eyes closed, hop backward on one foot for 5 hops.
2. After the last hop, hold your balance for 3 seconds.

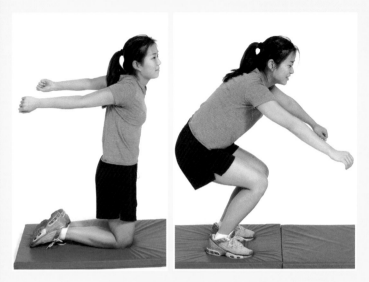

This activity focuses on power.

Knees to Feet (Power)

1. Kneel so that your shins and knees are on a mat. Hold your arms back. Point your toes straight backward.
2. Without curling your toes under you or rocking your body backward, swing your arms upward and spring to your feet.
3. Hold your position for 3 seconds after you land.

Double-Ball Bounce (Coordination)

1. Hold a volleyball in each hand. Beginning at the same time with each hand, bounce both balls at the same time, at least knee high.
2. Bounce both balls three times in a row without losing control of them.

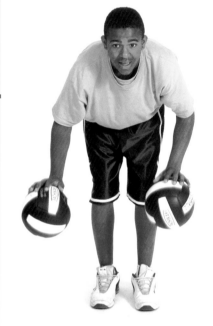

This activity focuses on coordination.

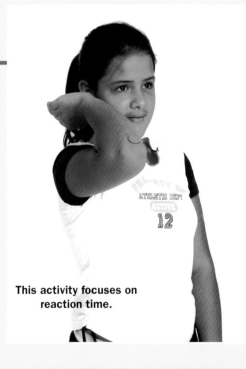

This activity focuses on reaction time.

Coin Catch (Reaction Time)

1. Point your right elbow in front of you. Your right hand, palm up, should be by your right ear. If you are left-handed, do this activity with your left hand.
2. Place a coin as close to the end of your elbow as possible.
3. Quickly lower your elbow and grab the coin in the air with your right hand before it touches the ground.

20

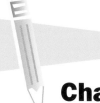

1 Chapter Review

Reviewing Concepts and Vocabulary

Number your paper from 1 to 5. Next to each number, write the word (or words) that correctly completes the sentence.

1. Physical activity done for the purpose of getting fit is called _____.
2. The _____ is a series of steps to help you achieve lifetime fitness.
3. Cardiovascular fitness is one part of _____ fitness.
4. A hypokinetic condition is a health problem caused by _____.
5. Body fatness is a _____.

Number your paper from 6 to 14. Next to each number, write the letter of the best answer.

Column I

6. muscular endurance
7. flexibility
8. agility
9. balance
10. coordination

11. reaction time
12. speed
13. physical activity

14. wellness

Column II

a. movement of body using larger muscles
b. ability to use body parts together
c. ability to cover a distance quickly
d. positive component of health
e. ability to use joints through a wide range of motion
f. ability to change body position quickly
g. ability to keep an upright position
h. ability to use muscles continuously without tiring
i. amount of time to start moving

Number your paper from 15 to 20. Write a short answer for each statement or question that follows.

15. What is physical fitness?
16. Why is fitness important for everyone?
17. How do health-related physical fitness and skill-related physical fitness differ?
18. Explain why a sports star may not possess the same levels of fitness in all areas of physical fitness.
19. What is the difference between power and strength?
20. Explain how the definition of health has changed over time.

Thinking Critically

Write a paragraph to answer the following question.

A friend of yours tells you she sees no reason to develop a plan for lifetime physical activity because she gets plenty of activity in school. She is on the basketball team and the track team. She also has physical education class five times a week. What would you tell her? Explain your answer.

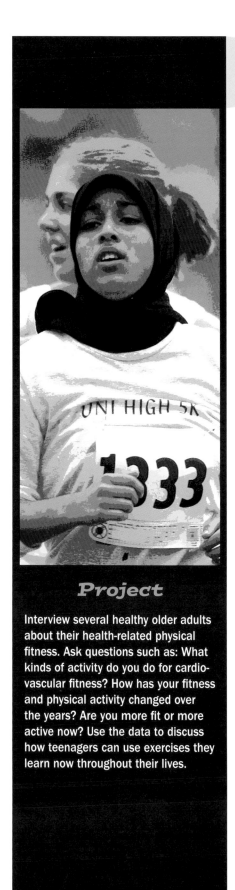

Project

Interview several healthy older adults about their health-related physical fitness. Ask questions such as: What kinds of activity do you do for cardio-vascular fitness? How has your fitness and physical activity changed over the years? Are you more fit or more active now? Use the data to discuss how teenagers can use exercises they learn now throughout their lives.

2

Safe and Smart Physical Activity

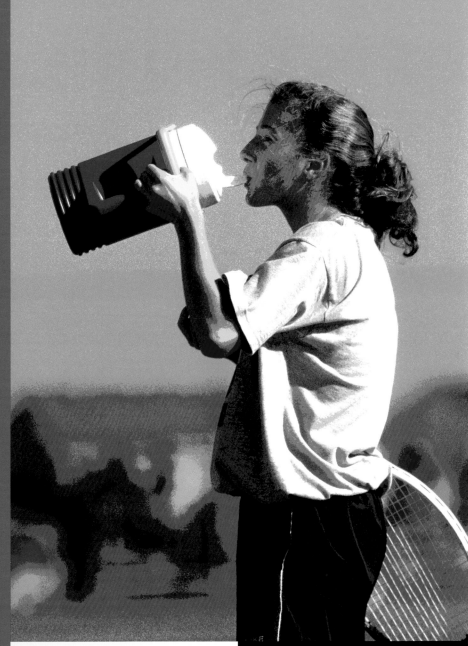

In this chapter...

Activity 1
Fitness Games

Lesson 2.1
Getting Ready

Self-Assessment
FITNESSGRAM 1—**Strength and Muscular Endurance**

Lesson 2.2
Physical Activity and Injury

Taking Charge
Building Self-Confidence

Self-Management Skill
Building Self-Confidence

Activity 2
Safe Exercise Circuit

Activity 1

FITNESS GAMES

Games are one of the most popular forms of physical activity. Generally young people play more games than adults, but games can be a fun way of being physically active to build fitness.

Getting Ready

Lesson Objectives

After reading this lesson, you should be able to

1. Explain how to prepare yourself for physical activity.
2. Explain how the environment affects physical activity.
3. Describe some steps for dressing for physical activity in normal environments.

Lesson Vocabulary

heat index (p. 24), humidity (p. 23), hyperthermia (p. 23), hypothermia (p. 24), PAR-Q (p. 23), windchill factor (p. 25)

 www.fitnessforlife.org/student/2/1

Whether you're a beginner or you've been physically active for some time, it's important for you to be prepared and to know how to exercise safely in all conditions. If you're a beginner, a first step is to be physically and medically ready. As a young person you probably won't have a problem with physical and medical readiness, but you should answer some simple questions about yourself just to be sure. Also, you should be ready for a variety of environmental conditions such as heat, cold, pollution, and altitude that may require a change in your exercise habits. In this lesson you will learn how to prepare yourself for physical activity.

 www.fitnessforlife.org/student/2/2

Medical Readiness

Before you begin a regular physical activity program for health and wellness, it is wise to assess your medical and physical readiness. Experts have developed a seven-item questionnaire called the Physical Activity Readiness Questionnaire (**PAR-Q**). If you answer "yes" to any of the seven questions, medical consultation is advised before beginning or continuing a program. You can access the PAR-Q online (see preceding Web icon), or your teacher can provide you with a copy. You may want to show the PAR-Q to your parents or other adults who are important to you. Older people are more likely to be at risk when doing exercise, so you may want to encourage them to answer the PAR-Q questions before they begin an exercise program.

If you are going to participate in an interscholastic sport or a program of similar intensity, such as preparing to participate in community sports or rigorous personal challenges, a medical examination is often required. Medical exams help make sure that you are free from disease and can help prevent future health problems. Also, you should answer the questions on the sports readiness questionnaire that is available from your teacher (also see preceding Web icon).

Later in life you should have a graded exercise test, sometimes called an exercise stress test, done by health professionals. These tests, done on a treadmill, can be helpful in identifying people who have a high risk of health problems such as heart attacks. Even seemingly fit athletes can be at risk. Outstanding baseball players, runners, and football players thought to be in good health have died from heart attacks. If these athletes had been tested, the heart attacks may have been prevented. Go to the Web address by the following icon to learn more.

 www.fitnessforlife.org/student/2/3

Readiness for Extreme Environmental Conditions

Environmental conditions play an important role in determining when and how strenuously you exercise. Whether you are just beginning a physical activity program or you have been exercising for a while, understanding how environmental conditions can affect your body during exercise is important. Your body is able to adapt to environmental factors such as heat, cold, and altitude. This is why people who have been exposed to an environment for a long time function better than those who have just become exposed. This chapter includes guidelines for adapting to weather and environmental factors, which will help you prevent injury and health problems. All people should follow these guidelines, but it is especially important for people new to exercise or new to an environment.

Hot, Humid Weather

Be careful when performing physical activity when the weather is hot and the **humidity** is high. **Hyperthermia,** or overheating, occurs when your body temperature rises too high. High environmental temperatures,

Heat index

As humidity increases, air can feel hotter than it actually is.
This chart shows how hot it feels as humidity rises.

Relative humidity (%)											
100	72	80	91	108	132						
90	71	79	88	102	122						
80	71	78	86	97	113	136					
70	70	77	85	93	106	124	144				
60	70	76	82	90	100	114	132	149			
50	69	75	81	88	96	107	120	135	150		
40	68	74	79	86	93	101	110	123	137	151	
30	67	73	78	84	90	96	104	113	123	135	148
20	66	72	77	82	87	93	99	105	112	120	130
10	65	70	75	80	85	90	95	100	105	111	116
0	64	69	73	78	83	87	91	95	99	103	107
	70	75	80	85	90	95	100	105	110	115	120

Air temperature (°F)

☐ Caution zone
■ Danger zone

Heat index chart.

especially when the humidity is high, can lead to hyperthemia. Exercise in the heat causes your body temperature to rise and you start to perspire (sweat). When sweat evaporates, the body is cooled. But when the humidity is high, evaporation is less effective in cooling the body and hyperthemia can occur. Hyperthermia causes three main conditions, which are described in table 2.1.

Follow these guidelines to prevent and cope with heat-related conditions:

▶ **Begin gradually.** As your body becomes accustomed to physical activity in hot weather, it becomes more resistant to heat-related injuries. Start with short periods of activity and gradually increase the time.

▶ **Drink water.** During hot weather your body perspires more than normally to cool itself. You need to drink plenty of water to replace the water your body loses through perspiration.

▶ **Wear proper clothing.** Wear porous clothing that allows air to pass through it to cool your body. Wear light-colored clothing; lighter colors reflect the sun's heat, while darker colors absorb heat.

▶ **Rest frequently.** Physical activity creates body heat. Periodically stop and rest in a shady area to help your body lower its temperature.

▶ **Avoid extreme heat and humidity.** You can use the heat index chart on this page to determine whether the environment is too hot and humid for activity. If the **heat index** is too high (danger zone), you should postpone or cancel activity. You should do physical activity in the caution zones only if you have adapted to hot environments, and follow all of the basic guidelines. The amount of time it takes to adapt to these conditions varies with each person.

▶ **Get out of the heat and cool the body if heat-related injury occurs.** Find shade; apply cool, wet towels to body; spray the body with water; drink water; and seek medical help if heatstroke occurs.

Cold, Windy, and Wet Weather

Exercising during cold, windy, and wet weather can be dangerous. Extreme cold can result in **hypothermia,**

Table 2.1

Heat-Related Conditions

Condition	Definition
Heat cramps	Muscle cramps caused by excessive exposure to heat and low consumption of water.
Heat exhaustion	A condition caused by excessive exposure to heat, characterized by paleness, cold clammy skin, profuse sweating, weakness and tiredness, nausea, dizziness, muscle cramps, and possible vomiting or fainting. Body temperature may be normal or slightly above normal.
Heatstroke	A condition caused by excessive exposure to heat, characterized by high body temperature (possibly as high as 106°); hot, dry, flushed skin; rapid pulse; lack of sweating; dizziness; or unconsciousness. This serious condition can result in death and requires prompt medical attention.

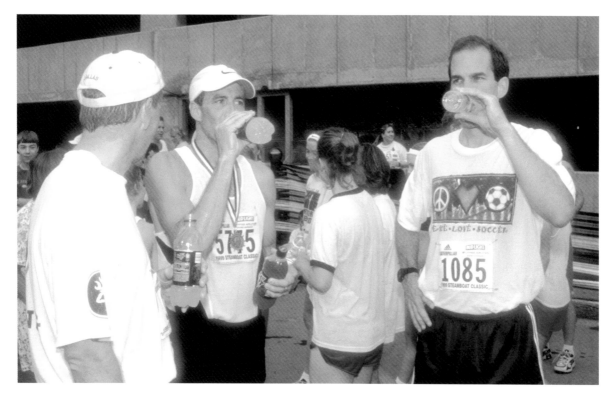

Wearing light-colored clothing and drinking water will help cool the body when exercising in hot weather.

FIT FACTS

Modern technology has produced clothing that is especially good for exercising in cold weather. A shirt made of wickable fibers such as polypropylene or Capilene absorbs moisture from the skin and transfers it (wicks it away) to the next layer of clothing. A windbreaker made of synthetic materials such as GORE-TEX blocks the wind but also allows body heat to be released. This type of garment is especially good for wearing as an outside layer in cold weather.

or excessively low body temperature. Hypothermia is accompanied by shivering, numbness, drowsiness, muscular weakness, and confusion or disorientation. Extreme cold can also cause a condition called frostbite. Frostbite occurs when a body part becomes frozen. Often a person with frostbite feels no pain, making this condition more dangerous. Follow these guidelines when exercising in cold, windy, and wet weather:

▶ **Avoid extreme cold and wind.** Before dressing for physical activity, use the chart on the next page to determine the **windchill factor.** Exercising when the temperature is cold and the wind is blowing is especially dangerous because the air feels colder. The windchill chart on the next page indicates the amount of time it would take to cause frostbite if the skin is exposed to

various windchill levels. Experts agree that if the time to frostbite is 30 minutes or less, activity should be postponed. If you are active when the windchill factor is high, be sure to dress properly and be aware of the symptoms of frostbite and hypothermia.

▶ **Dress properly.** Wear several layers of lightweight clothing rather than a heavy jacket or coat. The clothing closest to your body should be loose fitting and made from a fiber that wicks or transfers the moisture from the skin to the next layer of clothing. Silk, wool, and many synthetic garments are good (see FitFacts). Cotton tends to absorb water rather than transfer it away from the skin. Garments that are not absorbent—such as a plastic

Symptoms of Frostbite

❑ Skin becomes white or grayish yellow and looks glossy.
❑ Pain is sometimes felt early, but subsides later (often feeling is lost and no pain is felt).
❑ Blisters may appear later.
❑ The affected area feels intensely cold and numb.

 www.fitnessforlife.org/student/2/4

Temperature (°F)

Wind (mph)	30	25	20	15	10	5	0	−5	−10	−15	−20	−25
5	25	19	13	7	1	−5	−11	−16	−22	−28	−34	−40
10	21	15	9	3	−4	−10	−16	−22	−28	−35	−41	−47
15	19	13	6	0	−7	−13	−19	−26	−32	−39	−45	−51
20	17	11	4	−2	−9	−15	−22	−29	−35	−42	−48	−55
25	16	9	3	−4	−11	−17	−24	−31	−37	−44	−51	−58
30	15	8	1	−5	−12	−19	−26	−33	−39	−46	−53	−60
35	14	7	0	−7	−14	−21	−27	−34	−41	−48	−55	−62
40	13	6	−1	−8	−15	−22	−29	−36	−43	−50	−57	−64
45	12	5	−2	−9	−16	−23	−30	−37	−44	−51	−58	−65
50	12	4	−3	−10	−17	−24	−31	−38	−45	−52	−60	−67
55	11	4	−3	−11	−18	−25	−32	−39	−46	−54	−61	−68
60	10	3	−4	−11	−19	−26	−33	−40	−48	−55	−62	−69

Frostbite occurs in 30 minutes or less

Windchill chart.

or nylon shirt—should not be worn as the layer closest to the skin. A high collar on one of the inner layers is a good idea. The outer layer should be made of material that will stop the wind, such as nylon. Some garments made of synthetic fibers, such as porous windbreakers, stop the wind and allow heat to be released from the body (see FitFacts on the previous page). Wear a knit cap, ski mask, and mittens (they keep hands warmer than gloves do), as needed.

▶ **Avoid exercising in icy or cold, wet weather.** Special problems can occur during icy or cold, wet weather. Your shoes, socks, and pant legs can get wet, increasing the risk of foot injuries and falls. If exposure to cold is unavoidable, learn about steps you can take to help you survive.

Pollution and Altitude

Conditions other than weather, including air pollution and altitude, can influence the effectiveness and safety of exercise.

High levels of air pollution affect your breathing ability. Radio and television stations usually issue warnings when air

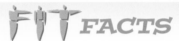

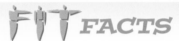
pollution levels are high. Avoid exercising outdoors during these times.

People who live at high altitudes are able to exercise with little trouble; however, people who live at lower altitudes might have trouble adjusting to higher altitudes. Even if you are physically fit, allow your body to adjust to higher altitudes by first exercising at low intensities for limited periods. For example, snow skiers should avoid hard skiing and limit the length of ski sessions for a day or two in order to become accustomed to the higher altitude.

General Readiness: Dressing for Physical Activity

Special environmental circumstances such as heat and cold require special dress for physical activity. Even under normal circumstances, the way you dress has a lot to do with your comfort and enjoyment. Consider these guidelines when dressing for physical activity:

▶ **Wear comfortable clothing.** Tight clothing can restrict your blood flow or limit your motion during vigorous exercise. Your body cools itself better if your clothing fits loosely.

▶ **Wash exercise clothing regularly.** Clean clothing is more comfortable than soiled clothing, and it reduces chances of fungal growth or infections.

▶ **Dress in layers when exercising outdoors.** You can remove layers of clothing as you become warmer while exercising and put them back on when you cool down.

▶ **Wear proper socks.** Thick sport socks provide a cushion, help prevent blisters, and absorb perspiration from your feet.

▶ **Wear proper shoes.** Most people can use a good pair of multipurpose exercise or sport shoes. However, if you plan to do special activities, you might prefer shoes designed for them. Try on shoes before buying them. When you try them on, wear the kind of socks you normally wear and walk to see how they feel. The shoes should not feel too heavy because extra weight makes exercise more tiring. Choose leather or cloth shoes. Vinyl or plastic shoes do not let air pass through to help cool your feet, so your feet perspire. Shoes do not have to be expensive. However, be sure to look for shoes with the features listed in the picture below.

▶ **Consider lace-up ankle braces.** Ankle braces can help prevent ankle injuries, especially for activities with quick changes in direction such as basketball and racquetball. Studies show that lace-up ankle braces reduce the number of ankle injuries among those who have a history of ankle injuries. Also consider wearing high-top shoes for ankle support.

The Warm-Up and Cool-Down

The time you spend doing physical activity on any given day is your daily physical activity session, or exercise session. A good, safe activity session has three stages: a warm-up, a workout, and a cool-down.

The Warm-Up

In chapter 1 you learned to perform exercises that can be used as a general warm-up or as a cool-down after your workout. In this chapter you will learn more about

why a warm-up and a cool-down are important. A warm-up is a series of activities that prepares your body for more vigorous physical activity, enhances performance, and helps prevent injury. A warm-up usually consists of a heart warm-up and a muscle stretching warm-up.

The heart is a muscle—one of the most important in your body. It needs to be warmed up. A heart warm-up consists of several minutes (at least 2) of walking, slow jogging, or a similar activity that prepares your heart for more vigorous activity. The heart warm-up increases the total body temperature as well as increasing muscle temperature and blood supply to the muscles. Warm muscles contract and relax more efficiently than cool muscles.

The muscle-stretching phase of the warm-up consists of exercises that slowly stretch the muscles to loosen and relax them. Most experts believe that warm, relaxed muscles are less likely to be strained or pulled than short, tight muscles.

The sample warm-up and stretch you performed in chapter 1 is useful for people doing moderate activity, including many of the activities in this book. People who participate in vigorous activities, especially sports, should design a personal warm-up to prepare them for that specific activity. Many lifestyle activities, such as walking, do not need a warm-up. However, you should do a warm-up for any activity that is vigorous or requires a lot of muscle stretching. Follow these guidelines to help you develop your own warm-up:

▶ Your heart warm-up should last at least 2 minutes and up to several minutes. It might include walking, slow jogging, slow swimming, slow bicycling, or a similar activity. Your goal is to gradually increase your heart rate and warm the large muscles of the body.

▶ Do your heart warm-up both before and after your muscle stretching warm-up. The first gets the muscles

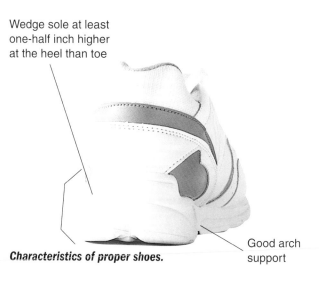

Wedge sole at least one-half inch higher at the heel than toe

Good arch support

Characteristics of proper shoes.

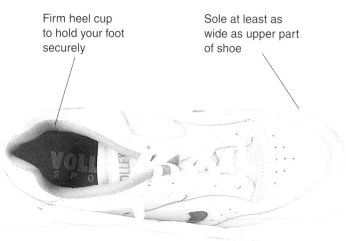

Firm heel cup to hold your foot securely

Sole at least as wide as upper part of shoe

ready for stretching and the second gets you ready for more vigorous activity after the stretching.

▶ Stretch slowly and easily. Do not bounce, jerk, or try to stretch too far. The warm-up is meant to get you ready for your workout; it is not the time for a flexibility workout.

▶ When preparing for sports or other vigorous activities, include a few slow, easy movements that are similar to the activity you will do. For example, if you are going to pitch for a baseball game, you should warm up your throwing arm. Start by making a few easy, short throws. Gradually work up to longer, harder throws as your arm muscles become warmer and more limber.

The Cool-Down

After a workout, your body needs to recover from the demands of physical activity. A cool-down usually consists of a heart cool-down and a muscle cool-down (stretch).

A heart cool-down consists of movements done at a slower pace than the workout. The heart cool-down helps prevent dizziness and fainting. Hard exercise causes an increased flow of blood to your muscles. For example, running causes more blood to be pumped to your arms and legs than to your head. If you suddenly stop running, the blood will pool in your legs, so your heart will have less blood to pump to the brain. As a result, you may feel dizzy or faint. But if you continue walking after a hard run, your muscles will squeeze the veins of your legs, helping the blood return to your heart. Your heart will then have more blood to pump to the brain, and you will be less likely to feel dizzy or faint.

Many experts agree that a muscle cool-down and stretch is beneficial after a workout. After your workout—for example, playing basketball or doing aerobic dance—gradually cool down the muscles by continuing to move around so that the blood does not pool in the legs, then slowly stretching the muscles used during the workout. Because the muscles are already warm, you may do stretches to increase flexibility at this time. Follow these guidelines when you cool down:

▶ Continue to move for several minutes after vigorous activity before stretching your muscles.

▶ Your muscle stretch can be the same stretching exercises you did as a warm-up, except that you may increase the intensity of each stretch because the muscles are now warm. Stretch slowly without bouncing. Stretch the muscle groups that you used vigorously in your workout.

Lesson Review
1. What are the many environmental factors that can make activity unhealthy or unsafe?
2. What are some of the guidelines for dressing properly for physical activity in normal environments?
3. Why should you perform a warm-up and a cool-down, and how can you perform them properly?

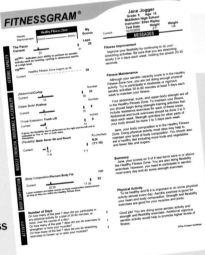

FITNESS Technology

FITNESSGRAM is a fitness self-assessment program developed by a group of experts at the Cooper Institute in Dallas, Texas. The program provides instructions for taking a variety of health-related physical self-assessments and includes a computer program that allows you to build a personal fitness profile by entering your data on the computer. You can find out more about FITNESSGRAM on the Internet (www.cooperinst.org) or by using the FITNESSGRAM software supplied by your teacher. In the self-assessment in this chapter you will perform two of the self-assessments in the FITNESSGRAM. In later chapters you will try the remaining tests. When all of your self-assessment scores have been entered using the software, you can print a personal fitness profile that will give you ratings for each part of health-related fitness and that can be used to help you in planning a personal fitness program. A sample FITNESSGRAM profile is shown here.

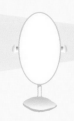

FITNESSGRAM 1—Strength and Muscular Endurance

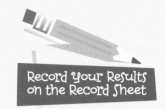

Record Your Results on the Record Sheet

FITNESSGRAM is a group of physical fitness assessments developed specifically for youth. In this activity you will perform two of the FITNESSGRAM assessments, the curl-up and the push-up. These two assessments are designed to measure strength and muscular endurance. You will perform the remaining FITNESSGRAM assessments in chapters 5 and 8.

For the FITNESSGRAM tests in this chapter and in chapters 5 and 8, you will record your scores and ratings on your record sheets supplied by your teacher. Later you will learn to interpret your ratings chart results for all your FITNESSGRAM assessments to provide a fitness profile. You can use this profile for personal fitness planning.

Curl-Up

1. Lie on your back on a mat or carpet. Bend your knees approximately 140 degrees. Your feet should be slightly apart and flat on the floor. Your arms should be straight and parallel to your trunk with palms of hands resting on the mat. Make sure you have extended your feet as far as possible from the buttocks while still allowing feet to remain flat on floor. The closer your feet are positioned in relation to the buttocks, the more difficult the movement.

2. Place your head on a piece of paper. The paper will assist your partner in judging if your head touched down on each repetition. Place a 4 1/2 inch strip (cardboard, rubber, or plastic) under your knees so that the fingers of both hands just touch the near edge of the strip. A partner can stand on the strip to keep it stationary or you can tape it down.

3. Keeping your heels on the floor, curl your shoulders up slowly and slide your arms forward so that the fingers move across the cardboard strip. Curl up until the fingertips reach the far side of the strip.

4. Slowly lower your back until your head rests on the piece of paper.

5. Repeat the procedure so that you do one curl-up every 3 seconds. A partner could help you by saying "up-down" every 3 seconds. You are finished when you cannot do another curl-up or when you fail to keep up with the 3-second count.

To avoid soreness, you may want to stop at 25 curl-ups, especially when your are testing yourself for

the first time. If you want to see whether you are in the high performance zone, you can retake the test when you have been active on a regular basis.

6. Record the number of curl-ups you have completed on your record sheet. Then find your rating in table 2.2.

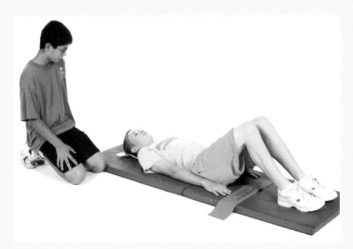

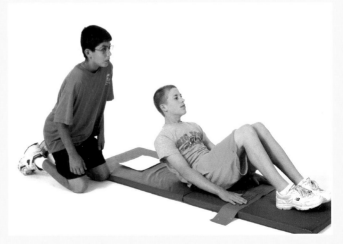

(continued)

29

Curl-Up (*continued*)

Table 2.2

Rating Chart: Curl-Up

	13 YEARS OLD		14 YEARS OLD		15 YEARS AND OLDER	
	Males	**Females**	**Males**	**Females**	**Males**	**Females**
High performance	41+	33+	46+	33+	48+	36+
Good fitness	21-40	18-32	24-45	18-32	24-47	18-35
Marginal fitness	18-20	15-17	20-23	15-17	20-23	15-17
Low fitness	17–	14–	19–	14–	19–	14–

Adapted with permission from *FITNESSGRAM*.

Push-Up

1. Lie facedown on a mat or carpet with your hands under your shoulders, your fingers spread, and your legs straight. Your legs should be slightly apart and your toes should be tucked under.

2. Push up until your arms are straight. Keep your legs and back straight. Your body should form a straight line.

3. Lower your body by bending your elbows until they are each parallel to the floor (at a 90-degree angle), then push up until the arms are fully extended. Do one push-up every 3 seconds. You may want to have a partner say "up-down" every 3 seconds to help you. You are finished when you fail to complete a push-up with proper form for the second time.

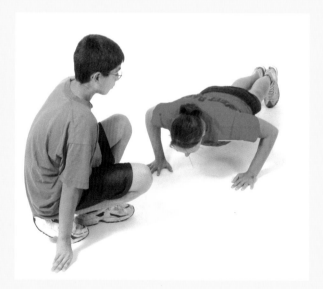

To avoid soreness you may wish to stop at 15 if you are female or 25 for males since these scores meet or exceed the good fitness zone for all ages. If you want to see if you are in the high performance zone, you can retake the test when you have been active on a regular basis.

4. Record the number of push-ups you performed on your record sheet. Then find your rating in table 2.3.

Table 2.3

Rating Chart: Push-Up

	13 YEARS OLD		14 YEARS OLD		15 YEARS OLD		16 YEARS AND OLDER	
	Males	Females	Males	Females	Males	Females	Males	Females
High performance	26+	16+	31+	16+	36+	16+	36+	16+
Good fitness	12-25	7-15	14-30	7-15	16-35	7-15	18-35	7-15
Marginal fitness	10-11	6	12-13	6	14-15	6	16-17	6
Low fitness	9–	5–	11–	5–	13–	5–	15–	5–

Adapted with permission from FITNESSGRAM.

Physical Activity and Injury

Lesson Objectives

After reading this lesson, you should be able to

1. List and describe some activity-related physical injuries.
2. List some guidelines for preventing injuries during physical activity.
3. Explain how to apply the RICE formula to the treatment of physical injuries.
4. Identify different types of risky exercises.

Lesson Vocabulary

biomechanical principles (p. 33), ligament (p. 33), microtrauma (p. 32), overuse injury (p. 32), side stitch (p. 32), tendon (p. 33)

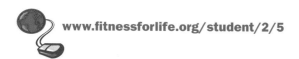

www.fitnessforlife.org/student/2/5

You know that physical activity has many advantages to your health and wellness. But if physical activity is not done properly, injury can sometimes result. Most injuries are minor but can be prevented if care is taken.

Before you start a physical activity program, be sure you are prepared to exercise and know how to exercise safely. In this lesson you will learn about some common minor injuries, as well as some basic precautions that you should take to avoid them. Some exercises are considered to be risky because they can lead to injury. You will learn about some of these risky exercises and about safer alternatives that you can use.

Common Injuries

If you have ever suffered an injury related to sports or exercise, you know that an injury can be quite painful even if it is not serious. Some of the more common minor injuries related to sports and exercise are sprains, strains, blisters, bruises, cuts, and scrapes. More serious but less common injuries include joint dislocations and bone fractures. The most common parts of the body injured in physical activity are the skin, feet, ankles,

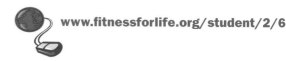

A sprain is an injury to ligaments. If a ligament is stretched, swelling and pain around the joint can result. A strain, or muscle pull, is an injury to tendons or muscles. A strain also can result in muscle pain and swelling.

knees, and leg muscles. Injuries to the head, arms, body, and internal organs such as the liver and kidneys are less likely.

www.fitnessforlife.org/student/2/6

One type of injury is called an **overuse injury.** These injuries occur when you repeat a movement so much that wear and tear occur to your body. You are most likely familiar with one very common overuse injury—a blister. Another example is shinsplints, which is a soreness in the front of the lower leg. It is probably caused by small muscle tears or muscle spasms from overuse of the muscles. Runner's heel is another overuse injury that results in soreness in the heel. The soreness is usually caused by running or jumping activities that require the heel to repeatedly hit the ground. These injuries are especially common among long-distance runners and people whose activities cause repeated impact on the feet.

A **side stitch** is a pain in the side of the lower abdomen that people often experience in sports, especially running activities. Side stitches are most common among people who are not accustomed to vigorous activity. A side stitch is not really an injury because the pain goes away if you stop the activity or continue at a more moderate pace. Unless the pain is extreme or persistent, a side stitch is nothing to worry about. To help relieve a side stitch, press firmly at the point of the pain with your hand while bending forward or backward.

Another type of injury is called **microtrauma.** *Micro* means small—so small it may not show up on an X ray or exam—and *trauma* is another word for injury. So a microtrauma is an invisible injury. Often these injuries do not cause immediate pain or soreness, but with repeated use, symptoms of the damage eventually appear. Many adults today are now experiencing back problems, neckaches, and stiff, painful joints caused by microtrauma done when they were younger. Some risky exercises that can cause microtrauma are discussed later in the chapter.

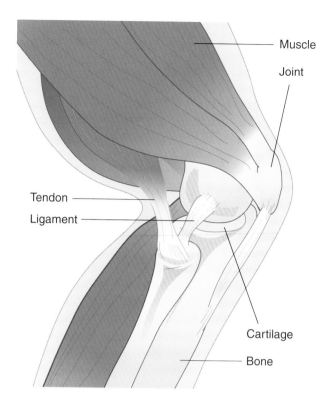

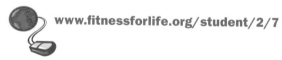

FIT FACTS

Anabolic steroids are illegal supplements taken by some athletes, including some teens. Those who take them are attempting to enhance their performance but they often have the opposite effect. Steroids have been shown to be an important cause of injury to tendons and ligaments. Leading sports medicine doctors indicate that steroid use causes athletes to miss many games and can result in career-ending injuries (see chapter 11 for more information).

Muscle
Joint
Tendon
Ligament
Cartilage
Bone

Tisues that are often injured.

Preventing Injuries

You probably know that your body is made up of about 206 bones that connect at joints. You can see in the diagram that ligaments hold the bones together at the joint. A **ligament** is made of tough tissues. The other type of tissue you see in the figure is a **tendon,** a tissue that connects muscles to bones.

When your muscles contract, they pull your tendons and make your bones move. The bones act as levers and work with your muscles to allow body movement. But when your muscles move the bones in your body, they exert a force on those bones. These forces can cause medical problems if you don't use correct techniques when doing physical activity.

The same principles used in physics and engineering to study forces can be applied to help living organisms function efficiently. These principles, called **biomechanical principles,** can help you use the levers of your body (your bones) to move efficiently and avoid injury to the joints and other body parts.

www.fitnessforlife.org/student/2/7

One important principle you should remember as you do physical activity is that you should not force your joints to move in ways that they were not designed to move. For example, you should avoid any movement that rotates your elbow or knee; the structure of these joints does not safely allow that kind of movement.

Another principle to keep in mind is that your movements should not overstress bones, tendons, ligaments, or muscles. Bending over and trying to touch your toes while both legs are straight has the possibility of injuring your back.

A third principle to remember is that you should balance the muscle development around a joint so that all

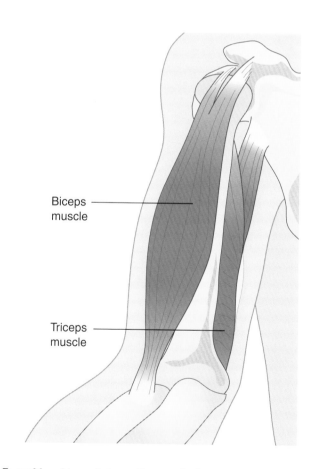

Biceps muscle

Triceps muscle

To avoid problems, balance the muscle development around a joint.

the muscles will develop properly. For example, look at the diagram of an upper arm. If you overdevelop your biceps muscle with no attention to your triceps, eventually you might be unable to fully extend your arm; your triceps will not be strong enough. Also you increase the risk of straining your triceps muscle because this weak muscle will be overstressed by the pull of the strong biceps.

As you perform your regular physical activity, keep those important biomechanical principles in mind. By understanding how your body works and by following some simple guidelines, you can reduce the risk of common injuries.

▶ **Start slowly.** The greatest number of injuries occur in beginners. If you haven't been exercising regularly, be sure to start slowly and gradually build up to more vigorous activity.

▶ **Listen to your body.** Injuries can occur when you ignore the signs and symptoms your body is giving you. If you experience pain, pay attention to it. Until you know what is causing the pain, slow your exercise or stop altogether. Most blisters and shinsplints can be avoided if people listen to their bodies.

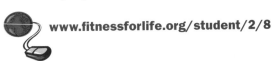

www.fitnessforlife.org/student/2/8

▶ **Warm up before activity and cool down after activity.** Follow the guidelines described earlier in this chapter.

▶ **Be fit!** One of the best ways to avoid injury is to be physically fit. A person with a fit heart and lungs and long, strong muscles is less likely to be injured than one who is unfit. Proper physical activity builds total physical fitness, which aids in injury prevention.

▶ **Use moderation.** Overuse is the cause of many minor injuries in physical activity. About 40 percent of

FIT FACTS

People just beginning a physical activity program sometimes get a type of soreness called Delayed Onset Muscle Soreness (DOMS). This soreness occurs 24 to 48 hours after a vigorous workout such as a sport practice. DOMS is caused by microscopic muscle tears. Unlike microtrauma, these muscle tears do not cause permanent damage. Beginning an exercise program gradually will help you avoid DOMS. It is alright to continue to exercise when you are sore, but if pain persists or is sharp rather than general in nature, stop exercising and seek medical advice.

regular runners and 50 percent of aerobic dancers experience injuries at some time. Injuries are usually caused by using a body part too intensely or for too long a period.

▶ **Dress properly.** Sometimes injuries are caused by improper dress. Poor shoes and socks can cause blisters or runner's heel. Make sure you dress properly, wear proper shoes, and replace them when they begin to wear down.

Simple Treatment of Minor Injuries

When injuries occur, it is often necessary to seek medical help. However, you can take immediate steps to reduce the pain or prevent complications of the injury. It is good to know first aid so that you know what steps to take when injuries occur. For muscle strains, sprains, and bruises, which are common in sports and other activities, you can follow the RICE formula (see p. 35). Each letter in the formula represents a step taken to treat a minor injury.

Risky Exercises

Some exercises are considered risky because they cause the body to move in ways that violate basic biomechanical principles. Doing these exercises may not cause immediate injury and pain. However, if they are done repeatedly over time, these exercises put you at risk for microtrauma. They can result in pain; joint problems; wear and tear injuries such as inflammation of tendons, bursa, or joints; and a wearing away of the joint cartilage. Microtrauma caused by doing risky exercises over time can result in crippling arthritis or back and neck pain, a leading medical complaint in our country.

In general, the exercises that follow should be avoided. In this lesson's activity, you will learn some safe alternative exercises. Some athletes might find it impossible to avoid potentially harmful exercises. For example, gymnasts must perform stunts that require back arching, and softball and baseball catchers must do full squats. It is especially important that these people do extra flexibility and strength exercises to prepare their bodies for these activities. They should carefully warm up and cool down. If pain occurs when exercising, they should get medical help immediately.

Hyperflexion Exercises to Avoid
Hyperflexion exercises bend your joints too far and overstretch your ligaments. *Hyper* means too much; *flexion*

The RICE Formula for Treating Injury

R is for rest.
After first aid has been given for the injury, the body part should be immobilized for two to three days to prevent further injury. In some cases, longer rest periods are required.

I is for ice.
A sprain or strain should be immersed in cold water or covered with ice in a towel or plastic bag. Ice for 20 minutes starting immediately after the injury to help reduce swelling and pain. Ice or cold should be applied several times a day for one to three days. Rubbing ice on the front of your leg can help relieve the pain of shinsplints.

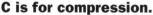

C is for compression.
Use an elastic bandage to wrap the injury to help limit swelling. For a sprained ankle, keep the shoe laced and the sock on the foot until compression can be applied with a bandage. The shoe and sock compress the injury. The compression should not be too tight and should be taken off periodically so as not to restrict blood flow.

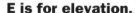

E is for elevation.
Raise the body part above the level of the heart to help reduce swelling.

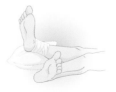

means to bend. The deep knee bend is an example of hyperflexion of the knee. Hyperflexion exercises cause you to use the joint in a way that it was not intended to be used. Other hyperflexing exercises to avoid include duckwalks, bicycles (also called shoulder stand), yoga ploughs, hands-behind-the-neck sit-ups, and knee pull-downs.

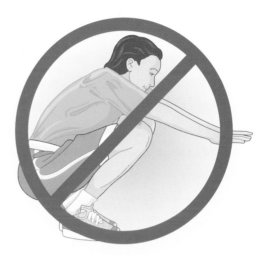

Avoid hyperflexion exercises (e.g., deep knee bends).

Back Hyperextension Exercises to Avoid
Hyperextension is the opposite of hyperflexion. Having some curve in the back is normal but arching the lower back more than normal is an example of hyperflexion. Some back arching exercises tend to stretch your abdominal muscles and can injure your spinal discs and joints. In addition, these exercises may shorten your back muscles, which are already too short in most people. People with swayback, weak abdominal muscles, a protruding abdomen, and back problems should be particularly cautious. You will learn more about

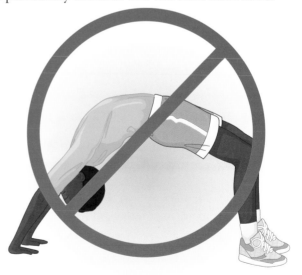

Avoid hyperextension exercises (e.g., back bends).

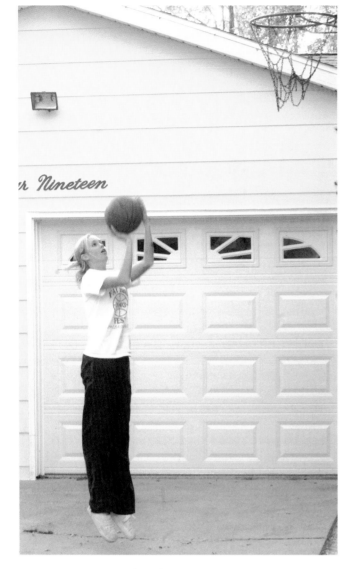

A good way to build self-confidence is to practice skills when others aren't watching so you don't feel awkward. Once you gain more confidence in your skills you'll be ready to get involved in a game.

swayback and other back problems in chapter 3. Risky hyperextension exercises include straight-leg sit-ups, back bends, rocking horses, cobras, prone swan positions, excessive upper back lifts, and incorrect weight-lifting positions with the back arched.

Other Hyperextension Exercises to Avoid

Some other exercises that hyperextend the spine are rear double-leg lifts, donkey kicks, landing from a jump with the back arched, wrestler's bridges, neck hyperextensions, neck circling to the rear, and backward trunk circling.

Joint Twisting, Compression, and Friction Exercises to Avoid

Exercises that cause the joints to bend too far or to bend in a way that they were not intended to move are

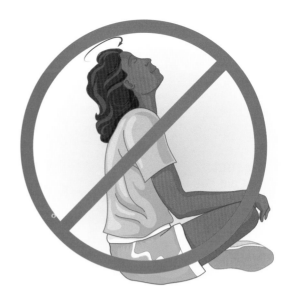

Avoid hyperextension and exercises that cause friction (e.g., neck circling to the rear).

also risky. They can result in injury to the joint and tissues around the joint. Some exercises also cause certain structures to rub against others, creating friction that causes wear and tear. Some exercises in this category are hurdle sits, heroes, double-leg lifts, sit-ups, standing straight-leg toe touches, standing windmill toe touches, and arm circling with palms down.

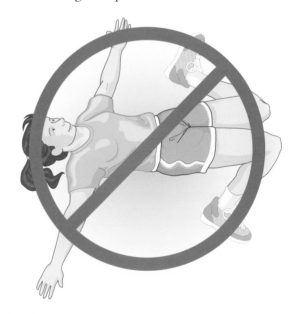

Avoid twisting or compressing joints (e.g., heroes).

Improper Strengthening or Stretching Exercises

Some exercises can result in muscle imbalance because they build muscles that are not especially in need of development rather than the muscles needed for good health and wellness. They are not risky but poor

Taking Charge: Building Self-Confidence

Self-confidence is having faith that you can be successful in some activity. If you think you will succeed in the activity, you have a higher level of self-confidence than if you are unsure about how well you will do. You are more likely to participate in an activity if your self-confidence level is high.

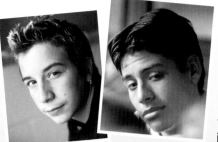

Tony is 6 feet tall and weighs 160 pounds. He looks like a natural athlete. In reality, Tony hardly ever takes part in any physical activity. Because he went through an awkward stage in his preteen years, Tony thinks that people laugh at the way he runs. "My arms and legs don't seem to work together when I run. I think that I look foolish."

Richard loves any kind of physical activity. Every day he shoots baskets or rides his bike. He is part of several teams. While Richard excels in sports, he is shy around strangers, especially when the strangers are female. "I can't think of anything witty or even halfway intelligent to say. Even when I try to talk, I get tongue-tied. It's easier for me to just avoid talking."

Tony and Richard both lack self-confidence, but in different situations. While Tony really wants to participate in physical activity and Richard wants to socialize with some girls, they both avoid getting into any situation that might require their involvement. Both need to find a way to build their self-confidence levels and be successful in these situations.

For Discussion

People who lack self-confidence may avoid trying new activities or experiences, or they may prematurely quit an activity. What are some reasons people lack self-confidence? How can they increase their confidence levels? Fill out the questionnaire provided by your teacher for this chapter to see how self-confident you are about taking part in physical activities. Consider the guidelines on page 38.

---

choices. For example, forward arm circling develops already strong pectorals, but backward arm circles with palms up are a better choice of exercise because they work on the weaker back muscles. Other improper exercises strengthen the already too strong muscles that go across the front of the hip joint. These exercises can cause injury to the discs, abdominal tears, tendon tears, and loose ligaments. Examples of this type of risky exercise include double-leg lifts and straight-leg sit-ups.

Safe Exercise Circuit

Look over the exercises on pages 39 and 40. These are safe exercises because they are less likely to cause microtrauma than the exercises just described. Read about these exercises before you perform the safe exercise circuit.

Lesson Review

1. What are some exercise-related physical injuries?
2. How can you prevent injuries during physical activity?
3. How can the RICE formula be used to treat physical injuries?
4. What are some different types of risky exercises?

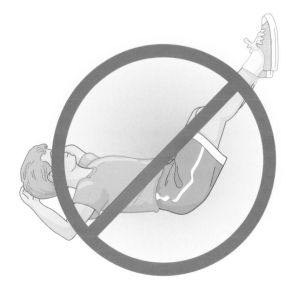

Avoid exercises that strengthen muscles that are already too strong (e.g., double-leg lift).

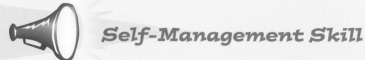

Self-Management Skill

Building Self-Confidence

A recent study of teenagers found that one of the best ways to determine who will be physically active is self-confidence. A person is self-confident if he or she thinks *I can do that* as opposed to *I don't think I can.* Some people are not very confident when it comes to physical activity because they think they are not very good or that others are better than they are. Research done in schools with teenagers shows that all people can find some type of activity in which they can be successful, regardless of physical ability. The most self-confident people are not always the best performers and some good performers lack self-confidence. We do know that people who think they can succeed in activity are nearly twice as likely to be active as those teens who don't think they can. Building self-confidence is a self-management skill that can be learned. You may want to assess your self-confidence using the worksheet supplied by your teacher. You can then use the following guidelines to help improve self-confidence if necessary.

▶ **Learn a new way of thinking.** A major reason why some people lack self-confidence is because they think that their own success depends on how they compare with others. Practicing a new way of thinking means setting your own standards of success, rather than comparing yourself to others. These guidelines are designed to help build self-confidence by developing a new way of thinking.

▶ **Set your own personal standards for success.** Assess yourself and set standards for success related to your own improvement. Comparing yourself to others is not necessary for your success, and it can contribute to low self-confidence.

▶ **Avoid competition if it causes you a problem.** Some people like to compete, but others do not. If competition makes you feel less confident in a physical activity, try to find noncompetitive activities such as walking, jogging, swimming, or other activities that allow you to feel good about yourself.

▶ **Set small goals that you are sure to reach.** Setting goals that are a bit higher than your current level is a good idea, but don't set them too high. As you reach one small goal you can set another. Reaching several small goals builds self-confidence, whereas not reaching one unrealistic goal can make you less confident.

▶ **Think and act on positive, not negative, ideas.** When you are involved in a physical activity, think of how you can improve. Talk to yourself about what you did well and what you can practice to improve in the future. Avoid negative self-talk such as berating yourself for what you did not do well or referring to yourself in negative terms.

▶ **Practice the skills of the activities in which you want to improve.** For example, if you want to be more confident in tennis, practice the skills specific to tennis.

Recognizing and Resolving Conflict in New Activities

This chapter was designed to help you prepare for participation in activity. Social interactions with other people can enrich your participation or, in some cases, lead to conflict. Conflict occurs when the actions or inactions of one person prevent, obstruct, or interfere with the actions of another person. For example, a new person in an exercise group may be ignored or fail to be included in the group's activities. In some cases, less-caring members of the group may belittle the new group member.

To keep self-confidence high and to ensure continued participation, you need to realize that a conflict exists. In this case, another person's actions prevent a new group member from enjoying an activity. Taking positive steps can help prevent and resolve potential conflict. For example, a new group member could start by introducing herself or himself to all members of the group, talking with group members before beginning the activity, sharing feelings with group members after the activity, or consulting with the group leader to get help. Using the self-management skills described previously can also be helpful. To help you learn more about appropriately recognizing and resolving conflict in physical activity, additional strategies are on pages 147, 191, and 315.

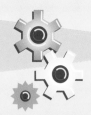

Activity 2

Safe Exercise Circuit

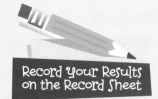
Record Your Results on the Record Sheet

You now know some risky exercises. If you have been doing any of them, you should substitute exercises such as the ones shown and described in this activity. If done properly, these exercises are safe to perform and give you the benefits of risky exercises without the risk.

The exercises presented are only a few of many safe exercises that you can substitute for risky ones. Additional safe exercises are described on your worksheet and throughout this book. Try each exercise, carefully following the directions. In chapters 11 and 12 you will learn more about the number of repetitions of exercises to perform. If you do this activity on your own, perform each exercise as many times as you can up to 15 times. If you are doing the exercises as part of a circuit in class, your teacher will tell you how many times to perform each exercise.

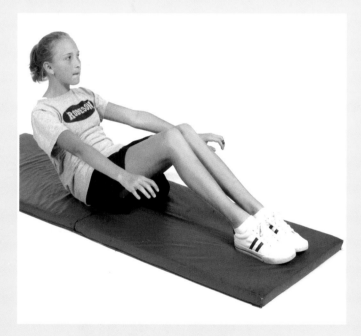

Curl-Up

The curl-up, sometimes referred to as the crunch, is a good substitute for the straight-leg sit-up, bent-knee sit-up, and hands-behind-the-head sit-up.

1. Lie on your back with your knees bent and your feet close to your buttocks.
2. Hold your hands and arms straight in front of you and curl your head, shoulders, and upper back off the floor.
3. Slowly roll back to the starting position.

 Caution: Do not hold your feet while doing a trunk curl.

As you improve, you might hold your arms across your chest. When you become very good, you might place your hands on your face (cheeks).

Reverse Curl

The reverse curl is a good substitute for the double-leg lift.

1. Lie on your back. Bend your knees, placing your feet flat on the floor. Place your arms at your sides.
2. Lift your knees to your chest, raising your hips off the floor.

 Caution: Do not lower your legs to the floor or hold your breath.

3. Return to the starting position.

This exercise can be made more difficult for the advanced exerciser by doing it on an inclined board with your head elevated.

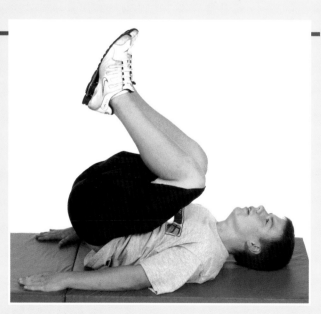

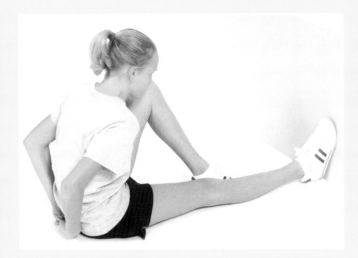

Back-Saver Hamstring Stretch

This is a safe exercise that can be substituted for the standing toe touch or the double-leg sit and reach.

1. Sit with your right foot against a wall and your left knee bent with your foot flat on the floor.
2. Clasp your hands behind your back and bend forward, keeping your lower back as straight as possible. Allow your bent knee to move sideways so that your trunk can move forward.
3. Stretch and hold.

Hip and Thigh Stretch

This exercise is a good substitute for the exercise commonly called the quadriceps stretch.

1. Kneel with your left knee directly above your left ankle.
2. Stretch your right leg backward so that your knee touches the floor. If necessary, place your hands on the floor for balance.
3. Press your pelvis forward and downward and hold for several seconds.

 Caution: Do not bend your front knee more than 90 degrees.

4. Repeat the exercise on the left side.

Knee-to-Nose Touch

This exercise is a good substitute for the donkey kick.

1. Kneel on all fours.
2. Pull your right knee toward your nose.
3. Extend your right leg and head to a horizontal position.

 Caution: Do not lift your leg higher than your hips. Do not hyperextend your neck and lower back.

4. Return to the starting position. Repeat the exercise with your left leg.

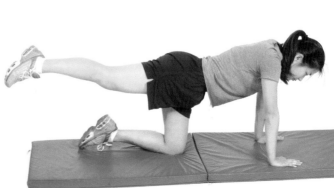

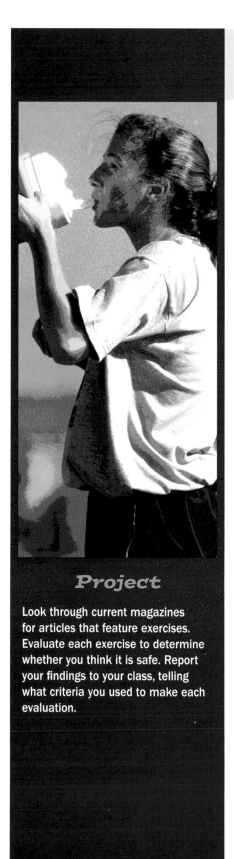

2 Chapter Review

Reviewing Concepts and Vocabulary

Number your paper from 1 to 5. Next to each number, write the word or words that correctly complete each sentence.

1. The rules of biology and physics that can be used to prevent injury to your joints are called _____.
2. Symptoms of frostbite include _____.
3. Invisible damage to the body resulting from repeating a movement often is a _____.
4. Some injuries related to sports and exercise are _____.
5. Numbness, shivering, low body temperature, and confusion are symptoms of _____.

Number your paper from 6 to 10. Next to each number, choose the letter of the best answer.

Column I	Column II
6. joint	a. connects muscle to bone
7. ligament	b. place where bones connect
8. tendon	c. pain in the lower abdomen
9. side stitch	d. holds bones together at a joint
10. hypothermia	e. body temperature becomes extremely low

Number your paper from 11 to 15. Write a short answer for each statement or question.

11. What are precautions you should take when getting ready to exercise in hot, humid weather?
12. What are the guidelines for exercising in wet, cold, or icy weather?
13. Why are self-assessments important tools when you plan for lifetime activity?
14. Explain how to follow the RICE formula when treating a minor injury.
15. What are some components of the warm-up and cool-down and why are they important?

Thinking Critically

Write a paragraph to answer the following question.

You are about to begin an exercise program with a group of friends. The leader of your group has selected some exercises for you to do. How can you determine whether the exercises are safe?

Project

Look through current magazines for articles that feature exercises. Evaluate each exercise to determine whether you think it is safe. Report your findings to your class, telling what criteria you used to make each evaluation.

2. Safe and Smart Physical Activity **41**

3

Benefits of Physical Activity

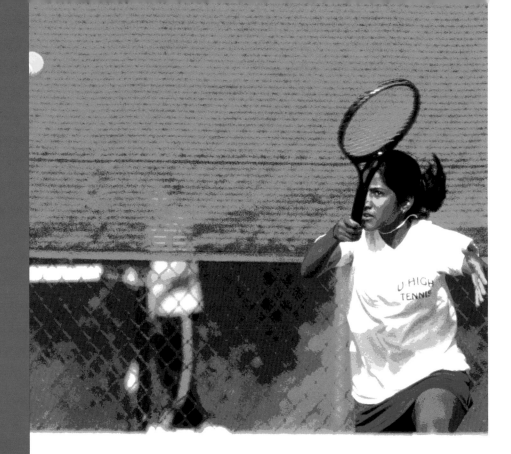

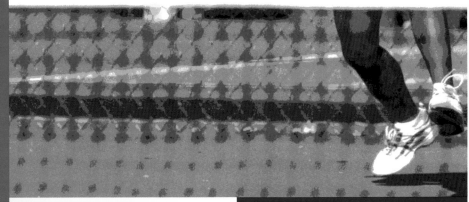

In this chapter...

Activity 1
Cooperative Games

Lesson 3.1
Health and Wellness Benefits

Self-Assessment
Healthy Back Test

Lesson 3.2
Healthy Back and Good Posture

Taking Charge
Reducing Risk Factors

Self-Management Skill
Reducing Risk Factors

Activity 2
Back Exercise Circuit

Activity 1

COOPERATIVE GAMES

Strangely enough, the concept of cooperative games grew out of the Vietnam War experience in the 1970s. Cooperative games are the opposite of war and competition. In these games, you have fun by playing for all you are worth, and everyone wins by cooperating with each other. Even when games are arranged so that teams compete, winning is not emphasized. Sometimes members of the opposite team have been known to change sides and try to help the losing team! The fun is in the play, not in the winning.

Lesson 3.1

Health and Wellness Benefits

Lesson Objectives

After reading this lesson, you should be able to

1. Describe some hypokinetic conditions.
2. List some benefits of physical activity that contribute to health and wellness.
3. Explain, using examples, how physical activity is related to hyperkinetic conditions.

Lesson Vocabulary

activity neurosis (p. 47), atherosclerosis (p. 43), blood pressure (p. 44), diabetes (p. 45), diastolic blood pressure (p. 44), eating disorders (p. 47), heart attack (p. 43), hyperkinetic conditions (p. 47), hypertension (p. 44), osteoporosis (p. 46), risk factor (p. 43), stroke (p. 44), systolic blood pressure (p. 44)

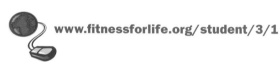

www.fitnessforlife.org/student/3/1

Prior to 1900 the leading cause of death was pneumonia. Many of the other leading causes of death were from infections caused by bacteria or viruses. Modern science found cures or vaccinations for many of these conditions, and now in the 21st century these diseases are no longer the leading health problems. Diseases such as heart disease (#1), cancer (#2), and stroke (#3) are now considered the leading health threats. These and many other diseases are considered to be hypokinetic conditions because they are caused in part from sedentary living. In this lesson you will learn more about how physical activity reduces your risk of hypokinetic conditions and increases your personal wellness.

Hypokinetic Diseases and Conditions

Sedentary living costs our nation $150 billion each year because of increased need for health care and loss of productivity. Approximately 250,000 people die prematurely because they are inactive. Reports of major health organizations, including the Office of the Surgeon Gen-

eral, indicate that regular physical activity is one of the best ways of reducing illness and increasing wellness in our society. Sometimes teenagers feel that these statistics are not relevant to them; they think illness happens only to old people. As you will see next, many hypokinetic diseases are now prevalent among teens and many teens are not active enough to resist these conditions.

Cardiovascular Diseases

Did you know that cardiovascular disease has been the leading cause of death in the United States each year since 1920? Cardiovascular disease is a primary or contributing cause of 60 percent of all deaths in our country. Currently about one in every four Americans has one or more forms of cardiovascular disease.

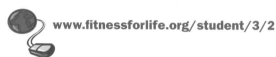

www.fitnessforlife.org/student/3/2

People get cardiovascular disease for many reasons, each one called a **risk factor.** The more risk factors you have, the more chance you have of getting a disease. Two kinds of risk factors exist: primary (most important) and secondary (less important). Sedentary, or inactive, living is one primary risk factor, so cardiovascular disease is considered a hypokinetic condition. Other primary risk factors that contribute to heart disease include smoking, high blood pressure, high fat levels in the blood, having too much body fat, or having diabetes. Secondary risk factors include stressful living and excessive alcohol use.

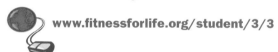

www.fitnessforlife.org/student/3/3

Various conditions are considered to be cardiovascular diseases. Coronary artery disease is a cardiovascular disease that is the number one cause of early death. Coronary artery disease exists when the arteries in your heart become clogged. Arteries are like pipelines that carry blood from the heart to all parts of your body. Clogging of the arteries is called **atherosclerosis.** It occurs when substances including fats, such as cholesterol, build up on the inside walls of the arteries. This build-up narrows the openings through the arteries. As a result, the heart must work harder to pump blood. Atherosclerosis can begin early in life but typically develops with age.

A **heart attack** occurs when the blood supply into or within the heart is severely reduced or cut off. As a result, an area of the heart muscle can die. The main reasons for heart attacks are arteries blocked by atherosclerosis, blood clots in narrowed arteries, spasms in the muscle of the artery, or a combination of these causes. During a heart attack, the heart may beat

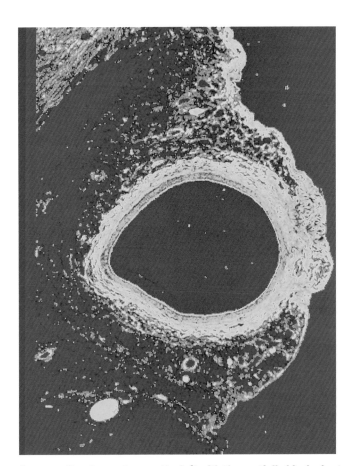 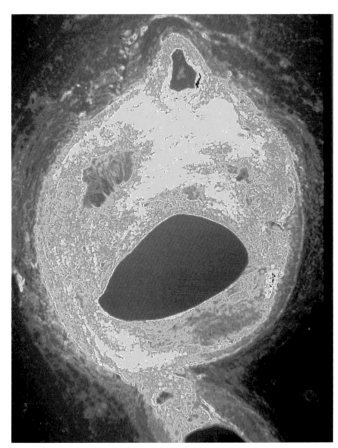

Compare the clear artery on the left with the partially blocked artery on the right.

abnormally or even stop beating. Medicines are often used to stabilize the heartbeat of someone in distress. Also, cardiopulmonary resuscitation (CPR) often is done to restore circulation of oxygen when the heart stops beating.

Stroke is another form of cardiovascular disease. It is the third leading cause of early death and occurs when oxygen in the blood supply to the brain is severely reduced or cut off. A blood clot or atherosclerosis can block any artery that supplies blood to the brain, causing a stroke. A stroke also can occur when an artery to the brain bursts. Because a stroke damages the brain, it can affect a person's ability to move, think, and speak. Some strokes are severe enough to cause death.

Each time your heart beats, it forces blood through your arteries, causing the blood to push against the artery walls. This force of blood against your artery walls is called **blood pressure.** When the doctor checks your blood pressure, he or she looks for two readings. The pressure in your arteries immediately after the heart beats—called **systolic blood pressure**—is the higher of the two readings. Your **diastolic blood pressure** is the lower of the two numbers and is the pressure in the artery just before the next beat of the heart. High blood pressure is

sometimes referred to as **hypertension.** It is a condition in which blood pressure is consistently higher than normal. It is not considered a leading cause of death as are coronary heart disease and stroke, but it is a primary risk factor for both of these conditions as well as many others. High blood pressure is a hypokinetic condition because regular physical activity is one way to help lower blood pressure. You can see the range of normal blood pressure in table 3.1. The table also shows the blood pressures for prehypertension, a new category that has recently been added. People in this range have higher than normal blood pressure and should start to take precautions to prevent even higher blood pressure. There are three stages of high blood pressure with stage 1 being the least severe and stage 3 the most severe. It is important to take your blood pressure when you are rested and relaxed. While a long-term effect of regular exercise is a decrease in blood pressure, involvement in exercise immediately before taking blood pressure will cause it to be higher than normal. Your blood pressure is also affected when you are excited or anxious.

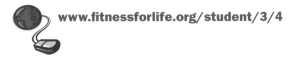 **www.fitnessforlife.org/student/3/4**

Table 3.1

Blood Pressure Readings

	Normal	Prehypertension	Stage 1	Stage 2	Stage 3
Systolic	<120	120-139	140-159	160-179	180+
Diastolic	<80	80-89	90-99	100-109	110+

The figure on this page illustrates some of the ways that regular physical activity reduces the risk of cardiovascular disease. An active person has arteries in the heart that are healthy and more likely to be free from atherosclerosis (see small pictures in the figure). The active person also has healthy arteries in the brain as well as in the muscles and other body organs, has a strong heart muscle capable of pumping adequate blood to the body, has fit blood low in fats such as cholesterol, and has blood pressure in the healthy range. Regular physical activity not only reduces risk of heart attack and stroke, it is often prescribed by medical doctors to help people recovering from these conditions.

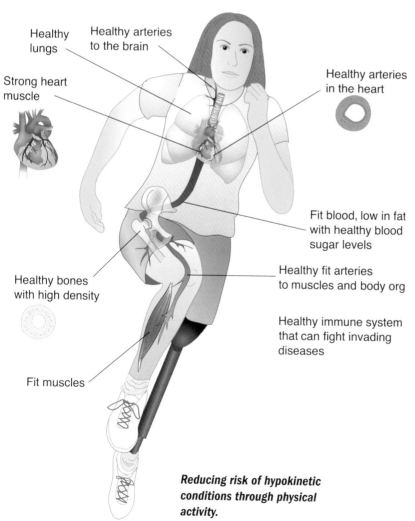

Healthy lungs

Healthy arteries to the brain

Strong heart muscle

Healthy arteries in the heart

Fit blood, low in fat with healthy blood sugar levels

Healthy fit arteries to muscles and body org

Healthy immune system that can fight invading diseases

Healthy bones with high density

Fit muscles

Reducing risk of hypokinetic conditions through physical activity.

Cancer

More than 100 different diseases characterized by the uncontrollable growth of abnormal cells are categorized as cancer. Cancer's uncontrolled cells invade normal cells, steal their nutrition, and interfere with the cells' normal functions.

Cancer is the second leading cause of death in the United States. When diagnosed early, many forms of cancer can be treated and even cured through surgery, chemical or radiation therapy, or medication. We know that the death rate from all forms of cancer is lower in active people than in inactive people. Certain forms of cancer, such as breast cancer and colon cancer, are considered hypokinetic conditions because people who are physically active are less likely to get them than people who are inactive. Many of the risk factors for heart disease are also risk factors for cancer. Getting regular physical exams is a good way to help prevent cancer. It is not clear why physical activity helps reduce the risk of cancer, but as shown in the figure one of the health benefits of activity is an immune system that is more capable of fighting diseases that invade the body.

Diabetes

When a person's body cannot regulate sugar levels, the person has a disease called **diabetes.** A person with diabetes will have excessively high blood sugar unless he or she gets medical assistance. Over time, diabetes can damage the blood vessels, heart, kidneys, and eyes. A very high level of sugar in the blood can cause coma and death. Several effective medical treatments exist to help diabetics regulate their blood sugar and lead normal lives.

One kind of diabetes—Type I—is not a hypokinetic condition. This condition is often hereditary and accounts for about 10 percent of all diabetics. Type I diabetics take insulin, a hormone made in the pancreas, to help control blood sugar levels.

The most common kind of diabetes—Type II—is a hypokinetic condition because people who are physically active are less likely to have it. As shown in the figure, active people are more likely to have blood with healthy sugar levels. Also, activity helps control body fat. Overfatness is considered to be a major risk factor for Type II diabetes. Diabetes has many of the same risk factors as heart disease.

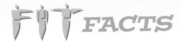

Type II diabetes used to be called adult-onset diabetes because adults got it, not teens and children. The name adult-onset is no longer used because in recent years the disease has become common among youth. Physical activity can reduce risk of Type II diabetes by helping young people keep body fat levels in the healthy range and by helping the body regulate blood sugar levels more effectively.

Obesity

A condition in which a person has a high percentage of body fat—called obesity—often is the result of inactivity, although many other factors may contribute. Having too much body fat contributes to other diseases such as heart disease and diabetes. Since 1980 the incidence of obesity among teens in the United States has increased from 5% to 14%, an increase of almost 300%, and there is a similar upward trend in other developed nations. You will learn more about obesity in chapter 13.

Osteoporosis

When the structure of the bones deteriorates and the bones become weak, a condition called **osteoporosis** exists. Osteoporosis is most common among older people, but it has its beginnings in youth. You develop your greatest bone mass—also called your peak bone mass—when you are young. As illustrated in the figure on the preceding page, those who exercise regularly develop stronger bones than those who are sedentary. It is especially important to do physical activities that cause you to bear weight, such as in walking and running, and that stress the bones, such as resistance training. If you do the right kind of activity when you are young, you will build a higher peak bone mass. As a result, if you lose bone mass as you get older, you will have stronger bones than if you hadn't exercised while young.

Lack of calcium in the diet, especially when a person is young, contributes to osteoporosis.

Women are more likely to have osteoporosis than men because, as a result of hormonal changes that take place in women later in life, calcium absorption becomes less efficient. For bone health throughout life, good nutrition, regular activity, and proper medical attention are necessary.

Other Hypokinetic Conditions

Evidence suggests that regular physical activity can enhance the function of the immune system, helping the body resist infections such as the common cold and the flu. Moderate activity has been shown to help reduce symptoms of some forms of arthritis. Being active can also help people avoid depression or reduce symptoms of depression. One-third of all adults report that they often feel depressed.

Physical Activity and Wellness

As you can see, physical activity plays an important role in the prevention of hypokinetic diseases and conditions. Therefore, physical activity is important to good health. But remember—health is more than freedom from disease; it also means being positively healthy. Two components of positive health identified as important national goals by the Healthy People 2010 report are helping all people have a sense of well-being, and helping them have a high quality of life. Some of the benefits

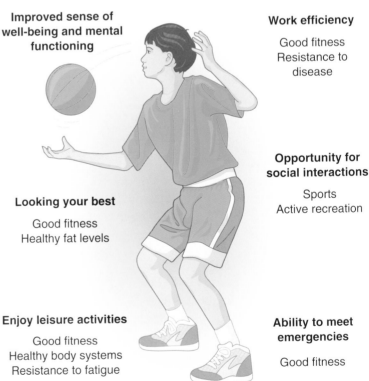

Improved sense of well-being and mental functioning

Work efficiency
Good fitness
Resistance to disease

Looking your best
Good fitness
Healthy fat levels

Opportunity for social interactions
Sports
Active recreation

Enjoy leisure activities
Good fitness
Healthy body systems
Resistance to fatigue

Ability to meet emergencies
Good fitness

Wellness and physical activity.

of physical activity that contribute to these two factors are illustrated in the figure on the previous page.

Hyperkinetic Conditions

You've probably heard the saying, "too much of a good thing can be bad." This saying can be true of physical activity. Just because some physical activity is good, more activity is not always better. In some cases people experience **hyperkinetic conditions**—health problems caused by doing too much physical activity.

Overuse Injuries

You learned in chapter 2 that overuse injuries occur when you do so much physical activity that your bones, muscles, or other tissues are damaged. It is easy to see that overuse injuries—for example, stress fractures, shinsplints, and blisters—are a type of hyperkinetic condition.

Activity Neurosis

Neurosis is a condition that occurs when a person is overly concerned or fearful about something. Excessive fear of high places is one type of neurosis. People with an **activity neurosis** are overly concerned about getting enough exercise and are upset if they miss a regular workout. In addition, they often continue physical activity when they are sick or injured. Runners and bodybuilders are more likely than other exercisers to experience activity neurosis. It is interesting that the risk of getting a cold or the flu is reduced if you are a regular exerciser but those who do excessive exercise have increased risk of getting a cold or the flu. Even those who do not have activity neurosis should avoid doing excessive exercise and reduce or avoid exercise when they are sick.

Body Image Disorder

This disorder occurs when a person tries to achieve an ideal body by doing excessive exercise. The ideal body is unrealistic and distorted. Teenaged boys and young adult men with body image disorder perform excessive resistance training and sometimes use dangerous supplements or substances such as steroids. Teenaged girls and young women often strive for extreme thinness, which is unhealthful and unrealistic. Several of the eating disorders described in chapter 13 are associated

FITNESS Technology

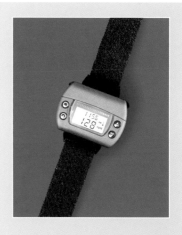

At one time it was thought that people with Type I diabetes should avoid physical activity. Now we know that physical activity can be helpful in managing diabetes. Most people with Type I diabetes take blood samples one or more times a day. These samples are used to test blood sugar levels. If blood sugar levels are high, people with diabetes take insulin to lower their blood sugar. People without diabetes automatically produce insulin in their bodies to keep blood sugar in normal range. In the past it was necessary to puncture the skin to take a blood sample. New technology has now been developed that allows some people with diabetes to wear a computer watch that automatically tests blood sugar levels without having to draw blood. The watch takes readings through the skin every 20 minutes. The watches are expensive and not accessible to all people with diabetes. However, with future refinement, this technology may improve the quality of life for people with diabetes and help them more effectively manage the disease. It is important for people with diabetes to know their blood sugar levels before exercise because activity reduces the blood sugar. A watch that monitors blood sugar can help them schedule exercise sessions.

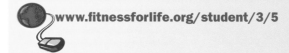
www.fitnessforlife.org/student/3/5

with body image disorders. People with body image disorders often need the help of an expert to overcome their problem.

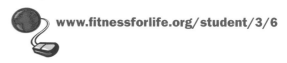
www.fitnessforlife.org/student/3/6

Eating Disorders

Several kinds of **eating disorders** result from an extreme desire to be abnormally thin. People with these conditions have dangerous eating habits and often resort to excessive activity to expend calories for fat loss. Eating disorders that abuse exercise are considered hyperkinetic conditions. You will learn more about eating disorders in chapter 13.

Lesson Review

1. What are three hypokinetic conditions? How can activity reduce the risk of getting these conditions?
2. What are some wellness benefits of physical activity?
3. How is physical activity related to hyperkinetic conditions? Give examples.

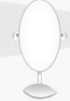

Healthy Back Test

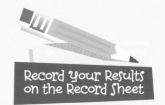

Record Your Results on the Record Sheet

Backache is a condition that is often caused by weak muscles. Use this self-assessment to test the muscles that help support your back. Each part focuses on a certain muscle group. If you do well on this assessment, you are likely to have a healthy back.

   If possible, work with a partner. As you complete each test, note the points you earn on your record sheet. When you complete all six tests, add your points to get your total score. Then use table 3.2 on page 50 to determine your risk of back problems.

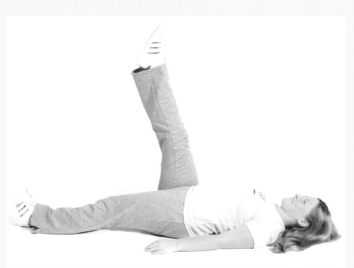

Single-Leg Lift (Supine)

1. Lie on your back on the floor. Lift your right leg off the floor as high as possible without bending either knee.
2. Repeat (this is a test not an exercise–there is a difference) using your left leg. Score 1 point if you can lift your right leg to a 90-degree angle to the floor. Score 1 additional point if you can lift your left leg to a 90-degree angle.

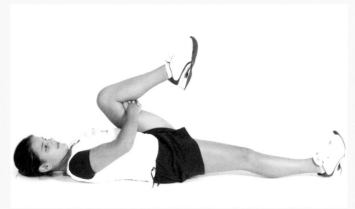

Knee to Chest

1. Lie on your back on the floor. Make sure your lower back is flat on the floor.
2. Keep your left leg straight and touching the floor. Bring your right knee up until you can hold it tightly against your chest. Grasp the back of the thigh.
3. Repeat using your left leg.
4. Score 1 point if you can keep your left leg touching the floor while you hold your right leg against your chest. Score 1 additional point if you can keep your right leg touching the floor while holding your left leg against your chest.

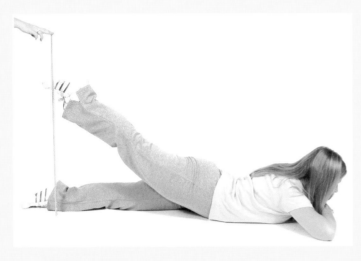

Single-Leg Lift (Prone)

1. Lie facedown on the floor. Lift your straight right leg as high as possible. Hold the position for a count of 10. Then lower your leg.
2. Repeat using your left leg.
3. Score 1 point if you can lift and hold your right leg 1 foot off the floor and hold the position for 10 counts. Score 1 point if you can lift your left leg 1 foot off the floor and hold for 10 counts.

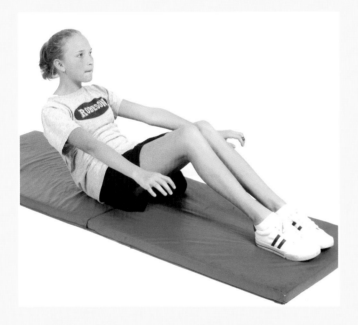

Curl-Up

1. Lie on your back with your knees bent 90 degrees and your arms extended.
2. Curl up by rolling your head, shoulders, and upper back off the floor. Roll up only until your shoulder blades leave the floor.
3. Score 1 point if you can curl up with your arms held straight in front of you and hold the position for 10 seconds without having to lift your feet off the floor.
4. Score an additional point if you can curl up with your arms across your chest and hold the position for 10 seconds.

Trunk Lift and Hold

1. Lie facedown on a padded bench or a bleacher with a towel on it (16 to 18 inches high). Your upper body (from the waist up) should extend off the bench.
2. Have your partner hold your ankles.
3. Place one hand over the other on your forehead with the palms facing away and your elbows extended to the sides.
4. Start with the upper body lowered and with the hands and elbows on the floor. Lift up slowly so that the upper body is even with the bench. Hold the position for a count of 10.
5. Score 1 point if you can lift the trunk even with the bench. Score an additional point if you can hold the upper body even with the bench for a count of 10.

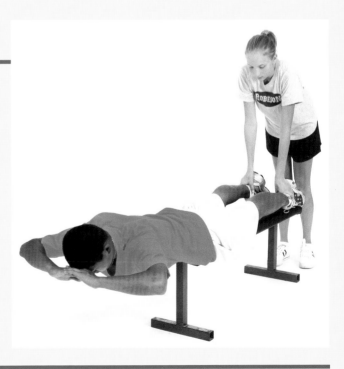

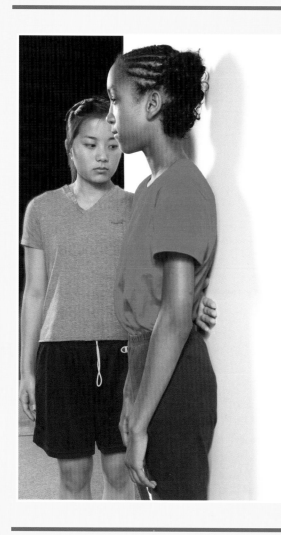

Back to Wall

1. Stand with your back to a wall so that your heels, buttocks, shoulders, and head are against the wall.
2. Try to press your lower back and neck against the wall without bending your knees or lifting your heels off the floor.
3. Have a partner try to place a hand between your back and the wall.
4. Score 2 points if you can press your back against the wall and hold it there for 10 seconds without bending your knees or moving your feet off the ground. Score 1 point if you can press your back against your partner's hand.

Table 3.2

Rating Chart: Healthy Back Test

Rating	Score
Healthy back	11-12
Average risk	9-10
Above average risk	6-8
High risk	<6

Lesson 3.2

Healthy Back and Good Posture

Lesson Objectives

After reading this lesson, you should be able to

1. Explain how good fitness helps your back work efficiently.
2. Describe some common posture problems.
3. List some biomechanical principles that will help you improve posture and avoid back problems.

Lesson Vocabulary

force (p. 53), kyphosis (p. 51), laws of motion (p. 53), lordosis (p. 51), ptosis (p. 51)

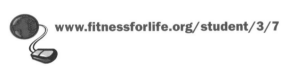

www.fitnessforlife.org/student/3/7

Each year as many as 25 million Americans seek a doctor's care for backache. According to some experts, next to the common cold, back pain is the leading medical complaint in the United States and will be experienced by 80 percent of all adults at some point in their lives. Although adults experience most of the back problems, young people do suffer from back pain. Studies show that back problems often begin early in life. In fact, recent evidence suggests that about one third of children in elementary school have had back pain and teens have almost as many back problems as adults. In this lesson you will learn how good fitness helps the back work efficiently. You will also learn how some back problems are related to poor posture.

Back Problems

Backache is considered a hypokinetic condition because weak and short muscles are linked to some types of back problems. Poor posture also is associated with muscles that are not strong or long enough. By building fit muscles to improve your posture, you can help reduce the risk of back pain and look your best. Even if you never experience back pain, a healthy back and good posture

are important so that you can function more efficiently in your daily activities.

How does good fitness help the back operate efficiently? Your body parts are balanced like blocks on your legs. Your chest hangs from your spine and is balanced over your pelvis. Your head sits on top of your spine, balanced over the other blocks in the stack. Because your spine is flexible and can move back and forth, the pull of your muscles keeps your body parts balanced. You might recall from the discussion of biomechanical principles in chapter 2 that if your muscles on one side are weak and long, while your muscles on the opposite side are strong and short, your body parts are pulled off balance.

One back problem that often occurs among teens is **lordosis,** which is too much arch in the lower back. Lordosis, also called swayback, results when the abdominal muscles are weak and the hip flexor muscles (iliopsoas) are too strong and too short (see figure on the next page). Lordosis is a problem that can lead to backache.

Even people who are relatively fit in other areas can lack fitness in the muscles related to back problems. One reason for this lack of fitness is that sports and games often overdevelop some muscles and neglect others. It is not unusual for basketball players, gymnasts, band members, and other active people to have weak back and abdominal muscles and short hamstring and hip flexors.

Posture Problems

Just as strong, long muscles contribute to a healthy back, they also are important to good posture. In the center picture of the figure on the next page, you can see some of the common posture problems associated with poor fitness. In addition to lordosis, **ptosis** (protruding abdomen) and **kyphosis** (rounded back and shoulders) are among the most common posture problems. You might recognize some of these problems with your own posture or that of others. The picture at the left illustrates how short, weak muscles contribute to posture problems. The picture at the right shows you what good posture looks like and illustrates how long, strong muscles are necessary.

Knowing what constitutes good posture helps improve your own posture. Good posture helps you look good, helps prevent back problems, and helps you work and play more efficiently. In chapter 4 you will get the opportunity to learn more about your posture using the self-assessment. You will check to see whether you have any of the problems shown in the center picture.

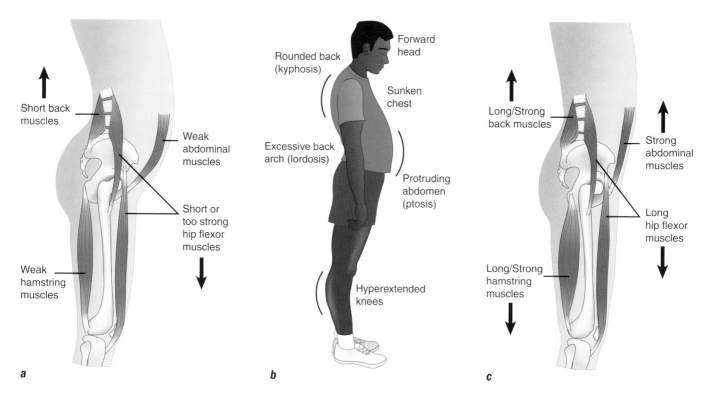

(a) Poor posture; (b) problems associated with poor posture; (c) good posture.

Back and Posture Improvement and Maintenance

Think back to the Healthy Back Test you did in the self-assessment earlier in this chapter. How did you do? If you didn't do well, avoid exercises that require you to arch your back or to lift inefficiently with your back muscles. Instead, use the Back Exercise Circuit in this chapter to help correct or prevent back problems. Because back problems are often related to poor posture, some exercises for improving posture have also been included. In addition, follow these biomechanical principles to help you improve your posture and avoid back problems:

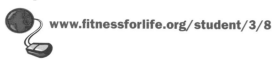

www.fitnessforlife.org/student/3/8

▶ **Use the large muscles of the body when lifting.** Let the strong leg muscles, not the relatively weak back muscles, do the work.

▶ **When lifting, keep your weight (hips) low.** Squatting with the back straight and the hips tucked helps keep weight low and makes lifting safer.

▶ **Divide a load to make it easier to carry.** For example, carrying two small suitcases, one in each hand, is easier than carrying one larger suitcase in one hand. A backpack is an efficient way to carry books. It is best to carry the backpack using both straps rather than over one shoulder. Avoid overloading your backpack or book bag. If you must carry your books in your arms, carry some in each arm. If you do carry your books in one arm, change arms from time to time.

▶ **Avoid twisting while lifting.** If you have to turn while lifting, change the position of your feet. It is especially important to avoid twisting your spine as you are straightening or bending it.

▶ **Push or pull heavy objects rather than lift them.** Heavy lifting can cause injury. Pushing or pulling an object is more efficient than lifting it.

▶ **Avoid a bent-over position when sitting, standing, or lifting.** The levers of your body, such as your spine, do not work efficiently when you are bent over. When sitting in a chair, sit back in the seat and lean against the backrest. Do not work for long periods of time in a bent-over position.

Taking Charge: Reducing Risk Factors

A risk factor is any action or condition that increases your chances of developing a disease. Some risk factors, such as your age, cannot be controlled or changed by you. Other uncontrollable risk factors, such as whether you are a male or female, are genetically controlled. Sometimes, you are able to control individual risk factors. For example, you can control your diet and physical activity. Your actions affect the probability of your getting a disease.

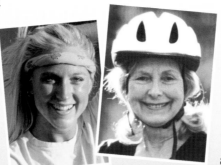

Brenda's family took a trip to the mountains last summer. Plans were made to hike, raft the rivers, and ride bikes and horses. Unfortunately, Brenda's mother did not get to enjoy all of the activities. "I never thought my mother had any health problems because she was always busy with work and taking care of the house. She never went to the doctor."

But Brenda's mother was a smoker. While she may have been "busy," she didn't really do much physical activity because she easily became short of breath.

Brenda's mother found that she couldn't keep up with the rest of the family. While hiking, she became so short of breath that she almost fainted. She fell far behind while trying to ride a bike. In the evenings, while the rest of the family did other things, Brenda's mother went to bed.

When they returned home, Brenda's mother went to her doctor. He recommended changes in her lifestyle. She was to stop smoking and get more exercise. He warned that she was at risk for heart disease and other health problems if she continued her present lifestyle.

For Discussion

What controllable risk factors for heart disease did Brenda's mother have? What can she do to reduce her risk? What can you do to decrease your risk for heart disease? Fill out the questionnaire on the worksheet supplied by your teacher to learn more about Brenda's mother's risk factors as well as your own. Consider the information on page 54.

Applying Biomechanical Principles

In chapter 2, you learned to avoid exercises that violate principles of biomechanics. These principles are based on **laws of motion.** In this chapter, you learned how to use biomechanical principles and laws of motion to move efficiently, to improve posture, and to avoid injury to your back. These principles and laws also apply when you use the body levers (the bones of the arms and legs) to apply **force.** For example, you apply force using the levers (leverage) when you throw or kick a ball and when you walk or run (see page 129). Efficient use of the body levers is also important in applying force when performing resistance exercises (see safety cautions in chapter 11), such as when you are putting the shot, throwing a javelin, or spiking a volleyball.

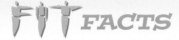

Why is it best to lift with the back straight? Simply touching your toes with the legs straight and the upper body leaning forward at the waist creates a force equal to 450 pounds on the back muscles and causes compression of the bones of the low back equal to 500 pounds. Lifting a 50-pound weight with the legs straight while bending at the waist increases the force on the back muscles to 750 pounds and causes compression on the bones of the back equal to 850 pounds.

Lesson Review

1. How does good fitness help your back operate efficiently?
2. What are some common posture problems?
3. What are some biomechanical principles that will help you improve your posture and avoid back problems?

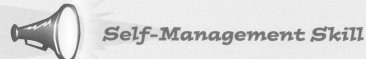

Self-Management Skill

Reducing Risk Factors

Of the 10 leading causes of death in our society, 6 can be considered hypokinetic conditions. Many of these conditions can be prevented if people change their lifestyles beginning early in life. You can take the following steps, even in your teen years, to reduce risk of hypokinetic conditions.

▶ **Be able to identify important risk factors.** If you are going to change your risks for disease you must be able to identify them. Use the questionnaire supplied by your teacher to identify your current risk factors. It is important that you continue to check your risk factors as you grow older because risk increases with age.

▶ **Learn about your family history.** Some risk factors are not in your control. Heredity is one of the factors over which you have no control. You can, however, check to see what diseases or conditions your parents or grandparents have had because you may inherit a tendency toward these conditions (for example, heart disease, diabetes, and some forms of cancer). If you have a family history of a disease, you will want to pay special attention to diseases over which you do have control.

▶ **Take steps to change the risk factors that are in your control.** Your gender and your age are other factors that you cannot control. Factors such as physical activity, what you eat, the use of tobacco, the use of alcohol, and your stress levels are factors you can control. Taking steps to alter these risk factors is especially important.

▶ **Take steps to change risk factors that are partially under your control.** Your blood pressure, the fat levels in your blood, your body's ability to regulate sugar, and your level of body fatness are all risk factors influenced by heredity but that can be modified with healthy lifestyle choices such as regular physical activity, proper eating, and proper medical care. If you have a family history of any of these risk factors, seek medical help and professional advice about how to make lifestyle changes to reduce your risk.

▶ **Use the self-management skills you learn in this book to make lifelong changes.** You will learn many self-management skills throughout this book. Use them to change the risk factors that you identify.

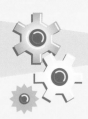

Activity 2

Back Exercise Circuit

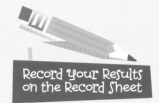

Record Your Results on the Record Sheet

You now know the importance of strong back muscles and good posture. The following exercises will help strengthen the muscles that support your back and improve your posture. You might want to include some of these exercises in your lifetime physical activity program.

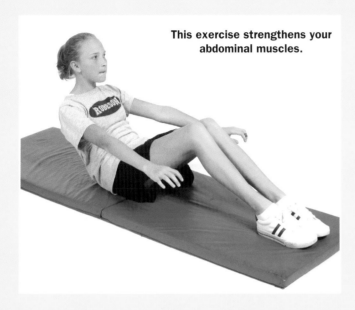

This exercise strengthens your abdominal muscles.

Curl-Up

1. Lie on your back with your knees bent and your feet close to your buttocks.
2. Hold your hands and arms straight in front of you and curl your head and shoulders up only until your shoulder blades leave the floor.
3. Slowly roll back to the starting position. Repeat the exercise up to 10 times.

Trunk Lift (Table or Bench)

1. Lie facedown on a table (or bench). Slide forward until your upper body extends over the edge at the waist. With a partner holding your legs, allow the upper body to lower.
2. From the low position, lift your upper body until it is even with the edge of the table.

 Caution: Do not lift any higher.

3. Lower to the beginning position. Repeat the exercise up to 10 times.

Safety Tip: As you do these exercises, move only as far as the directions specify.

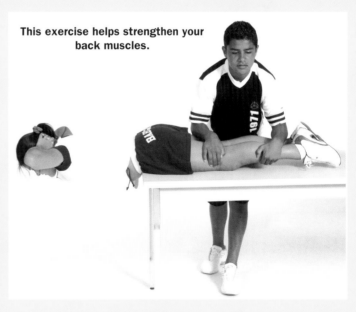

This exercise helps strengthen your back muscles.

55

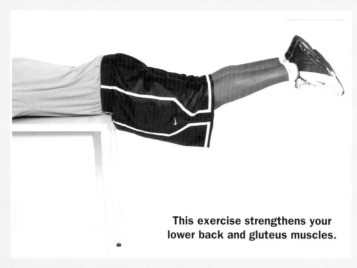

This exercise strengthens your lower back and gluteus muscles.

Double-Leg Lift (Table or Bench)

1. Lie facedown on a table (or bench) with your leg extending off the end. With a partner holding your upper body, lower the legs to the ground. If you have no partner, grasp under the edge of a table.

2. Lift your legs until they are even with the top of the table.

 Caution: Do not lift any higher. You might lift one leg at a time until you are able to lift both legs at once.

3. Lower to the starting position. Repeat the exercise up to 10 times.

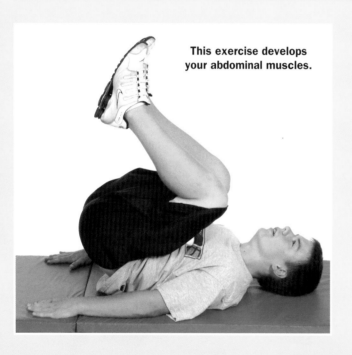

This exercise develops your abdominal muscles.

Reverse Curl

1. Lie on your back. Bend your knees, placing your feet flat on the floor. Place your arms at your sides.

2. Lift your knees to your chest, raising your hips off the floor.

3. Return to the starting position. Repeat the exercise up to 10 times.

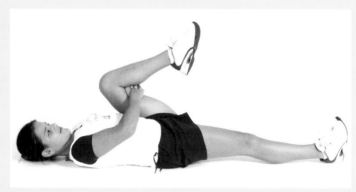

This exercise helps prevent and correct lordosis and backaches.

Knee to Chest

1. Lie on your back. Bend your right knee to your chest.

2. Grasp your thigh under the knee with your arms. Pull it down tightly against your chest. Keep your left leg flat on the floor.

3. Return to the beginning position. Repeat with your left leg.

4. Pull both thighs to your chest and hug them. Repeat the exercise up to 10 times.

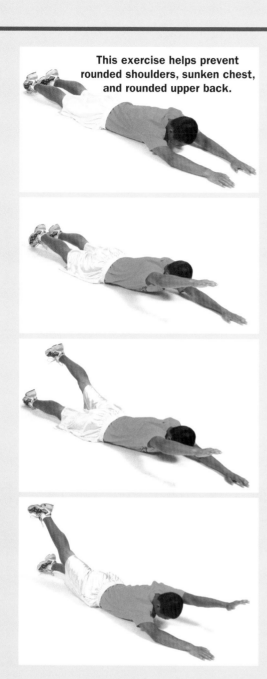

This exercise helps prevent rounded shoulders, sunken chest, and rounded upper back.

Arm and Leg Lift

1. Lie facedown with your arms stretched in front of you.
2. Raise your right arm and then lower it. Raise your left arm and then lower it. Finally, raise both arms and then lower them.
3. Raise your right leg and then lower it. Raise your left leg and then lower it.
4. Raise your right arm and right leg and then lower them. Raise your left arm and left leg and then lower them.
5. Raise your left arm and your right leg and then lower them. Raise your right arm and left leg and then lower them.
6. Repeat all the steps up to 5 times.

 Caution: Do not arch your back during this exercise.

Single-Leg Hang

1. Lie on your back on a table (or bench). Bend your knees to your chest.
2. Grasp your right leg under your knee with your arms. Lower your left leg so that your thigh remains on the table while your knee and the rest of your leg hang over the edge of the table. Have a partner push your left leg down if it comes up. Hold this position for several seconds.
3. Return to the starting position, and repeat the exercise with the other leg. Repeat the exercise 10 times with each leg.

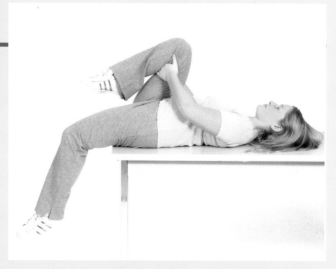

This exercise stretches your iliopsoas (hip flexor) muscle.

57

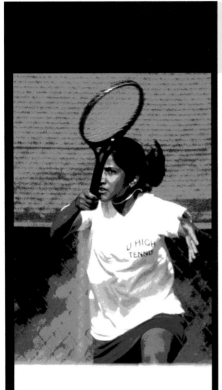

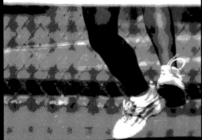

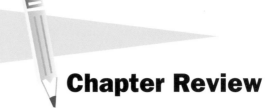

3 Chapter Review

Reviewing Concepts and Vocabulary

Number your paper from 1 to 8. Next to each number, write the letter of the best answer.

Column I
1. osteoporosis
2. atherosclerosis
3. hypertension
4. obesity
5. diabetes

6. lordosis
7. kyphosis

8. ptosis

Column II
a. having a high percentage of body fat
b. swayback
c. bones deteriorate and become weak
d. protruding abdomen
e. blood pressure is consistently higher than normal
f. rounded shoulders
g. the body cannot regulate blood sugar level
h. substances build up inside artery walls

Thinking Critically

Write a paragraph to answer the following question.
Why is inactivity a primary risk factor for many different diseases?

Unit Review on the Web

 www.fitnessforlife.org/student/3/9

Unit I review materials are available on the Web at the address listed above.

Project

Conduct a survey. A recent study showed that approximately one in four adults does not participate in regular leisure-time physical activity. What percentage of students at your school participate in leisure-time physical activity? Conduct a survey to find out. You might also poll those who respond to your survey to find out why they do or do not exercise.

Unit II

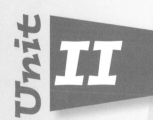

Becoming and Staying Physically Active

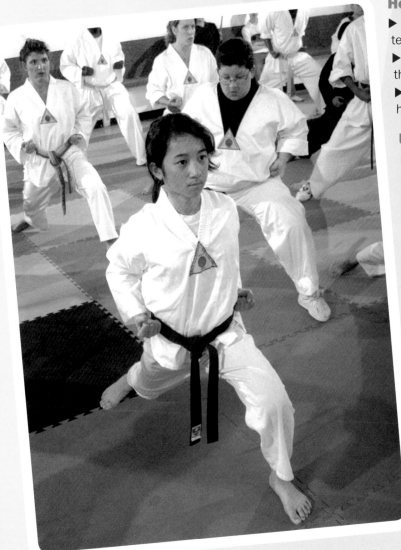

Healthy People 2010 Goals

▶ Increase daily moderate physical activity of teens.

▶ Improve fitness, health, and wellness through lifestyle change.

▶ Increase information to teens concerning healthy lifestyle change.

Unit Activities

▶ Line Exercise

▶ Circuit Workout

▶ Fitness Trail

▶ Elastic Band Exercise Circuit

▶ School Stepping

▶ Walking for Wellness

4

How Much Is Enough?

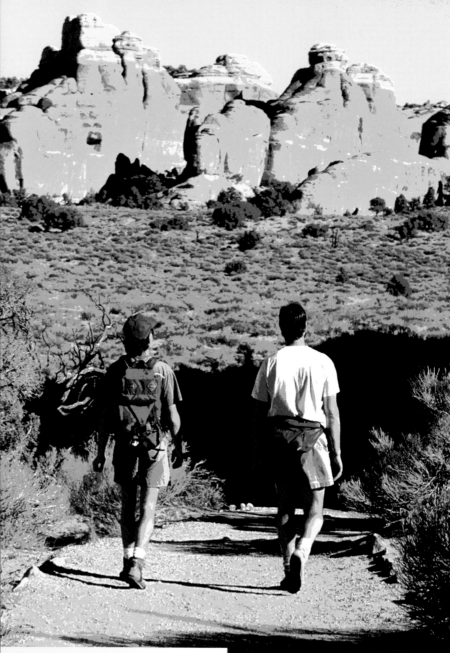

In this chapter...

Activity 1
Line Exercise

Lesson 4.1
How Much Physical Activity Is Enough?

Self-Assessment
Assessing Your Posture

Lesson 4.2
How Much Fitness Is Enough?

Taking Charge
Choosing a Good Activity

Self-Management Skill
Choosing a Good Activity

Activity 2
Circuit Workout

Activity 1

LINE EXERCISE

Music adds to the enjoyment of exercise. Line exercise is a form of group exercise that is done to music and is fun and easy to learn. It can be done in a relatively small space and produces many health and wellness benefits. After you have tried a planned line exercise routine you can create routines of your own.

How Much Physical Activity Is Enough?

Lesson Objectives

After reading this lesson, you should be able to

1. Name and discuss the three basic principles of exercise.
2. Explain how the FITT formula helps you build fitness.
3. Explain how to use the Physical Activity Pyramid to plan a physical activity program.

Lesson Vocabulary

FITT formula (p. 62), frequency (p. 62), intensity (p. 62), principle of overload (p. 61), principle of progression (p. 61), principle of specificity (p. 62), target ceiling (p. 62), target fitness zone (p. 62), threshold of training (p. 61), time (p. 62), type (p. 62)

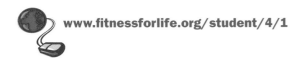

www.fitnessforlife.org/student/4/1

How much physical activity is enough? This question might seem very simple, but the answer can be complicated, especially if you are just beginning an activity program. In this lesson you will develop an understanding of several basic exercise principles as a good first step in answering the "how much is enough" question.

Basic Principles of Physical Activity

Mia has been exercising for several months. Every day she does the same physical activities for about 15 minutes. Her activity program has not changed since she started. Initially Mia saw some positive results from her program. She no longer was tired at the end of her exercise, and a self-assessment showed that her cardiovascular fitness had improved. However, lately Mia is disappointed because her strength does not seem to be improving as it did at first. She has noticed improvement in her cardiovascular fitness but her flexibility has not improved as much as she would like. Mia wants to know whether she is doing something wrong. A look

at the three basic principles of exercise might give some clues about what Mia might do differently.

Principle of Overload

The **principle of overload,** the most basic law of physical activity, states that the only way to produce fitness and health benefits through physical activity is to require your body to do more than it normally does. An increased demand on your body (overload) forces it to adapt. Your body was designed to be active; so if you do nothing (underload), your fitness will decrease and your health will suffer.

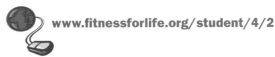

www.fitnessforlife.org/student/4/2

If Mia is not overloading when she exercises, she will not gain fitness and health benefits. Mia will need to increase the amount of her physical activity if she expects to continue improving her strength and flexibility.

Principle of Progression

The **principle of progression** states that the amount and intensity of your exercise should be increased gradually. After a while your body adapts to an increase in physical activity (load) and your activity becomes too easy. When this happens, increase your activity slightly.

Notice in the following diagram that the minimum amount of overload you need to build physical fitness is your **threshold of training.** Activity above your threshold builds fitness and promotes health and wellness benefits. Having exercised for several months at the same level, Mia might now be exercising below her threshold of training for some of the parts of fitness.

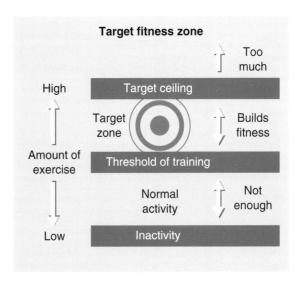

It is possible to exercise too much and to go above your upper limit of activity, also called your **target ceiling.** Ideally you should do exercise that is above your threshold of training and below your target ceiling. This correct range of physical activity is called your **target fitness zone.**

When you do physical activity in your target fitness zone, you build fitness and other benefits. However, when you go above your target ceiling, you increase the chances of injury and you can develop muscle soreness. The principle of progression provides the basis for rejecting the "no pain, no gain" theory. If you have pain when you exercise, you are probably overloading too quickly for your body to adjust.

Principle of Specificity

The **principle of specificity** states that the specific type of exercise you do determines the specific benefit you receive. Different kinds and amounts of activity produce very specific and different benefits. For example, Mia jogs around the track several days a week but she does not do stretching exercises as often as she should. Mia may also need to increase the resistance she uses for the exercises that she does to improve strength. An activity that promotes health benefits in one part of health-related fitness may not be equally good in promoting high levels of fitness in another part of fitness. Finally, exercises for specific body parts, such as the calf muscles, may provide benefits only for those body parts. For example, if Mia does only exercises for the calf muscles, she will not build the muscles in her back or shoulders.

FITT Formula

You know that you must do more physical activity than normal to build fitness. You also know that you should gradually increase your physical activity in order to stay within your target fitness zone. But how much physical activity do you need?

You can use the **FITT formula** to help you apply the basic principles of exercise. Each letter in the word FITT represents an important factor for determining how much physical activity is enough:

▶ **Frequency refers to how often you do physical activity.** For physical activity to be beneficial, you must do it several days a week. As you will see later, **frequency** depends on the type of activity you are doing and the part of fitness you want to develop. For example, to develop strength you might need exercise two days a week, but to lose fat daily activity is recommended.

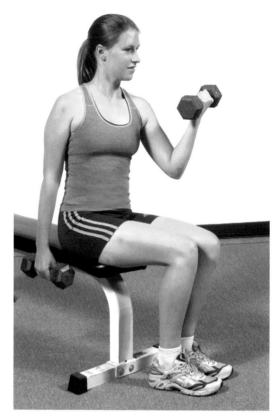
Biceps curls are a good way for Mia to improve her strength.

▶ **Intensity refers to how hard you perform physical activity.** If the activity you do is too easy, you will not build fitness and gain other benefits. But remember—extremely vigorous activity can be harmful if you do not work up to it gradually. **Intensity** is determined differently depending on the types of activity you do and the type of fitness you want to build. For example, counting heart rate can be used to determine the intensity of activity for building cardiovascular fitness, while the amount of weight you lift can be used to determine the intensity for building strength.

▶ **Time refers to how long you do physical activity.** The length of **time** you should do physical activity depends on the type of activity you are doing and the part of fitness you want to develop. For example, to build flexibility you should exercise for 15 seconds or more for each muscle group, while to build cardiovascular fitness you need to be active continuously for a minimum of 20 minutes or more.

▶ **Type refers to the kind of activity you do to build a specific part of fitness or to gain a specific benefit.** One **type** of activity may be good for building one part of fitness but may not work to build another part of fitness. For example, active aerobics is a type of activity that builds cardiovascular fitness but it does little to develop flexibility.

Throughout this book, you will learn how to apply the FITT formula to different activities that build specific parts of physical fitness. Each type of activity has its own formula. For simplicity we will use the phrase FIT formula. The final T will not be used when describing the frequency, intensity, and time for each type of activity.

The Physical Activity Pyramid

The Physical Activity Pyramid on page 64 can help you understand the concept of specificity and will help you see which types of activity are best for your fitness, health, and wellness. Different types of activity in the pyramid build different parts of fitness and produce different health and wellness benefits. For optimal benefits you should perform activities from all parts of the pyramid each week. As you can see, those activities at or near the bottom of the pyramid may need to be done more frequently than those near the top of the pyramid.

Lifestyle Physical Activity

Lifestyle physical activity, the bottom area of the pyramid, should be performed daily or nearly every day. Examples of this kind of activity include doing yard work or climbing stairs. This kind of activity is associated with many of the benefits of activity described in chapter 3. Lifestyle activity is helpful in controlling your level of body fat and building cardiovascular fitness, and it is well suited for people of all abilities.

Active Aerobics

Aerobic activity, which you will learn about in chapter 8, is also associated with many of the health and wellness benefits described in chapter 3. It is especially beneficial for building high levels of cardiovascular fitness and helps in controlling levels of body fat. You should perform aerobic activity three to six times a week.

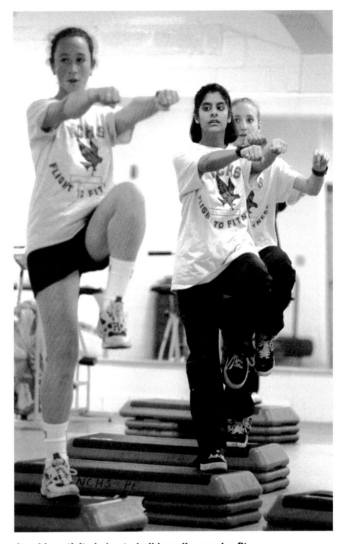

Aerobic activity helps to build cardiovascular fitness.

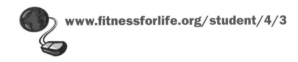

www.fitnessforlife.org/student/4/3

Active Sports and Recreation

Active sports and recreation are associated with many health and wellness benefits if done moderately or vigorously. It is helpful in maintaining many parts of fitness and in building skills. You can substitute active sports or recreation for some of the aerobic activities you do three to six times a week.

Exercise for Flexibility

To build and maintain flexibility, you should perform flexibility exercises at least three days and as many as every day of the week. Exercising in this way builds flexibility and produces such benefits as better performance, improved posture, and reduced risk of injury.

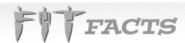

FACTS

The word *aerobic* means "with oxygen." It is a scientific term that has been used for decades. In 1968 Dr. Ken Cooper wrote a book popularizing the term. The book *Aerobics* helped the average person understand how much activity is necessary to provide fitness and health benefits. In Brazil, no equivalent of the word *aerobics* exists, so Brazilians refer to active aerobic activity as "Cooper." Dr. Cooper founded the Cooper Institute, a world-famous health and fitness research institution in Dallas, Texas.

Level 4

Limit Sedentary Living

- Watching TV
- Playing computer games
- Surfing the Internet

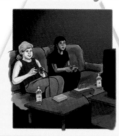

Avoid inactive periods of two hours or more during the day (or during waking hours).

Level 3

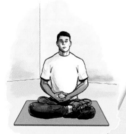

Flexibility Activities

- Stretching
- Yoga
- Gymnastics

F = 3-7 days/week
I = Moderate stretch
T = 15 to 60 seconds, 1 to 3 sets

Muscle Fitness Activities

- Resistance training
- Calisthenics
- Wall climbing

F = 2-3 days/week
I = Moderate to vigorous resistance
T = 8 to 12 reps, 1 to 3 sets

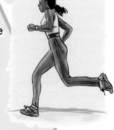

Level 2

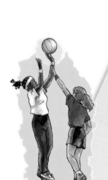

Active Sports and Recreational Activities

- In-line skating
- Basketball
- Tennis
- Canoeing
- Hiking
- Dancing

F = 3-6 days/week
I = Moderate to vigorous (increased heart rate)
T = 20 or more minutes

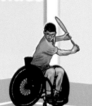

Active Aerobic Activities

- Biking
- Jogging
- Running
- Step aerobics
- Aerobic dance
- Swimming
- Treadmill
- Stair stepper

F = 3-6 days/week
I = Moderate to vigorous
T = 20 or more minutes

Level 1

Lifestyle Physical Activities

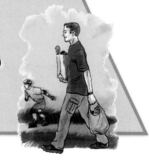

- Walk rather than ride
- Take the stairs
- Do yard work
- Play golf
- Go bowling
- Play active games

F = All or most days of the week
I = Moderate (equal to brisk walking)
T = 30 or more minutes

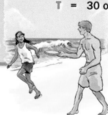

Accumulate moderate activity from the pyramid on all or most days of the week, and vigorous activity at least three days a week.

Eating well helps you stay active and fit.

Fitness Technology: ACTIVITYGRAM

You can now use computer technology to monitor or log your own physical activity. *ACTIVITYGRAM* is a computer program that helps you keep track of your physical activity over a three-day period. You enter the activity you performed for every 30-minute block of time during the day from 7 A.M. to 11 P.M. or whenever you go to bed. You also record the type of activity you do (from the pyramid) and whether the activity was rest, light, moderate, or vigorous. The computer will print a report showing the total number of minutes of activity each day, the amount of activity done at each level of the pyramid, and the amount of moderate and vigorous activity performed. Ask your instructor for more details on *ACTIVITYGRAM*.

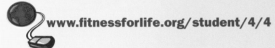

www.fitnessforlife.org/student/4/4

Exercise for Strength and Muscular Endurance

To develop strength, exercise for muscle fitness at least two days a week. You will need to exercise at least three days a week to improve muscular endurance. The exercises you do for strength and muscular endurance also produce such benefits as better performance, improved body appearance, a healthier back, good posture, and stronger bones.

Inactivity and Sedentary Living

We need to take time to recover from daily stresses and prepare for new challenges, so periods of rest and sleep are important to good health. Some activities of daily living—such as studying, reading, and even watching moderate amounts of television—are appropriate. But general inactivity or sedentary living is discouraged during the hours when you are awake. Choices from active areas of the pyramid should exceed those from the inactivity area. The information in the space below each level of the pyramid summarizes the amount of time you should perform activity from each level of the pyramid.

In the chapters that follow you will learn more about the Physical Activity Pyramid and how much physical activity from each area of the pyramid you need for building specific fitness and benefits to your health and wellness. You will see that the frequency, intensity, and time of activity will vary for each type of activity.

Lesson Review

1. What are the three basic principles of exercise?
2. How does the FITT formula help you build physical fitness?
3. How can you use the Physical Activity Pyramid to begin planning a physical activity program?

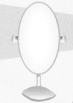

Assessing Your Posture

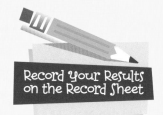
Record Your Results on the Record Sheet

You need to practice good posture at all times. You can use this self-assessment to determine whether your posture is as good as it should be. Wear exercise clothing or a swimsuit when taking this self-evaluation. Work with a partner to determine each other's scores. Write your results on your record sheet.

1. Stand sideways next to a string hanging from at least 1 foot above your head. The string should be weighted at the bottom so that it hangs straight. Position yourself so that the string aligns with your ankle bone.

2. Have your partner answer "yes" or "no" to each question that follows.

   ▶ Head: Is the ear in front of the line?
   ▶ Shoulders: Are the shoulders rounded? Are the tips of the shoulders in front of the chest?
   ▶ Upper back: Does the upper back stick out in a hump?
   ▶ Lower back: Does the lower back have excessive arch?
   ▶ Abdomen: Does the abdomen protrude beyond the pelvic bone?
   ▶ Knees: Do the knees appear to be locked or bent backward?

3. Now stand with your back to the string so that the string is aligned with the middle of your back.

   ▶ Head: Is more than one half of the head on one side of the string?
   ▶ Shoulders: Is one shoulder higher than the other?
   ▶ Hips: Is one hip higher than the other?

4. Add the total number of "yes" answers. Check the score against table 4.1. Do you think your posture is as good as it should be? How might you improve your posture all of the time, not just when standing?

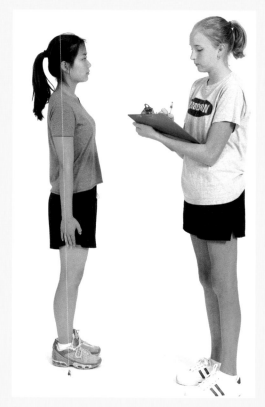

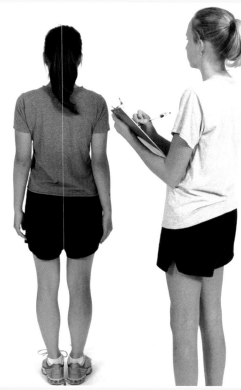

Posture test.

Table 4.1

Rating Chart: Good Posture Test

Score ("yes" answers)	Rating
0-1	Good posture
2-4	Posture can use some improvement
5+	Posture definitely needs improvement

How Much Fitness Is Enough?

Lesson Objectives

After reading this lesson, you should be able to

1. Discuss fitness ratings and how they apply to your physical activity program.
2. Identify factors that contribute to fitness.
3. Describe several factors to consider when creating a personal physical activity program.

Lesson Vocabulary

criterion-referenced health standards (p. 67), maturation (p. 67)

www.fitnessforlife.org/student/4/5

You now know that physical activity is necessary to build each of the different parts of fitness. But exactly how much fitness do you need? In this lesson you will learn some ways to decide how much fitness is enough for you.

Fitness Rating Categories

Sometimes people judge their fitness by comparing themselves to others. If they score higher on a fitness test than most other people, they consider themselves fit. This type of comparison creates several problems. First, it suggests that only a few can be fit. Second, it suggests that only high test scores are adequate for fitness.

Most experts agree that you should judge your fitness using standards of health and wellness, also called **criterion-referenced health standards,** rather than using standards that require you to compare yourself to others. Health and wellness standards require you to have enough fitness to

▶ reduce risk of health problems,

▶ achieve wellness benefits,

▶ work effectively and meet emergencies, and

▶ be able to enjoy your free time.

During this course you will learn to do self-assessments that you can use to determine whether your fitness is as good as it should be and whether you are fit enough to meet the important goals listed above. You will use one of the four categories shown in the Fitness Rating box on the next page to rate each of the five parts of health-related physical fitness. If you achieve the good fitness category, you will have achieved basic health and wellness standards of physical fitness.

Factors Influencing Physical Fitness

Physical activity is the most important thing you can do to improve and maintain health-related physical fitness. Physical activity is something that you can control. You can choose the kinds of activities you want to do and schedule a regular time to do them. But as the diagram on page 69 shows, physical activity is not the only factor that contributes to physical fitness. Other important factors contributing to physical fitness are **maturation,** age, heredity, the environment, and lifestyle choices including nutrition and stress management. You will learn more about nutrition in chapter 14 and stress management in chapter 17.

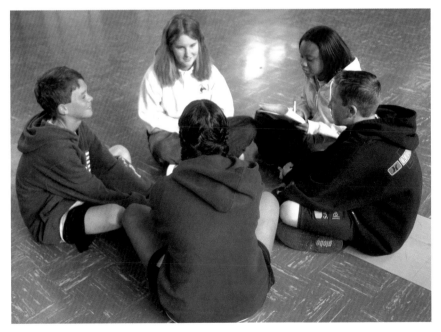

Your fitness should be compared to the criterion-referenced health standards rather than to your friends' fitness.

Fitness Rating

High Performance Rating

Most experts agree that reaching a high performance rating is not necessary for good health, for meeting normal daily emergencies, or for performing daily activities. However, if you want to be an athlete or perform a job such as being a firefighter, soldier, or police officer, a high performance rating increases your chance of success.

Good Fitness Rating

A good fitness rating indicates that you have the necessary level of fitness needed to live a full, healthy life. In fact, achieving a good fitness rating is the goal of most people. However, to maintain this level of fitness, you will have to continue to be physically active.

Marginal Fitness Rating

Moving from the low to the marginal rating shows important progress in fitness. However, if you have marginal ratings you should continue to work for a good fitness rating.

Low Fitness Rating

If you have low fitness ratings, you have an above-average risk of developing the health problems described in chapter 3. You might not look your best, feel your best, or work and play most efficiently.

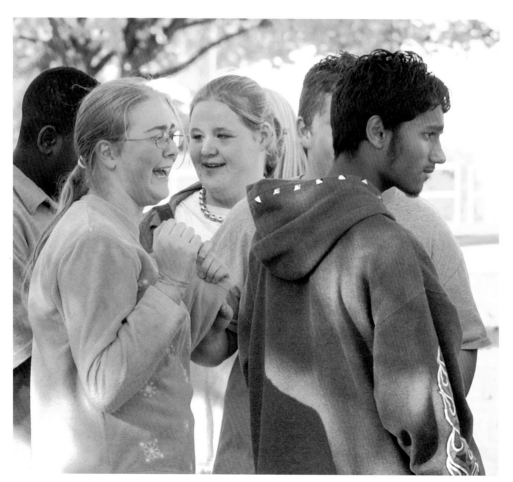

Your friends (and other environmental factors) can indirectly affect your physical fitness.

68

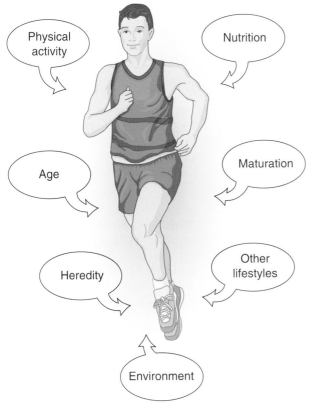

Factors that influence physical fitness

- Physical activity
- Nutrition
- Age
- Maturation
- Heredity
- Other lifestyles
- Environment

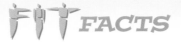

FIT FACTS

The amount of medicine prescribed for an illness is often referred to as a dose. The amount of activity you need to get health benefits is sometimes referred to as an exercise prescription and is measured in doses. To a certain point, people who do more doses get more benefits, but too many doses can be harmful. Following the FIT formula for each type of physical activity can help you get just the right number of doses to achieve good health and fitness.

Maturation

Physical maturation refers to becoming physically mature or fully grown and developed. In the early teens, maturation begins because of hormones that promote growth and development of tissues such as muscle and bone. Some people mature earlier than others. Early developers often do better on physical fitness tests than those who mature later.

Age

Studies show that older teens perform better on fitness tests than younger teens. In the same class, those who are older will typically do better than those who are younger. This difference is mostly because the older you are, the more you have grown and the more mature you are likely to be. However, sometimes younger people mature earlier than those who are older, and therefore could have an advantage on physical fitness tests.

Heredity

Heredity plays a role in determining the physical characteristics we inherit from our parents that influence how we do on different physical fitness tests. For example, some people have more of the muscle fibers that help them run fast, and others have more of the muscle fibers that help them run a long time without fatigue. Still others have more fat cells because of heredity. Fortunately, fitness is composed of many different parts. Your heredity

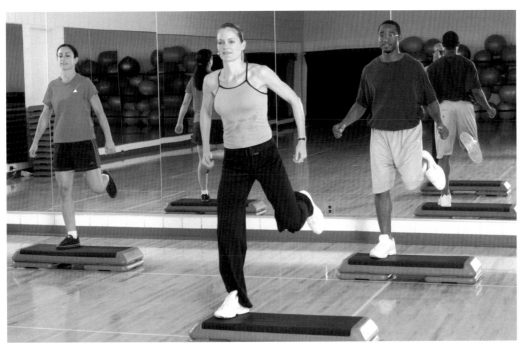

Find an activity you enjoy and will be able to do later in life.

Taking Charge: Choosing a Good Activity

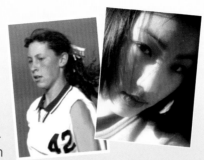

You can help yourself be active by choosing activities you are likely to do both now and throughout your life. One way to evaluate an activity is to find out the number of people who participate and how long they stay involved.

At a recent high school reunion, the alumni enjoyed seeing their former classmates again. Everyone remembered Norma as an active participant in sports. She played soccer, basketball, and softball. What a surprise when her classmates discovered 10 years later that Norma did very little physical activity! The closest she got to participating in any sport was to watch her son's T-ball games. According to Norma, "It was too hard to find people who wanted to play the team sports I once enjoyed."

Kim Lea was the opposite of Norma. In high school she'd always go to the games and cheer for the teams, but she never dreamed of taking part in a sport. Kim Lea would be the first to admit that she was the original couch potato. Now Kim Lea goes biking with her two children. She also organizes the neighborhood aerobics class. "Every Tuesday and Thursday morning we all get together and talk while we work out. No one cares how we dress or how good we are at doing the exercises, and we all seem to be energized as we go on to our next activities."

For Discussion

Why was it no longer feasible for Norma to continue participating in the same sports she played in high school? What might help her get involved in a physical activity again? Why do you think Kim Lea started to participate in activities? Fill out the questionnaire provided by your teacher to find out what factors determine the popularity of an activity. Consider the guidelines on page 71.

---

will partly determine the parts of fitness in which you will do well and not so well. Each person will have some areas in which heredity enables better performance and some areas in which it will be harder to perform well.

Environment

Where you live (city, suburbs, country), your school environment, availability of places to play and do other types of physical activity, and even your social environment including the friends you choose have an effect on your fitness. You will learn more about environmental factors in chapter 16.

Anyone Can Succeed

Because many factors contribute to physical fitness, it is possible for some people who do relatively little physical activity to achieve relatively good fitness scores while they are in their teens. These people probably matured early and have inherited physical characteristics that help them to do well on physical fitness tests. They may conclude that they do not need to do physical activity. This idea may be true if they only care about doing well on fitness tests while they are young, but it will not be true for a lifetime. As people get older, physical maturation and age no longer result in a fitness advantage. Sooner or later physical inactivity starts to catch up with even those who have a hereditary advantage. Regular physical activity and healthy lifestyle choices

are absolutely necessary if fitness, health, and wellness are to occur for a lifetime.

Just as some people have fitness advantages because of age, maturation, and heredity, others have disadvantages. Even if these people do physical activity, they may find it hard to get high fitness scores, and therefore they become discouraged. If you are one of these people, avoid comparing yourself to others. Try to achieve a good fitness rating rather than worrying about getting a high performance rating. Good fitness is something that all people can accomplish, but it may be harder for some than others to reach this rating. Studies show that people who were good in sports in school, but are not active later in life, die earlier and are less healthy than those who do regular activity all of their lives, even if they were not especially good performers when they were young.

Anyone can do physical activity. No matter who you are, physical activity is important to good health and wellness as well as fitness development. With regular physical activity all people can achieve good fitness ratings in all parts of fitness.

Lesson Review

1. What are the four fitness ratings? How do they apply to your physical activity program?
2. Identify several factors that contribute to fitness.
3. Describe the factors you should consider in selecting a good personal physical activity.

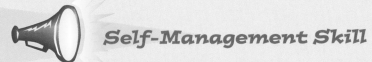

Self-Management Skill

Choosing a Good Activity

We know that the most active people in our society are those who have a special activity they enjoy. For example, some people love tennis, golf, running, or some other activity and participate on a regular basis. Others like variety and choose cross-training. These people do a variety of activities but are very regular in their participation. They might not have become as active as they are if they were not able to do the activities they especially enjoy. Follow these guidelines to help you find a physical activity that is especially good for you:

▶ **Consider your physical fitness.** How well you do in an activity depends on all parts of fitness, health-related as well as skill-related. Choose activities that match your abilities in both kinds of fitness.

▶ **Consider your interests.** If there is an activity that you really enjoy or always wanted to do, don't avoid it just because it doesn't match your fitness profile. However, be aware that it may take you longer than others to learn the activity even with practice. Finding an activity that is fun is very important.

▶ **Consider an activity that you can do with others.** Try to find others of your own ability so that you won't be discouraged if you do not learn the activity as quickly as you would like.

▶ **Consider the benefits of the activity.** As you progress through this book you will learn a lot about the benefits of different activities. Selecting activities from each area of the pyramid is a good idea if you want to get optimal fitness, health, and wellness benefits.

▶ **Practice, practice, practice.** Becoming skilled in a sport or activity increases your enjoyment. If you choose an activity that is new to you, there is no substitute for practice. Taking lessons in the particular sport or activity can help you because it makes your practice more productive.

▶ **Consider activities that do not require high levels of skill.** Some activities do not require high levels of any part of skill-related fitness. Of activities in the Physical Activity Pyramid, sports provide the most benefits to skill-related fitness, but they also require relatively high levels of it. In addition, most sports require you to have good skills as well as to have good skill-related fitness. Sport skills such as throwing, catching, hitting, and kicking are different from skill-related fitness abilities such as agility, balance, and coordination that help you learn skills more easily. Learning skills of sports requires a lot of practice if you are to perform them well. Lifestyle and aerobic activities generally require fewer skills than sports. Even people with relatively low scores on most or all parts of skill-related fitness can find a lifestyle or aerobic activity that can be enjoyed. Jogging, walking, and cycling are only a few of these activities. Because they also do not require many skills, extensive practice is not necessary to perform them. You may want to consider one of these activities if you are not willing to take the time necessary to learn more complicated activities. In chapter 9 you will learn more about which sports and activities are best for improving the various parts of health-related physical fitness.

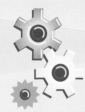

Activity 2

Circuit Workout

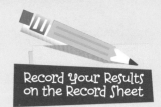
Record Your Results on the Record Sheet

Circuit training consists of several different exercises done consecutively. You move from one exercise station to the next. At each station, you complete an exercise. When you have completed the exercises at all stations, you have completed the exercise circuit. Many kinds of exercise circuits exist. This one is designed to help you build all parts of health-related physical fitness.

You can use circuit training to increase your exercise overload. As you improve in a certain exercise, you can increase the number of times you complete it. In other words, you can increase the repetitions. If you try to complete the circuit more quickly, take extra care to do each exercise properly.

For a total fitness circuit such as this one, exercises for all parts of physical fitness and all body parts should be included. You may use a variety of equipment at the exercise stations. If no special equipment is available, you can perform calisthenics at each exercise station. Circuit training is usually planned by an exercise specialist, but you can learn to plan your own circuit course. Try the starter circuit training workout described here. Record your results on your worksheet. You can start by performing the circuit one time. You may increase the number of times you perform it as you improve.

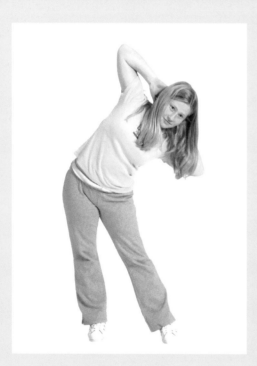

Side Stretch

1. Stand with your feet shoulder-width apart.
2. Clasp your hands behind your neck.
3. Bend your trunk sideways to the left as far as possible.
4. Repeat the exercise to the right.

Safety Tip: While doing the Side Stretch, do not twist your body, bend forward, or push your hips sideways.

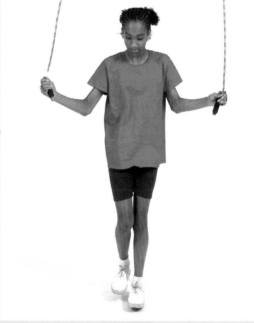

Jump Rope

Use either the jog step or the two-foot jump.

1. For the two-foot jump, jump on both feet simultaneously with each rope swing. Beginners should jump twice with each rope swing. This second jump is a small bounce.
2. For the jog step, jog or step from one foot to the other foot.

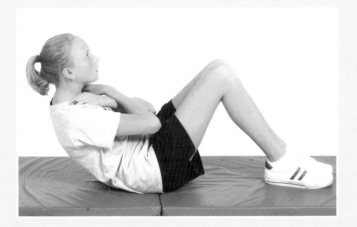

Curl-Up

1. Lie on your back with your hands folded across your chest.
2. Bend your knees at a 90-degree angle.
3. Flatten your back, then roll your head and shoulders forward and upward. Roll far enough to feel tension in the abdominal muscles. Your shoulder blades should come up off the floor, but do not lift your back off the floor.
4. Return to the starting position.

Bench Step

1. Step up to a bench with your right foot, then up with your left foot.
2. Step down with your right foot, then down with your left foot.
3. Repeat this 4-count (up, up, down, down) stepping at an even rhythm about 25 times per minute.

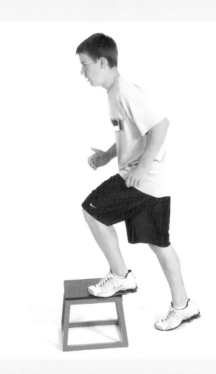

Inchworm

1. Support your body with your arms and feet in a push-up position.
2. Slowly walk your feet forward as far as possible while your hands remain stationary on the floor.
3. Slowly walk your hands forward, away from your feet, until you are again in the push-up position.

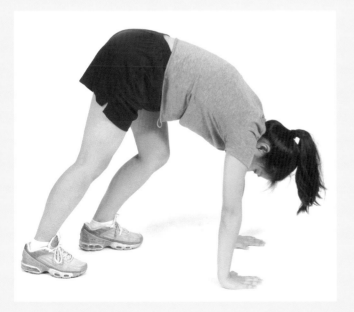

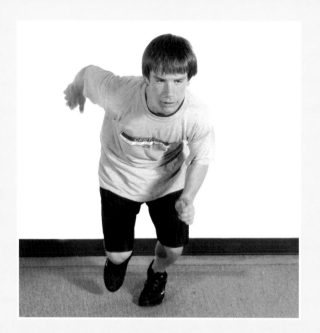

Sprint the Line

1. Run from one line to another 10 yards away.
2. Walk back and repeat the sprint.

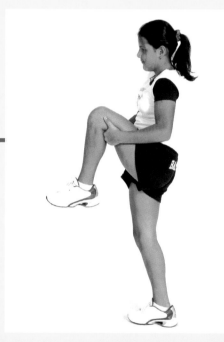

Knee Lift

1. Stand with your feet together and arms at your sides.
2. Raise your left knee as high as possible, grasping your thigh with your hands.
3. Pull your knee against your body while keeping your back straight.
4. Return to the starting position and repeat the exercise with your right knee.

Jog in Place

Jog in place at a rate of 120 steps a minute.

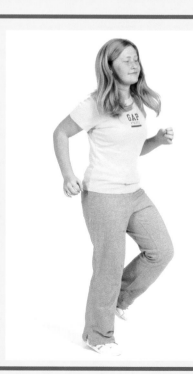

Table 4.2

Circuit Workout

Exercise	Repetitions
Side Stretch	15 within 2 min
Jump Rope	60 jumps/min for 2 min
Curl-Up	5-10 within 2 min
Bench Step	50 within 2 min
Inchworm	5-15 within 2 min
Sprint the Line	6 within 2 min
Knee Lift	5 on each leg within 2 min
Jog in Place	120 steps/min for 2 min

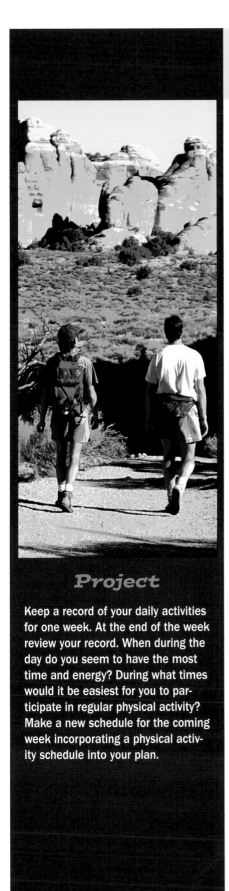

4

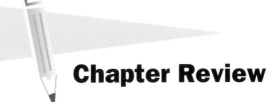

Chapter Review

Reviewing Concepts and Vocabulary

Number your paper from 1 to 4. Next to each number, write the word or words that correctly complete the sentence.

1. For optimal benefits, you should perform activities from _____ parts of the Physical Activity Pyramid each week.

2. The minimum amount of overload needed to achieve physical fitness is called _____.

3. If you are exercising in your target fitness zone, you are between your threshold of training and your _____.

4. If you achieve a _____ fitness rating, you probably are at the level of fitness needed to live a full, healthy life.

Number your paper from 5 to 10. Next to each number, choose the letter of the best answer.

Column I
5. target ceiling
6. frequency
7. intensity
8. progression
9. specificity
10. overload

Column II
a. how hard you perform physical activity
b. increasing exercise gradually
c. the upper limit of your physical activity
d. how often you exercise
e. doing more exercise than you normally do
f. exercise for one fitness part

Number your paper from 11 to 15. Write a short answer for each statement or question.

11. How do age and maturation affect physical fitness?

12. Why should you develop a lifetime physical activity plan even if you are in the good fitness zone now?

13. Explain why your physical activity program should include activities from all parts of the Physical Activity Pyramid.

14. Why should you not exercise above your target ceiling?

15. Explain why you should not compare yourself to others when assessing your fitness levels and needs.

Thinking Critically

Write a paragraph to answer the following question.

A friend tells you that he thinks it is important for everyone to attain a high performance fitness rating. He says that if a good rating is the goal for all people, then a high performance rating must be even better for everyone. How would you respond? Explain your answer.

Project

Keep a record of your daily activities for one week. At the end of the week review your record. When during the day do you seem to have the most time and energy? During what times would it be easiest for you to participate in regular physical activity? Make a new schedule for the coming week incorporating a physical activity schedule into your plan.

5

Learning Self-Management Skills

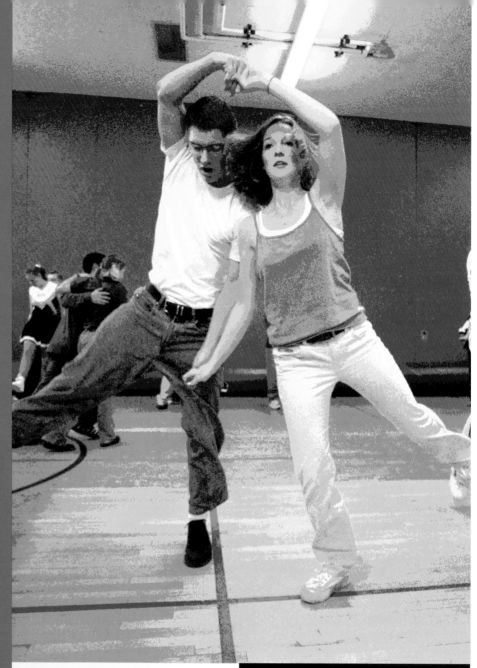

In this chapter...

Activity 1
Fitness Trail

Lesson 5.1
Learning Self-Management Skills

Self-Assessment
***FITNESSGRAM* 2—Body Composition and Flexibility**

Lesson 5.2
Goal Setting

Taking Charge
Setting Goals

Self-Management Skill
Setting Goals

Activity 2
Elastic Band Exercise Circuit

Activity 1

FITNESS TRAIL

A fitness trail is a physical fitness workout in which you follow a varied path and stop at exercise stations along the way. You jog from station to station and perform the exercise described on the posted sign, using the number of repetitions recommended for your fitness status. These stations are designed for a complete workout—a warm-up and cool-down with flexibility, strength, and endurance exercises in between. Jogging between stations takes care of the cardiovascular component.

Learning Self-Management Skills

Lesson Objectives

After reading this lesson, you should be able to

1. Describe the stages of physical activity change.
2. Describe several different self-management skills.
3. Explain how you can use self-management skills for living a healthy life.

Lesson Vocabulary

determinants (p. 77), motor skill (p. 78), self-management skills (p. 78), skill (p. 78), sport skill (p. 78)

www.fitnessforlife.org/student/5/1

In chapter 3 you learned about the benefits of physical activity, and in chapter 4 you learned about how much physical activity you have to do to get those benefits. In this chapter you will learn how to become active if you are not already active and how to stay active if you are currently active on a regular basis.

Stages of Physical Activity

Some people are more active than others. Look at the figure at the bottom of the page. It shows the five stages of physical activity. The least active is the couch potato.

Couch potatoes are totally sedentary. More than 40 percent of all adults over 18 are included in this stage because they do no regular physical activity. You might think there are no teen couch potatoes. It is true that fewer teens than adults exist in this category, but 14 percent of teens can be classified here. In an ideal world, all people would be active exercisers, but sometimes people move slowly from one stage to the next. For example, a couch potato might read about the importance of physical activity and start to think about being active but take no action. A person like this would move from being a couch potato to being an inactive thinker. An inactive thinker does little physical activity but is thinking about becoming active. At the next stage a person starts planning to be active. For example, the inactive thinker might visit an exercise facility or buy a new tennis racket. The person has now become a planner, even though he or she is not yet active. The next stage is actually becoming active. The activator goes to the exercise facility to do exercise or plays tennis with a friend. The ultimate goal is to help all people progress to the stage of the active exerciser. When this stage is reached, a person is active on a regular basis for a long time.

Many factors are involved in determining who will be active and who will not. Some of these factors, sometimes called **determinants,** that account for why some people are active and some are not include skill level, fitness level, self-confidence, barriers to physical activity, and attitude toward activity. All of these determinants, as well as many others, will be discussed in this chapter and throughout this book.

Activity Levels of Teens

We know from viewing the Physical Activity Pyramid that many different kinds of activity exist. It is possible to be at a different stage for one type of activity than for

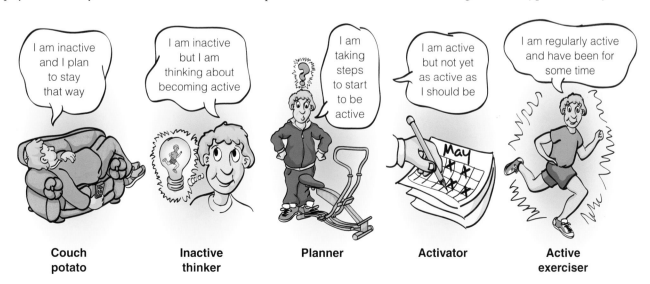

Couch potato	Inactive thinker	Planner	Activator	Active exerciser
I am inactive and I plan to stay that way	I am inactive but I am thinking about becoming active	I am taking steps to start to be active	I am active but not yet as active as I should be	I am regularly active and have been for some time

another. For example, some people do active sports regularly but may not do stretching or muscle fitness exercises. A national survey of teens shows the percentage of teens who are classified as active exercisers for each of the different types of physical activity. The chart here shows that many teens are not active exercisers. You may be interested to know that girls are less active than boys in all types of activity other than flexibility exercises. And as teens progress through school they become less active. For example, ninth graders are twice as likely to do moderate activity as twelfth graders, and one in three teens who is an active exerciser in the ninth grade is no longer an active exerciser by the twelfth grade.

So how do you become more active if you are not as active as you should be? Or if you are active now, how do you avoid becoming an adult couch potato? Experts have studied these questions extensively and have learned that people who learn **self-management skills** and use them regularly are likely to be active and stay active.

You already know what a **sport skill** is. Examples of a **skill** are throwing, catching, hitting a tennis or golf ball, and kicking a soccer ball. In fact, sport skill is one type of self-management skill. Learning sport skills helps you to be active for a lifetime. Teachers and coaches help you learn these skills, and with practice you improve your skills. Other types of self-management skills are shown in table 5.1. All of the self-management skills can help you no matter what your current stage of physical activity. However, some are especially useful in helping you to get started. They can help people who are couch potatoes or who are thinking about becoming more active. Other self-management skills help you to plan to be active. Finally, some are most useful in helping you continue to be an active exerciser and avoid dropping out.

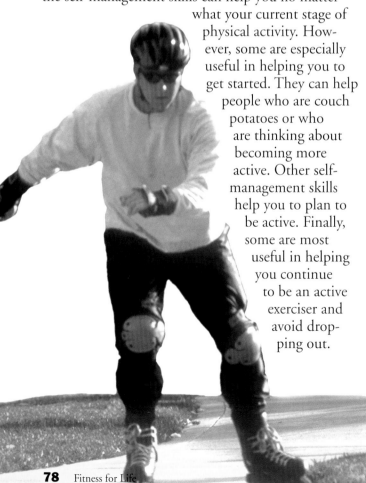

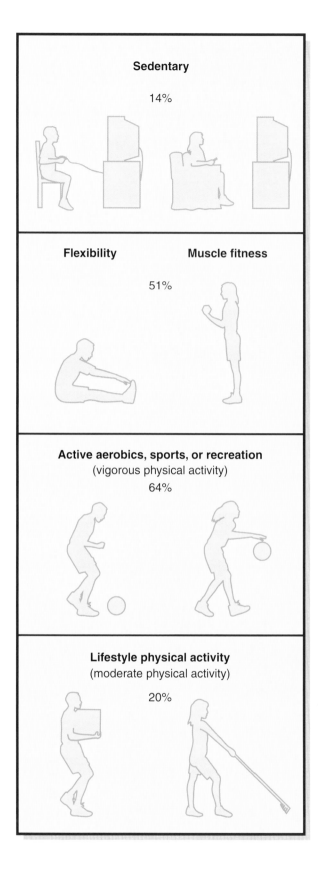

Sedentary

14%

Flexibility   **Muscle fitness**

51%

Active aerobics, sports, or recreation
(vigorous physical activity)
64%

Lifestyle physical activity
(moderate physical activity)
20%

FIT FACTS

Skills and skill-related physical fitness are different things. Skill is the ability to do a specific task such as throwing, catching, and kicking. Skills are also called sport skills or **motor skills** because they are frequently used in sports and because "motor" nerves cause muscles to contract, allowing you to perform skills. The six parts of skill-related fitness are abilities that influence the learning of motor skills. For example, if you have good coordination, it will help you learn to catch or kick a ball more quickly and better than someone without good coordination. Most experts agree that if you practice, you can learn motor skills regardless of your skill-related fitness.

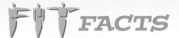

FIT FACTS

Who is most active? National surveys indicate that many factors are associated with physical activity among teens, including age, gender, ethnicity, and socioeconomic status. Young teens are more active than older teens. Boys do more moderate, vigorous, and muscular fitness activities than girls. Hispanic and African American teens are less active than other ethnic groups; this is probably related to socioeconomic status. People in lower socioeconomic groups are less active than those in higher socioeconomic groups. A national health goal is to increase opportunities for all people to be active.

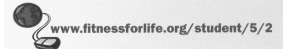
www.fitnessforlife.org/student/5/2

Table 5.1

Self-Management Skills for Active Living, Health, and Wellness

Skill	Definition
Self-assessment	This skill allows you to test your own fitness to help you see where you are and to help you get to where you want to be. *Chapter 1*
Building self-confidence	This skill helps you build the feeling that you are capable of being active for life. *Chapter 2*
Identifying risk factors	This skill helps you identify, assess, and reduce health risks. *Chapter 3*
Choosing good activities	This skill helps you select activities that are best for you personally. *Chapter 4*
Goal setting	This skill helps you set realistic and practical goals for being active and achieving physical fitness. *Chapter 5*
Building positive attitudes	This skill allows you to identify and build attitudes that will help you to be active throughout life. *Chapter 6*
Self-monitoring	This skill helps you learn to keep records (or logs) to see whether you are in fact doing what you think you are doing. *Chapter 7*
Finding social support	This skill helps you find ways to get the help and support of others (your friends and family) to adopt healthy behaviors and to stick with them. *Chapter 8*
Building performance skills	These skills help you to be good at and enjoy sports and other physical activities. *Chapter 9*
Building intrinsic motivation	This skill helps you learn to enjoy physical activity for your own personal reasons rather than because others think it is good for you. *Chapter 10*
Preventing relapse	This skill helps you stick with healthy behaviors even when you have problems getting motivated. *Chapter 11*
Managing time effectively	This skill helps you learn to schedule time efficiently so that you will have more time for important things in your life. *Chapter 12*
Building positive self-perceptions	This skill helps you think positively about yourself so you can stay active for a lifetime. *Chapter 13*
Learning to say "No"	This skill helps keep you from doing things you don't want to do, especially when you are under pressure from friends or other people. *Chapter 14*
Thinking critically	This skill helps you find and interpret information that will be useful in making decisions and solving problems. *Chapter 15*
Finding success	This skill helps you find success in physical activity. *Chapter 16*
Overcoming competitive stress	This skill helps you prevent or cope with the stresses of competition or the tension you feel when performing some types of activity. *Chapter 17*
Overcoming barriers	This skill helps you find ways to stay active despite barriers such as lack of time, unsafe places to be active, and weather. *Chapter 18*

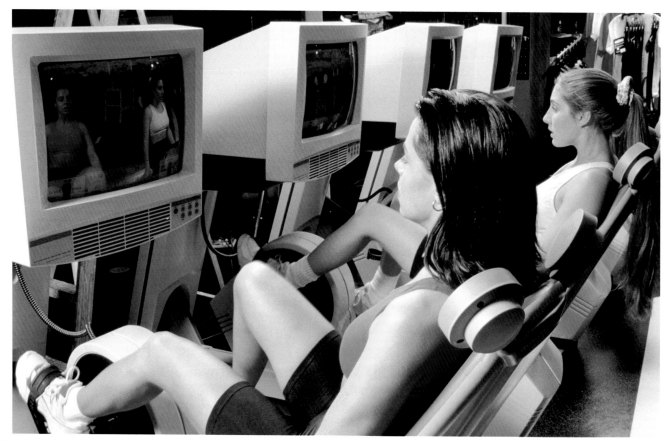

Several manufacturers have developed interactive video games that require moderate to vigorous activity to do well at the game. Using one of these games is a great way to enjoy playing video games while maintaining a healthy level of physical activity.

You have already learned about several self-management skills such as self-assessment, building self-confidence, reducing risk factors, and choosing good activities in chapters 1 through 4. In this chapter you will learn about goal setting, and in the remaining chapters you will learn about other self-management skills. A major purpose of this book is to help you to live an active, healthy life. To accomplish this goal it is important for you to learn about and practice each of the self-management skills listed in table 5.1.

Lesson Review

1. What are the five stages of physical activity?
2. What are some self-management skills?
3. How can you use self-management skills for living a healthy life?

Fitness Technology: Active Video Games

Research has shown that the average teen spends more time watching television and playing computer games than in school (as many as 4 hours a day). This includes weekend time when teens do not attend school but spend considerable time playing video games or watching television. Research has also shown that watching television and playing video games are associated with inactivity and greater risk of obesity. One study has shown that inactive video games, especially violent ones, increase aggressive behavior. Several manufacturers have developed interactive video games that require moderate to vigorous activity to do well at the game. Examples are bicycle exercisers, resistance machines, and steppers that allow you to score points while you exercise. In one exercise game you are a self-powered aircraft that fights fires. People who use these active computer games can get fit and enjoy the game at the same time, and they may reduce aggressive behavior rather than increase it.

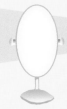

Self-Assessment

FITNESSGRAM 2—Body Composition and Flexibility

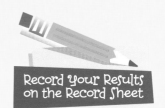

Record your Results on the Record Sheet

In this self-assessment you will perform two additional tests from *FITNESSGRAM:* the body mass index and the back-saver sit and reach. The body mass index (BMI) is an indicator of your body composition. It is one of two methods for assessing body composition in *FITNESSGRAM*. You will do this assessment now so that you can complete your report, but you will also measure skinfolds when you study body fat later. The back-saver sit and reach measures flexibility of the lower back and the muscles on the back of the thigh (hamstrings). After you record your results on the record sheet, complete your record sheet.

Body Mass Index

1. Measure your height in inches without shoes.
2. Measure your weight without shoes. If you are wearing street clothes (as opposed to light-weight gym clothing), you can subtract 2 pounds from your weight.

3. Use the body mass index chart to determine your BMI. You can also calculate your BMI using the formula: BMI = weight in kilograms/(height in meters)^2.
4. Consult table 5.2 to find your BMI rating. Record the results on your record sheet.

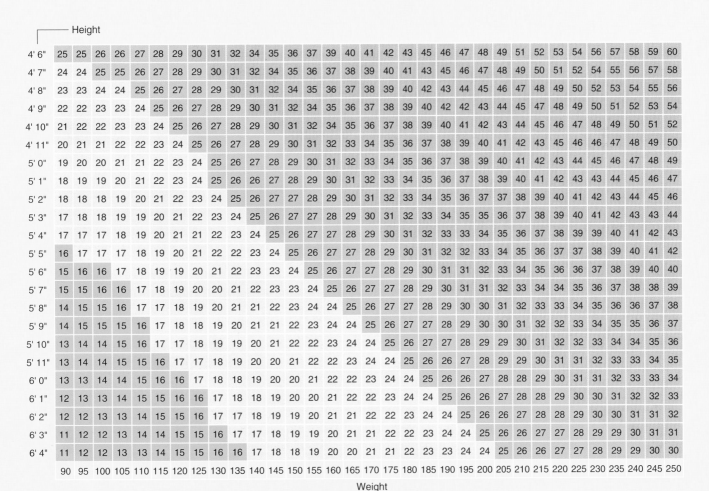

Low   Good fitness zone   Marginal   Obese

(continued)

Body Mass Index (*continued*)

Table 5.2

Rating Chart: Body Mass Index

	13 YEARS OLD		14 YEARS OLD		15 YEARS OLD		16 YEARS OLD		17 YEARS OLD		18 YEARS OLD	
	Males	Females	Males	Females	Males	Females	Males	Females	Males	Females	Males	Females
High performance	16.6-19.9	17.5-21.0	17.5-20.9	17.5-21.5	18.1-21.5	17.5-21.5	18.5-22.0	17.5-21.5	18.8-21.9	17.5-21.5	19.0-22.4	18.0-21.9
Good fitness	20.0-23.0	21.1-24.5	21.0-24.5	21.6-25.0	21.6-25.0	21.6-25.0	22.1-26.5	21.6-25.0	22.0-27.0	21.6-26.0	22.5-27.5	22.0-27.3
Marginal fitness	23.1-26.0	24.6-27.0	24.6-26.5	25.1-27.5	25.1-27.0	25.1-27.5	26.6-27.5	25.1-27.5	27.1-28.0	26.1-27.5	27.6-28.5	27.4-28.0
Low fitness	26.1+	27+	26.6+	27.6+	27.1+	27.6+	27.6+	27.6+	28.1+	27.6+	28.6+	28.1+

Adapted by permission from *FITNESSGRAM*.

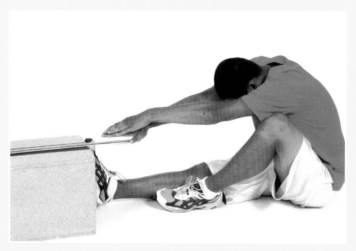

Table 5.3

Rating Chart: Back-Saver Sit and Reach

	13-14 YEARS OLD		15 YEARS AND OLDER	
	Males	Females	Males	Females
High performance	10+	12+	10+	14+
Good fitness	8-9	10-11	8-9	12-13
Marginal fitness	6-7	8-9	6-7	10-11
Low fitness	5–	7–	5–	9–

Adapted by permission from *FITNESSGRAM*.

Back-Saver Sit and Reach

1. Place a measuring stick such as a yardstick on top of a 12-inch-high box. Have the stick extend 9 inches over the box with the lower numbers toward you.
2. To measure flexibility of your right leg, fully extend it and place your right foot flat against the box. Bend your left leg with the knee turned out and your left foot 2 to 3 inches to the side of your straight right leg.
3. Extend your arms forward over the measuring stick. Place your hands on the stick, one on top of the other, with the palms facing down. The middle fingers should be together with the tips of one finger exactly on top of the other.
4. Lean forward and reach with the arms and fingers four times. On the fourth reach, hold the position for 3 seconds and observe the inch mark below your fingertips. Then record your score to the nearest inch.
5. Repeat the test with the left leg straight. Consult table 5.3 and write the results on your record sheet.

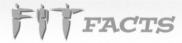

Some companies have developed a flexibility box that adjusts for each person's arm and leg length. The fitness ratings in this book and for the *FITNESSGRAM* back-saver sit and reach test using a box and a measuring stick. If your school has an adjustable testing box, you may want to test yourself both ways to see whether you get a difference.

Goal Setting

Lesson Objectives

After reading this lesson, you should be able to

1. Explain how goal setting can help you plan your fitness program.
2. Identify some guidelines you should follow when setting goals.

Lesson Vocabulary

goal setting (p. 83), long-term goals (p. 83), short-term goals (p. 84)

www.fitnessforlife.org/student/5/3

Suppose you wanted money for a specific purpose. It might be to buy a CD player, a bicycle, or a car. Or you might want to go on a trip or need money for college. Most likely you would develop a plan to get money. You might decide to babysit after school or work on weekends. You would identify your goal—to make money—and then develop a plan to reach it.

Successful people use **goal setting** as part of their overall planning to achieve success; they decide ahead of time what they plan to accomplish and then establish how they will go about doing it. You can use goal setting to plan your personal fitness program. In this lesson you will learn how to use long-term goals and short-term goals to plan your personal program.

Long-Term Goals

Goals that take months or even years to accomplish are called **long-term goals.** For example, if your goal is to save money for college, you might have to work on weekends and summers all through high school. When you plan your fitness program, you will want to consider two types of long-term goals: long-term physical activity goals and long-term physical fitness goals.

Long-Term Physical Activity Goals

When setting physical fitness goals, long-term goals are usually set for more than one month and up to several months or even a year. An example of a long-term phys-

ical activity goal would be to spend at least 30 minutes a day in activities from the Physical Activity Pyramid each week for the next two months. You should examine your long-term goals periodically to see whether you need to adjust them in any way.

Obviously, long-term goals are sometimes hard to accomplish because they require a lot of effort and dedication. For this reason, you are more likely to succeed if you perform activities you enjoy. Fun activities not only build fitness but they also enrich life.

Long-Term Physical Fitness Goals

Setting long-term fitness goals is a good idea, especially if the goals are consistent with your long-term physical activity goals. If you do the right kind of physical activity, your fitness will improve automatically. For example, a person who meets a long-term activity goal of doing at least 30 minutes of physical activity each day for two months would no doubt meet a long-term fitness goal to improve fitness by the end of the two-month period.

Long-term fitness goals are important because they increase the probability that fitness improvement will occur. Of course, doing the right kind of activity and doing it regularly (meeting long-term activity goals) is critical to meeting long-term physical fitness goals.

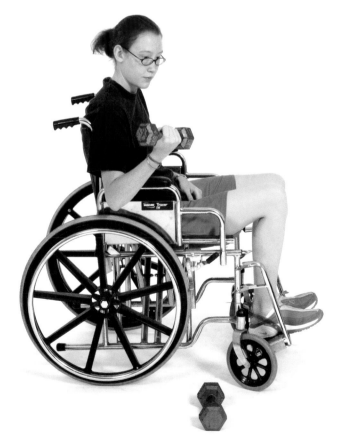

Goal setting is a great way to improve your overall fitness.

Short-Term Goals

Short-term goals can be reached in a short period of time, such as a few days or a few weeks. You might set a series of short-term goals to help accomplish a long-term goal. For example, to meet your long-term goal of making money, you may set a short-term goal of finding a job. After completing this short-term goal, you can re-examine your long-term goal, decide on the next step, and establish your next short-term goal.

Short-Term Physical Activity Goals

Most physical activity goals make good short-term goals. Walking 30 minutes a day for the next two weeks is a short-term activity goal. It can be accomplished in a short time—two weeks—and with effort virtually anyone can accomplish it. Your participation, rather than your performance, determines whether you meet the goal.

Short-Term Physical Fitness Goals

Although physical activity goals are good short-term goals, achieving fitness takes time. A realistic short-term fitness goal is one that can be accomplished in four to six weeks because it takes at least this many weeks of regular exercise to produce fitness improvement. An example of a short-term fitness goal would be to move from the marginal fitness zone to the good fitness zone on a fitness assessment such as the back-saver sit and reach test of flexibility. This goal could be realistically reached in four to six weeks.

Short-Term Physical Activity Versus Short-Term Physical Fitness Goals

Each year millions of Americans set unrealistic short-term fitness goals. One reason is that many people choose short-term goals that cannot be accomplished in the time allotted. This explains why so many people waste their money on products that claim to give them quick fat loss or fast muscle gain. These products do not work because fitness does not come quickly.

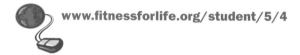

www.fitnessforlife.org/student/5/4

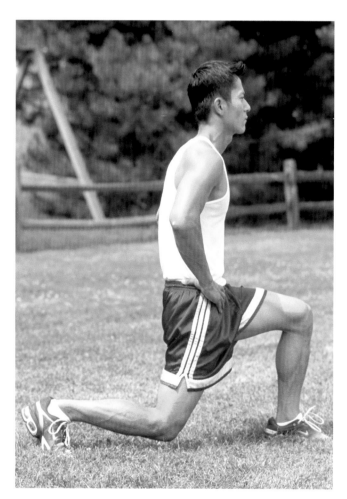

Proper stretching is a good way to increase your flexibility and help you reach your fitness goals.

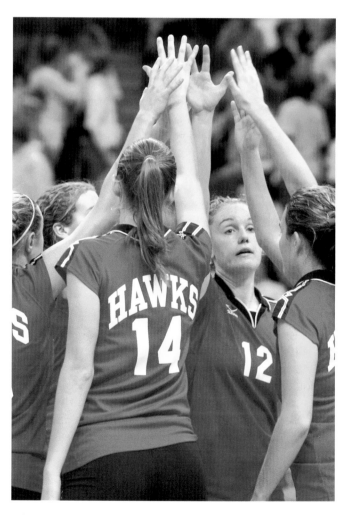

It is also important to set team goals as well as individual goals.

Taking Charge: Setting Goals

Chances are good that you have heard someone say something such as: "I know I should exercise, but I'm tired of setting goals and never reaching them. Sometimes I feel like a failure." The key to reaching goals is to set the right goals for you.

As the physical education teacher passed the weight room, he couldn't help noticing Kevin, who was struggling to do one more biceps curl. Anyone could see that he was discouraged. "What's up, Kevin?" Mr. Booker asked.

Kevin put down the weights and pushed up the sleeves on his T-shirt. "Look at my arm. I've been doing biceps curls and bench presses for two weeks. I wanted my arms to be at least an inch bigger by the end of the month." He shook his head. "It doesn't look like I'm going to reach my goal. I might as well give up."

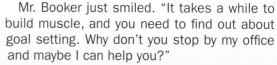

Mr. Booker just smiled. "It takes a while to build muscle, and you need to find out about goal setting. Why don't you stop by my office and maybe I can help you?"

Kevin decided to go talk to Mr. Booker the next day.

For Discussion

Was the goal Kevin set a realistic one? What kinds of advice do you think Mr. Booker gave Kevin about goal setting? What kind of goal did Kevin set? What other kinds of goals do you think Kevin should set for himself? What else could Kevin do to make sure that he set realistic goals for himself? You can use the goal-setting worksheet supplied by your teacher to plan some realistic goals for yourself. Consider the guidelines on page 86.

If you are a beginner, you should focus on short-term activity goals rather than fitness goals. If you meet your short-term activity goals, you are making progress toward getting fit. Set goals for increasing activity in one or more areas of the Physical Activity Pyramid. Both long-term activity and long-term fitness goals are appropriate for beginners. If you are a more advanced exerciser who has been active for several months, you may want to set both short-term activity and short-term fitness goals. Because a long-term exerciser has had continuous involvement in activity, short-term gains in fitness are more likely than for beginners.

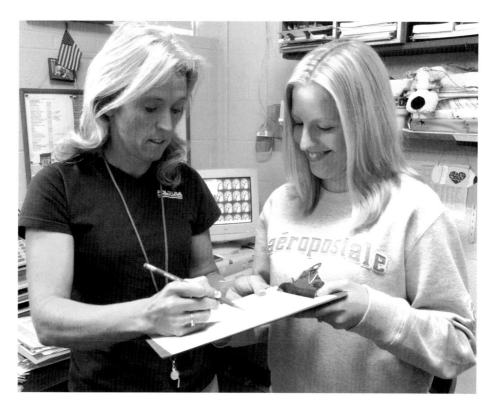

Your physical education teacher can help you set realistic goals.

Lesson Review

1. How can you use long-term and short-term goals to plan your fitness program?
2. What are some guidelines you should follow when setting goals? Be sure they are appropriate for your level.

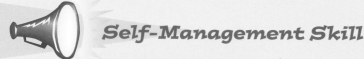

Self-Management Skill

Setting Goals

Now that you know more about the different types of activity and fitness goals, you can begin developing some goals of your own. Follow these guidelines to help you as you identify and develop your personal goals:

▶ **Be realistic.** Realistic goals are ones that can be accomplished easily by those willing to give effort but that are difficult enough to be challenging. Set goals you know you can attain. People who set goals that are too difficult doom themselves to failure before they begin.

▶ **Be specific.** Vague or very general goals are difficult to accomplish. Specific goals help you determine whether you have accomplished what you set out to do.

▶ **Personalize.** A realistic goal for one person can be unrealistic for another. Base your goals on your own individual needs and abilities. Meeting health standards or setting your own performance standards makes more sense than trying to be like others.

▶ **Put your goals in writing.** Writing down a goal represents a personal commitment and increases the chances that you will meet that goal. You will get the chance to write down your goals as you do the activities in this book.

▶ **Know your reasons for setting your goals.** Those who set goals for reasons other than their own personal improvement often fail. Ask yourself *why* when setting goals. Make sure you are setting goals for yourself based on your own needs and interests.

▶ **Consider goals for all parts of fitness.** If you want to reap the health and wellness benefits described in this book, you will have to set goals for all parts of health-related fitness. A realistic goal is to reach the good fitness zone for all parts. You may want to focus first on the parts of fitness in which you need improvement rather than trying to do everything at once.

▶ **Self-assess periodically and keep logs.** Doing self-assessments will help you set your goals and determine whether you have met them. Keeping logs will help you determine whether you have met physical activity goals.

▶ **Focus on improvement.** Set goals at one level higher than your current fitness level. For example, if you are in the low fitness zone, aim for the marginal zone. If you are very far from moving to the next zone, set smaller, short-term goals.

▶ **Set new goals periodically.** Achieving a personal goal is rewarding. You feel good. Congratulate yourself for your accomplishment. Now you can set a new goal.

▶ **Revise if necessary.** Set smaller, more realistic goals rather than goals that are too difficult. If you do find that your goal is too difficult to accomplish, don't be afraid to revise the goal. It is better to revise your goal than to quit being active because you did not reach an unrealistic goal.

▶ **Reward yourself.** If you decide to walk every day for two weeks and you accomplish your goal, tell someone! Your effort deserves credit. Keeping an activity log is a good way to reward yourself.

▶ **Participate in activities with others who have similar abilities.** Friends can keep friends going and can give each other a pat on the back whenever a goal is achieved.

▶ **Consider maintenance goals.** An active, fit person cannot continue to improve in fitness forever. At some point enough is enough. Following a regular workout schedule and maintaining fitness in the good fitness zone are reasonable goals for fit and active people.

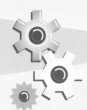

Activity 2

Elastic Band Exercise Circuit

Record Your Results on the Record Sheet

Elastic band exercises are an inexpensive way of providing resistance for building strength and muscular endurance. In this type of exercise, you use elastic bands to provide overload to the muscles. The first people to use elastic band exercises used old bicycle inner tubes or pieces of surgical tubing. You might try using these yourself. The size and thickness of the band you use will depend on your current fitness level.

In this activity you will get the opportunity to try several elastic band exercises and to develop some of your own. You will learn more about muscle fitness in chapters 11 and 12.

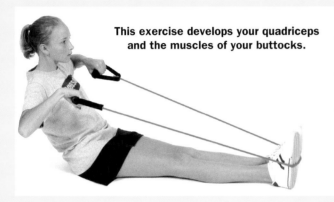

This exercise develops your quadriceps and the muscles of your buttocks.

Two-Leg Press

1. While sitting on the floor, loop the band under the balls of your feet with the ends held with your hands.
2. Begin with your knees near your chest. Press out with your legs against the band to straighten your legs.
3. Return to the starting position. Repeat the exercise 7 to 10 times. Do 1 to 3 sets.

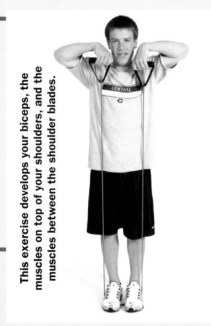

This exercise develops your biceps, the muscles on top of your shoulders, and the muscles between the shoulder blades.

Upright Row

1. While standing, loop the band under your feet.
2. Hold the band with both hands, your palms facing you. Gradually pull up on the band, keeping your elbows high. Pull until your hands reach your chin or as far as you can pull.
3. Lower your hands to the starting position. Repeat the exercise 7 to 10 times. Do 1 to 3 sets.

Arm Curl

1. While standing, loop the band under your feet.
2. With your palms facing up, pull your hands to your chest. Keep your elbows against your sides.
3. Return to the starting position. Repeat the exercise 7 to 10 times. Do 1 to 3 sets.

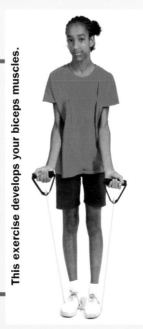
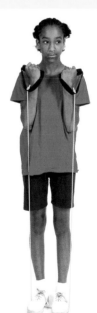

This exercise develops your biceps muscles.

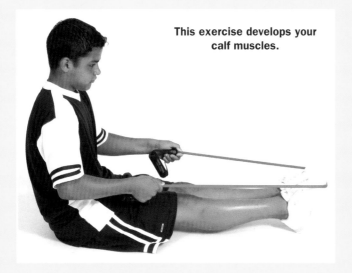

This exercise develops your calf muscles.

Toe Push

1. Sit on the floor and loop the band under your toes. Hold the ends with your hands.
2. Push with your feet by pointing your toes against the band.
3. Return to the starting position. Repeat the exercise 7 to 10 times. Do 1 to 3 sets. To make the exercise more difficult, hold the band closer to your feet.

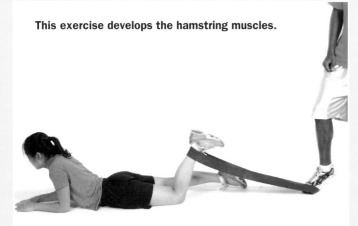

This exercise develops the hamstring muscles.

Leg Curl (Prone)

1. Lie on the floor facedown and loop the band behind one heel.
2. Have a partner stand on the ends of the bands.
3. Pull backward on the band with your heel until your leg is bent at a 90-degree angle.
4. Perform the exercise with your other leg. Complete 7 to 10 repetitions with each leg. Do 1 to 3 sets.

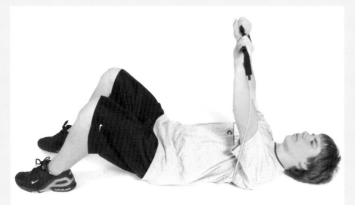

This exercise develops your pectoral and triceps muscles.

Arm Press

1. Lay the band on the floor. Lie down so that the band is under your back. Grab the ends of the band.
2. With your arms bent, press up against the band. Return to the starting position. To make the activity more difficult, hold the band closer to your shoulders.
3. Repeat the exercise 7 to 10 times. Complete 1 to 3 sets.

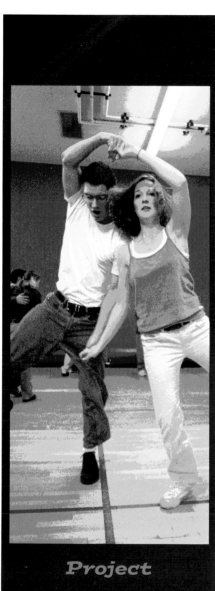

Project

Investigate locations in your school and community that have facilities and equipment for various types of physical activity. Compile a directory of phone numbers, addresses, Internet addresses, facilities, and equipment. Distribute the directory to class members or post it on a Web site that other students can access.

5

Chapter Review

Reviewing Concepts and Vocabulary

Number your paper from 1 to 5. Next to each number, choose the letter of the best answer.

Column I
1. couch potato
2. inactive thinker
3. planner
4. activator
5. active exerciser

Column II
a. just bought exercise equipment
b. is active most days of week
c. is sometimes active
d. is thinking about becoming active
e. is sedentary

Number your paper from 6 to 15. Next to each number, write the word (or words) that correctly completes the sentence.

6. Deciding to walk 30 minutes a day for the next two months is an example of a _____-term goal.

7. Performing 30 push-ups by next week is an example of a _____-term goal.

8. Being able to run a mile in 6 minutes six months from now is an example of a _____-term goal.

9. Deciding to do flexibility exercises three days a week for the next week is an example of a _____-term goal.

10. A skill that helps you change your behavior is called _____.

11. A type of fitness that helps you learn skills is called _____.

12. A term used to describe throwing, kicking, and catching is _____.

13. A self-management skill that enables you to test your own fitness is called _____.

14. A self-management skill that enables you to keep track of the things you have accomplished is called _____.

15. The self-management skill that helps you get the help of friends and family is called _____.

Thinking Critically

Write a paragraph to answer the following question.

What suggestions would you give a friend who is just beginning a physical activity program and wants to set some goals?

6

Lifestyle Physical Activity and Positive Attitudes

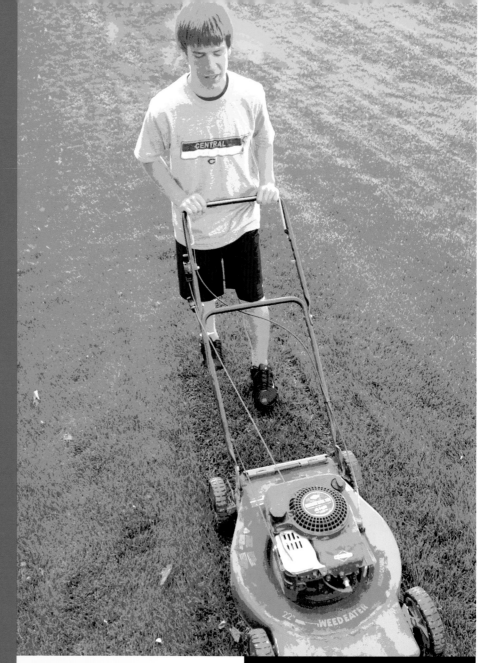

In this chapter...

Activity 1
School Stepping

Lesson 6.1
Activities for a Lifetime—Choices From the Pyramid

Self-Assessment
Walking Test

Lesson 6.2
Attitudes

Taking Charge
Building Positive Attitudes

Self-Management Skill
Building Positive Attitudes

Activity 2
Walking for Wellness

Activity 1

SCHOOL STEPPING

Walking is a popular physical activity that you can engage in for a lifetime. In recent years pedometers have become familiar tools for use during walking and jogging workouts (see Fitness Technology later in this chapter). Pedometers can be used to set and measure goals and monitor progress pertaining to total steps taken, distance covered, or even calories burned. This activity uses pedometers to monitor distance covered as you walk or jog around your school campus for a specific amount of time. If pedometers are not available for your use, an alternative option is provided. Follow the instructions on the Activity Worksheet provided for this chapter.

Activities for a Lifetime— Choices From the Pyramid

Lesson Objectives

After reading this lesson, you should be able to

1. Describe various types of lifestyle physical activities.
2. Describe the FIT formula for lifestyle physical activities.

Lesson Vocabulary

MET (p. 91), moderate physical activity (p. 92)

 www.fitnessforlife.org/student/6/1

In chapter 4 you learned about the many activities in the Physical Activity Pyramid. While it is good to choose activities from each of the levels of the pyramid, public health experts place a high priority on the first level, lifestyle physical activity.

What Are Lifestyle Physical Activities?

Lifestyle physical activities are activities that all people can do regardless of age or physical ability. You can

perform them at home or at work, and they are of moderate intensity. This means that they take four to seven times as much energy as being sedentary. Lifestyle physical activities include housework such as mopping, yard work such as raking the leaves or mowing the lawn, and work-related activities such as carpentry or bricklaying. Walking (rather than driving) and climbing stairs (rather than taking an elevator) are also considered lifestyle activities because they can be done at home, at work, or at school.

 www.fitnessforlife.org/student/6/2

Some activities often thought of as recreational in nature are also classified as lifestyle physical activities. Bicycling is a good example. You can bicycle for recreation but you can also bicycle to school or work. Activities such as golf, bowling, and social dancing are not activities that people typically do at home or at work, but they are of moderate intensity. For this reason they are placed at the bottom level of the pyramid. Table 6.1 includes examples of lifestyle physical activities.

You will notice in table 6.1 that the activities are rated using the term **MET**. The word MET comes from *metabolism*, a word that refers to the use of energy to sustain life. The term can be used to help you determine the intensity of an exercise. One MET represents the energy you expend while resting. Very light activities such as typing require 2 METs, or twice as much energy as when resting. Lifestyle activities require energy expenditures of 4 to 7 METs. Vigorous activities require much more energy (8 to 12 times as much as being sedentary).

Moderate-intensity sports such as golf are considered to be lifestyle physical activities.

Pyramid diagram:
- Rest or inactivity
- Exercise for flexibility
- Exercise for strength and muscular endurance
- Active aerobics
- Active sports and recreation
- Lifestyle physical activity — Level 1

Table 6.1

Examples of Lifestyle Physical Activities

Activity	Description	METs
Walking	Slow	3.0-4.0
	Brisk	4.0-5.5
Yard work	Pushing hand mower	6.0-7.0
	Pushing power mower	4.0-5.0
	Raking leaves	3.0-4.0
	Shoveling	5.0-7.0
	Chopping wood	6.0-7.0
Recreational	Bicycling (slow)	3.0-5.0
	Bicycling (brisk)	5.0-7.0
	Bowling	3.0-3.5
	Golf (walking)	3.5-4.5
	Social dance	3.0-6.0
Occupational work	Bricklaying	3.5
	Carpentry	5.5
	Heavy assembly work	5.5
Housework	Mopping floors	3.0-4.0
	Ironing	3.0
	Making beds	3.0
	Hanging the wash	3.5

Table 6.2

The FIT Formula for Getting Health and Wellness Benefits From Lifestyle Physical Activities

FIT formula	Threshold of training	Target zone
Frequency	Most days of week	Daily, or most days of week
Intensity	Moderate activity equal to brisk walk 200+ calories/day (4 METs)	Moderate activity equal to brisk walk 200+ calories/day (4-7 METs)
Time	30 min in bouts of 10+ min	30 min to several hr in bouts of 10+ min

Why Should I Do Lifestyle Physical Activities?

Experts used to think that the health benefits described in chapter 3 required vigorous physical activity. We now know that most of those health benefits can be achieved by doing moderate or lifestyle physical activities. As people grow older, they are less likely to participate in vigorous sports and games. The most popular activities among adults 18 and over are walking, biking, yard work, and home calisthenics. If you establish the habit of doing lifestyle physical activity early in life, you are more likely to continue to be active as you grow older. Consider doing some lifestyle physical activity as part of your daily routine. For example, you might walk or ride a bicycle to get to school.

How Much Lifestyle Physical Activity Is Enough?

Experts from the American College of Sports Medicine (ACSM), United States Centers for Disease Control and Prevention, and the Surgeon General of the United States indicate that, at a minimum, all teens and adults should do 30 minutes of **moderate physical activity** (4 to 7 METs) on most, if not all, days of the week. They

use brisk walking as an example of how much physical activity is necessary to reduce risk of disease and to promote wellness. Walking is just one example. Any of the activities in table 6.1, or other activities of moderate intensity, are also appropriate. Table 6.2 illustrates the FIT formula for lifestyle physical activities.

While your goal should be to accumulate at least 30 minutes of moderate activity each day, more is even better. For some of the many health benefits of physical activity an hour or more is recommended. Thirty minutes was chosen as a minimum value because if you do that amount you get many of the benefits without a lot of effort. Experts now agree that it is best to get your 30 minutes in bouts or activity sessions lasting at least 10 minutes each. In other words, you could do three 10-minute bouts, one 20-minute and one 10-minute bout, or other combinations that equal 30 minutes a day. Just accumulating 30 minutes in shorter bouts is better than doing nothing, but it does not give you the amount of activity recommended by the health officials.

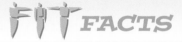

A health goal for the nation is to increase the percentage of teens who do moderate lifestyle physical activity at least five days a week to 35 percent. Currently 27 percent of teens do lifestyle activity at least five days a week.

Counting Physical Activity Calories

As shown in table 6.2, you can use METs or minutes to determine how much lifestyle activity you should perform. We know that for best results the activity should be of an intensity equal to brisk walking. Another way to determine whether you perform enough lifestyle activity is to count the calories you expend each day. Notice in table 6.2 that the FIT formula for calorie counting suggests that, as a minimum (threshold), you should expend at least 200 calories a day in physical activity. This would amount to 1,000 to 1,400 calories each week based on 5 to 7 active days a week. For optimal benefits to health and wellness (target zone), you should expend 2,000 to 3,500 calories a week from the Physical Activity Pyramid. You can also count the more vigorous activities discussed in chapters 7 and 8 in meeting this total. Consult table 13.4 on page 231 for a list of the calories expended in a wide variety of physical activities.

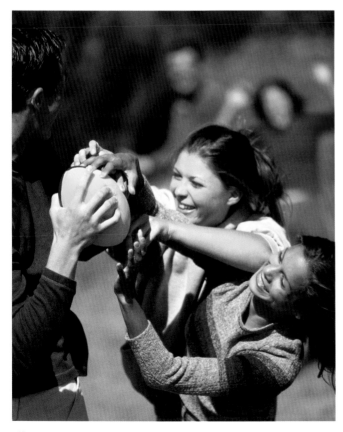
Lifestyle physical activities also include fun, active games.

FITNESS Technology

Walking is the most popular form of lifestyle physical activity. One method of self-monitoring walking is with a pedometer. A pedometer is a small battery-powered device that can be worn on your belt. The pedometer counts each step you take and displays the counts on a meter. You simply open the face of the pedometer and see how many steps you have taken. Some experts believe that if you walk at least 10,000 steps each day, you will be in the target zone for lifestyle physical activity. Other experts are concerned that you could reach 10,000 steps without doing any sustained activity such as bouts of 10 or more minutes. On the other hand, some people can do a brisk walk of 30 minutes each day and still not reach a 10,000-step count. The President's Active Lifestyle Award, presented by the President's Council on Physical Fitness and Sports, requires girls to perform 11,000 steps a day and boys to perform 13,000 steps a day for several weeks to earn the award. Still, the pedometer is an easy way to see how much activity you are doing. You may have the opportunity in school to wear a pedometer to monitor your own activity levels.

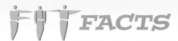
www.fitnessforlife.org/student/6/3

FIT FACTS

You can find out more about the President's Council on Physical Fitness and Sports Active Lifestyle Award by logging on to www.fitness.gov.

Lesson Review

1. What does the term MET mean? How is it useful?
2. What are some types of lifestyle physical activity? How do they benefit you?
3. What is the FIT formula (threshold of training and target zone) for getting health and wellness benefits from lifestyle physical activities?

Walking Test

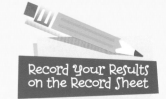

Record Your Results on the Record Sheet

Many of the self-assessments you perform in this course require very intense physical activity. The cardiovascular fitness self-assessments, such as the mile run, can be good assessments but they are not for everyone. Beginners and people who do not enjoy running may prefer doing another type of assessment. The walking test gives you an alternative to the mile run, the PACER, and the step test.

If you are a very active person and are quite fit, the mile run or PACER may be best for estimating your cardiovascular fitness, but the walking test is also a good test. The test is especially good for people who are beginners, who haven't been doing a lot of recent activity, and who are regular walkers. It is also good for older people and for those who cannot do running tests because of joint or muscle problems. Try all of the assessments, because you will have a better overall view of your fitness by using results from various assessments.

Because you are walking, a warm-up is not necessary. The walk itself is a warm-up. Some people prefer to do some preliminary walking and a warm-up stretch before this test.

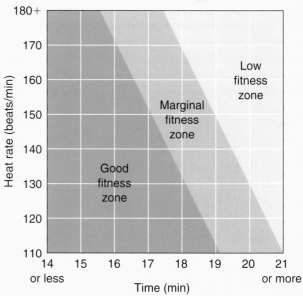

Rating Chart: Walking Test (females).

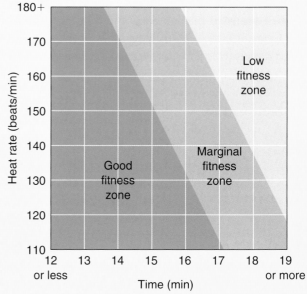

Rating Chart: Walking Test (males).

Adapted from the *One Mile Walk Test* with permission of author James M. Rippe, M.D.

1. Walk a mile at a fast pace (as fast as you can while keeping approximately the same pace for the entire walk).

2. Immediately after the walk, count your heart rate for 15 seconds. Calculate your one-minute heart rate by multiplying by 4. Record your rate on your record sheet.

3. Locate your walking rating using the appropriate chart. Record your rating.

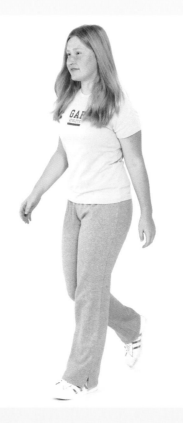

Lesson 6.2

Attitudes

Lesson Objectives

After reading this lesson, you should be able to

1. List some negative attitudes about physical activity and describe how to change them into positive attitudes.
2. List some reasons why people like to exercise.
3. Explain how you can help others have a positive attitude toward physical activity.

Lesson Vocabulary

attitude (p. 95)

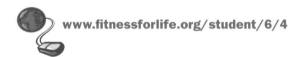 www.fitnessforlife.org/student/6/4

Attitude is another word for your feelings about something. Your attitude about physical activity can affect your well-being throughout life. In this lesson, you will learn about attitudes people have about physical activity and how to change negative attitudes to positive ones. Having a positive attitude is the key to success in fitness.

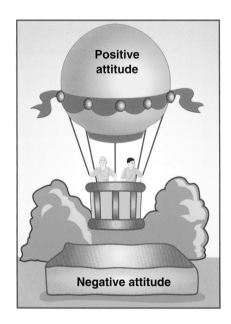

Active people have more positive than negative attitudes.

Change Negative Attitudes

The following list shows you some negative attitudes and positive alternatives. Follow these guidelines:

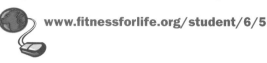 **www.fitnessforlife.org/student/6/5**

▶ **Negative: "I don't have the time." Positive: "I will plan a time for physical activity."** If you planned time for physical activity, you would feel better, function more efficiently, and actually may have more time to do other things you want to do.

▶ **Negative: "I don't want to get all sweaty." Positive: "I'll allow time to clean up afterward."** Sweating is a natural by-product of a good workout. Allow yourself time to change before exercising, and shower and change afterward. Focus on how good you will feel.

▶ **Negative: "People might laugh at me." Positive: "I don't care what people think. When they see how fit I get, they'll wish they were exercising, too."** Don't let other people's opinions affect you. Find friends who are interested in getting fit. Those who do laugh may be jealous of your efforts and results.

▶ **Negative: "None of my friends work out, so neither do I." Positive: " I'll ask my friends to join me and we'll all work out together."** Talk with your friends. Some of them may be interested in working out or doing lifestyle activities together.

▶ **Negative: "I get nervous and feel tense when I am in sports and games." Positive: "Everyone gets nervous. I'll stay calm and do the best I can."** Many athletes need to learn techniques to reduce their stress levels. You will learn some of these techniques in chapter 17.

▶ **Negative: "I'm already in good condition." Positive: "Physical activity will help keep me in good condition."** Use the self-assessments in this book, and then take an honest look at yourself. Are you as fit as you thought? Physical activity can help you get in shape and stay in shape.

▶ **Negative: "I'm too tired." Positive: "I'll just do a little to get started, and as I get more fit, I'll do more."** You'll probably find that physical exertion actually gives you more energy. Begin slowly and gradually increase the amount of activity you do.

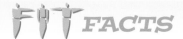

Active teens have more positive attitudes than negative attitudes. This is called a positive balance of attitudes.

Increase Positive Attitudes

Following is a list of reasons people like to be physically active. Think about these attitudes and how you might make some of them your own.

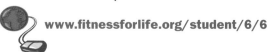
www.fitnessforlife.org/student/6/6

▶ **"Physical activities are a great way to meet people."** Many activities provide opportunities to meet people and strengthen friendships. Aerobic dance and team sports are examples of good social activities.

▶ **"I think physical activity is really fun."** Many teenagers do activities because they are fun. Participating in activities you enjoy also helps reduce stress.

▶ **"I enjoy the challenge."** Sir Edmund Hillary was asked why he climbed Mt. Everest. "Because it was there," he replied. Many people welcome challenges.

▶ **"I like the rigor of training."** Some people enjoy doing intense training. Winning and competition can be secondary for people who enjoy training.

▶ **"I like competition."** If you enjoy competition, sports and other physical activities provide ways to test yourself against others. You can even compete against yourself by trying to improve your score or your time in an activity.

▶ **"Physical activities are my way of relaxing."** Physical activity can help you relax mentally or emotionally after a difficult day—for example, after a day of difficult schoolwork.

▶ **"I think physical activity improves my appearance."** Physical activity can help build muscle and control body fat. However, remember that regular activity cannot completely change your appearance.

▶ **"Physical activity is a good way to improve my health and wellness."** As you learned in chapter 3, regular physical activity helps you resist illness and improves your general sense of well-being.

▶ **"Physical activity just makes me feel good."** Many people just feel better when they exercise and have a sense of loss or discomfort when they do not.

Sensitivity to Others

The way others react can affect an individual's personal feelings about physical activity. Your positive reactions can help others change negative feelings about physical activity. Consider the following suggestions when you interact with others in physical activity.

▶ **Instead of laughing, provide encouragement.** Do you remember how difficult it is to start something new or different? You can encourage others by saying such words as, "Good to see you exercising. Way to go!"

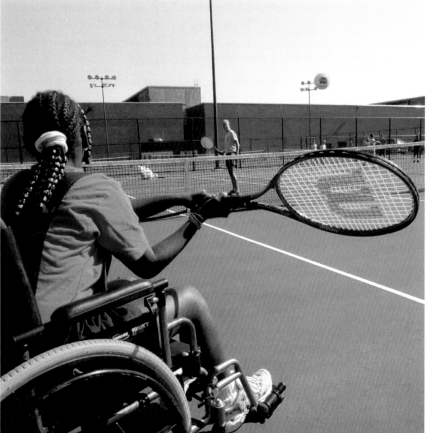

Physical activity makes you feel good.

Taking Charge: Building Positive Attitudes

Many people have both positive and negative feelings about exercise and physical activity. Some use negative feelings as an excuse to avoid being active. To become and stay physically active, they need to increase their positive feelings and decrease negative feelings.

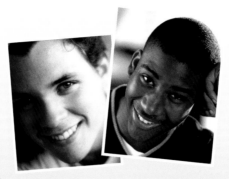

"Allen, I don't want to play tennis now." Matt put the tennis rackets down. Then he led Allen into the family room. "Anyway," he said, "a good TV show is on."

"I think you just don't want to lose to me in tennis again," Allen said.

"You're right," Matt admitted. "I hate losing."

"You win sometimes, Matt. The competition is what makes tennis fun."

"Not when I lose," Matt replied.

Allen thought for a minute. "How about taking a jog around the block?" he asked. "There will be no winner or loser."

"I don't want to get all sweaty," Matt replied. "I'd rather relax watching TV."

"Oh, come on, Matt. Jogging will help you relax. We need to stay in shape."

Matt smiled at Allen. "I guess I could stand to get sweaty once in a while. It does make me feel more alive." He jumped up and headed for the front door. "C'mon! Let's go for a run!"

For Discussion

What does Allen like about being physically active? What does Matt like and not like about physical activity? How could Matt change his negative attitudes and become more active? What are some positive attitudes that keep people active? What are some other negative attitudes that keep people from being active, and how can those attitudes be changed? Fill out the questionnaire provided by your teacher to find out more about your own attitudes toward physical activity. Consider the guidelines on page 98.

▶ **Try to make new friends through participation in physical activities.** Introduce yourself to others and offer to help other people when it seems appropriate.

▶ **Don't hesitate to ask for help from others.** Start or join a sport or exercise club. You and your friends can combine socializing with physical activity by starting or joining an activity club. Check with your school's activity coordinator concerning the rules for setting up an activity club.

▶ **Be sensitive to people with special needs.** Some people need certain accommodations or modifications when performing physical activity. People with no special needs can help by participating with those who have special challenges and by being sensitive to their needs.

▶ **Be considerate of cultural differences.** The popularity of physical activities varies from culture to culture. What is popular in one culture is not necessarily popular in another. Activities such as field hockey and curling are not popular in the United States but are very popular in other countries. What one person enjoys may not be so enjoyable to another. Learning to accept cultural differences will help all people to enjoy activity and can lead to better interpersonal understanding.

Lesson Review

1. What are some examples of negative attitudes toward physical activity? How would you change them into positive attitudes?
2. What are some reasons why people enjoy physical activity?
3. How can you help others have a positive attitude toward physical activity?

Self-Management Skill

Building Positive Attitudes

Most of us have had both positive and negative attitudes about physical activity at one time or another. Experts have shown that people who have more positive attitudes than negative ones are likely to be active. You can take the following guidelines to try to build positive attitudes and get rid of negative ones:

▶ **Assess your attitudes.** Make a list of your positive or negative attitudes. You can use the attitudes listed in this lesson to help you or you can use the worksheet provided by your instructor.

▶ **Identify reasons for negative attitudes.** Your self-assessment will help you identify negative attitudes. Once you have identified them, ask yourself why you feel negative. If you can find the reason, it may help you change. For example, you may not have liked playing a sport when you were young because you did not like a coach or another player. Maybe you can find a situation that will make an activity more fun.

▶ **Find activities that bring out fewer negative attitudes.** People have different attitudes and feelings about different activities. You may not like team sports but you might like recreational activities. List your negative attitudes, then ask yourself whether activities exist for which you do not have these negative feelings. If so, consider trying these activities.

▶ **Choose activities that accentuate the positive.** If you really like certain activities and have good feelings about them, focus on these activities rather than ones you don't like as much.

▶ **Change the situation.** You may not feel positively about an activity because of things unrelated to the activity. For example, if you hated playing basketball because you had too little time to get dressed and groomed after participating, maybe you can find a situation in which you can do the activity and also have more time to shower and dress.

▶ **Be active with friends.** Activities are more fun when you do them with friends. Sometimes just participating with other people you enjoy is enough to change your feelings about an activity.

▶ **Discuss your attitudes.** Just talking about your attitudes can sometimes help. Sometimes people think that they are the only people who have problems in certain situations. Talking about it with others can help change the situation to make it more fun for everyone concerned.

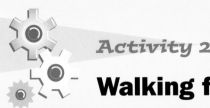

Activity 2

Walking for Wellness

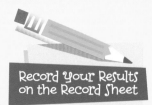

Record Your Results
on the Record Sheet

The Surgeon General of the United States has recommended every American get at least 30 minutes of physical activity on all or most days of the week. The type of activity recommended is lifestyle physical activity, described in this chapter. One of the activities most often performed to meet the minimum recommendation is walking. A group of weight control experts has recommended that people perform at least 60 minutes of daily activity to maintain a healthy body fat level. Most agree, however, that 30 minutes of brisk walking would be a good place to start. This walking for wellness activity provides various walking opportunities. You can try one or more of the activities on your own or do one of them in class as directed by your instructor.

Pedometer Walking

Wear a pedometer during a 30-minute walk. Keep track of how many steps you take in 30 minutes. Some experts feel that people who take 10,000 steps in a day will have done enough activity to meet the Surgeon General's recommendation. Other experts indicate that teens should accumulate as many as 13,000 to 14,000 steps in a day. In addition to wearing the pedometer in class, you might want to wear one for several days to see how many steps you take in a typical day. Pedometers are a good way to help you self-monitor your activity. A worksheet is available to use in recording your steps.

Calculating Steps Per Mile

The word mile comes from a Latin phrase, *milia passuum,* which means 1,000 paces (or 2,000 steps) for a soldier. Most people doing a brisk walk take about 2,000 steps a mile, but the number of steps you take depends on your height. Taller people take longer steps than shorter people. In this activity you will count your steps for a walk around the track (1/4 mile). You can use a pedometer if you have one. Continue to walk multiples of 1/4 mile until you have walked 3 miles. How many minutes did it take you? How many steps did you take for the full 3 miles (multiply your steps for the 1/4 mile times 12)?

Counting Calories

After you do your walk you can calculate the calories you expended. Use table 6.3 to determine caloric expenditure. First determine the calories you expend each minute of brisk walking by looking at the number under your body weight. Multiply this number by the total number of minutes you walked. Did you expend 200 or more calories as recommended earlier in the chapter?

Table 6.3

Calories Expended in Walking (per Minute)

Weight (lb)	Cal/min
<100	2.3
101-125	2.9
126-150	3.5
151-175	4.1
176-200	4.7
201+	5.2

Group Walk

Walk in a group with four or five other people. Walk in a single file line at a brisk pace for 30 minutes. The person at the front of the line will determine where you will walk. Follow the leader, and change leaders every 3 minutes. The last person in line will need to walk faster than the rest of the group to move to the front of the line. The new leader will then determine where the group will walk. Be sure that the leaders late in the walk keep you near your starting place so that you have time to return during the last few minutes of the walk. Try to keep a steady pace during the walk.

Weekly Walking

Keep track of your walking each day of the week for one week. Use the worksheet provided by your instructor to monitor the minutes you walk each day. Do you walk 30 minutes a day on a typical day?

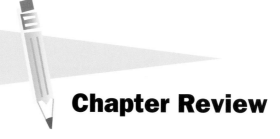

6 Chapter Review

Reviewing Concepts and Vocabulary

Number your paper from 1 to 6. Next to each number, write the word (or words) that correctly completes the sentence.

1. Activity equal to brisk walking is considered to be _____ physical activity.

2. Activities at the base of the Physical Activity Pyramid are called _____.

3. You should perform _____ minutes of physical activity on all or most days of the week.

4. A device worn on your belt that counts steps is called a _____.

5. You can change your _____ about physical activity from negative to positive.

6. A term that is used to describe intensity of activity is called a _____.

Number your paper from 7 to 10. Next to each number, choose the letter of the best answer.

Column I	Column II
7. yard work	a. bowling
8. recreational	b. mowing
9. occupational work	c. carpentry
10. housework	d. mopping

Number your paper from 11 to 20. On your paper, list the answers for each question.

11-15. What are some of the reasons why people are physically active? List five positive attitudes.

16-20. What are some of the reasons why people are not physically active? List five negative attitudes.

Thinking Critically

Write a paragraph to answer the following question.

Teens are often more vigorously active than adults. For this reason some people say that teens should begin to do lifestyle or more moderate activity so that they will stay active later in life. Do you think you will become more or less active as you grow older? Do you think your attitudes toward activity will change? What types of activity do you think you will do?

Unit Review on the Web

 www.fitnessforlife.org/student/6/7

Unit II review materials are available on the Web at the address listed above.

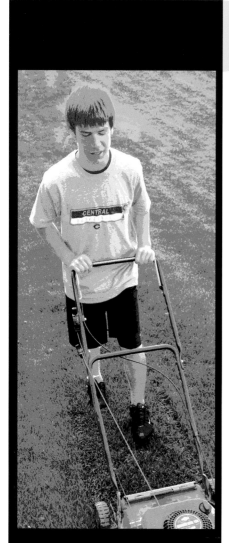

Project

What do the people you know think about physical activity? Develop a list of questions and ask at least six people to answer them. Try to interview people from several different age groups. Analyze your results. Then develop a plan to improve any negative attitudes you found.

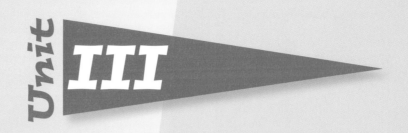

Physical Activity Pyramid:

Level 2 Activities

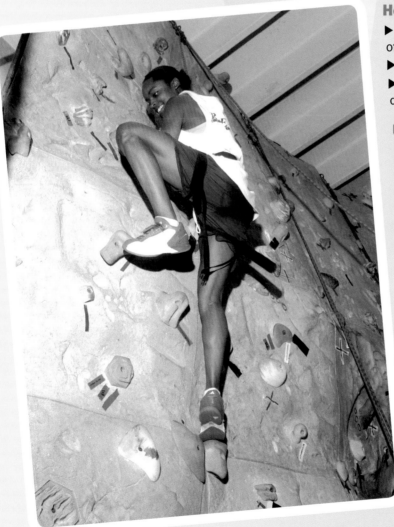

Healthy People 2010 Goals

▶ Increase regular vigorous physical activity of teens.

▶ Improve cardiovascular fitness.

▶ Reduce risk of a variety of heart diseases.

Unit Activities

▶ Aerobic Dance Routine

▶ Cardiovascular Fitness: How Much Activity Is Enough?

▶ Step Aerobics

▶ Jogging: Biomechanical Principles and Guidelines

▶ Orienteering

▶ The Sports Stars Program

7

Cardiovascular Fitness

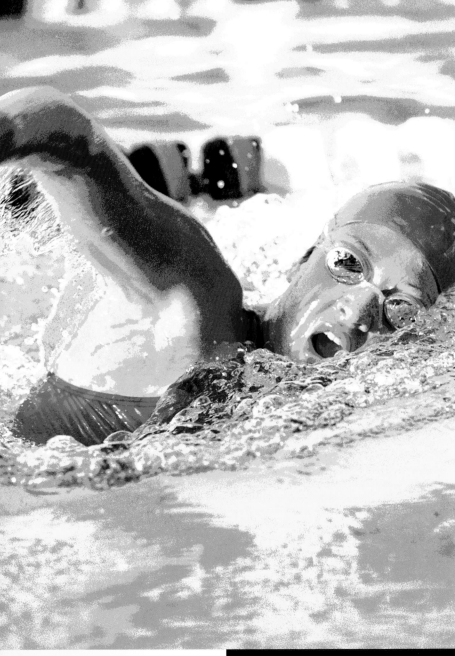

In this chapter...

Activity 1
Aerobic Dance Routine

Lesson 7.1
Cardiovascular Fitness Facts

Self-Assessment
Cardiovascular Fitness—Step Test and One-Mile Run

Lesson 7.2
Building Cardiovascular Fitness

Taking Charge
Learning to Self-Monitor

Self-Management Skill
Learning to Self-Monitor

Activity 2
Cardiovascular Fitness: How Much Activity Is Enough?

Activity 1

AEROBIC DANCE ROUTINE

Aerobic dance is a type of exercise routine that is also a form of aerobic exercise. Aerobic dance routines are developed by combining a variety of steps and arm movements performed to music. The key to getting a good aerobic workout during the routine is to keep moving at a regular pace. Many young people enjoy aerobic dance because they can get a good workout while listening to music they enjoy.

Cardiovascular Fitness Facts

Lesson Objectives

After reading this lesson, you should be able to

1. Describe the benefits of cardiovascular fitness to health and wellness.
2. Explain the relationship between physical activity and good cardiovascular fitness.
3. Describe and demonstrate some methods you can use to assess your cardiovascular fitness.
4. Determine how much cardiovascular fitness is enough.

Lesson Vocabulary

artery (p. 104), cardiovascular system (p. 103), cholesterol (p. 104), fibrin (p. 104), high-density lipoprotein (HDL) (p. 104), lipoproteins (p. 104), low-density lipoprotein (LDL) (p. 104), respiratory system (p. 103), vein (p. 106)

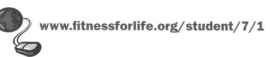

www.fitnessforlife.org/student/7/1

Of the 11 parts of fitness, cardiovascular fitness is the most important because those who have it receive many health and wellness benefits, including a chance for a longer life. The activity that you do to improve your cardiovascular fitness will make you look better, too. The boy in the figure can run a long distance because he has good cardiovascular fitness. When doing regular physical activity, to improve your cardiovascular fitness requires fitness of the heart, lungs, blood, blood vessels, and muscles, as shown in the figure. In this lesson you will learn how proper physical activity improves cardiovascular fitness. You will also learn how to assess your own cardiovascular fitness.

Benefits of Physical Activity and Cardiovascular Fitness

Looking good is important to most people, and you most likely are one of them. Doing regular physical activity can help you look better by controlling your weight, building muscle, and developing good posture. In addition, regular physical activity produces changes in body organs such as making your heart muscle stronger and your blood vessels healthier. These changes result in improved cardiovascular fitness and wellness, as well as a reduction in risk of hypokinetic diseases.

Regular physical activity benefits two vital body systems. Your **cardiovascular system** is made up of your heart, blood vessels, and your blood. Your **respiratory system** is made up of your lungs and the air passages that bring air, including oxygen, from outside of the body into the lungs. In your lungs, oxygen enters your blood while carbon dioxide is eliminated. The cardiovascular and respiratory systems work together to bring your body cells the materials they need to function and to rid the cells of waste. Exercise helps these systems function more effectively (with the most benefits possible) and efficiently (with the least amount of effort).

Heart

Because your heart is a muscle, it benefits from exercise and activities such as jogging, swimming, or long-distance hiking. Your heart acts as a pump to supply

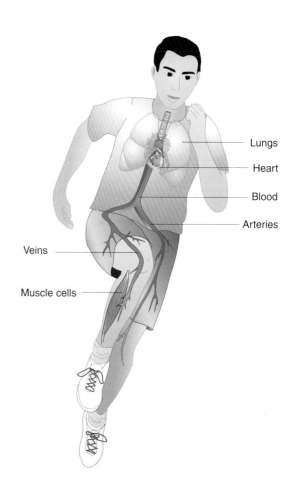

Lungs
Heart
Blood
Arteries
Veins
Muscle cells

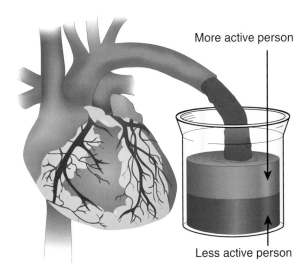

More active person

Less active person

blood to your body cells. When you do vigorous physical activity, your muscle cells need more oxygen and they produce more waste products. Your heart must pump more blood to supply the increased amount of oxygen and to remove the waste products. If your heart is unable to pump enough blood, your muscles will be less able to contract and they will become fatigued more quickly.

Your heart's ability to pump blood is very important when doing physical activity, especially for an extended length of time. Your heart has two ways to get more blood to your muscles—by beating faster or by sending more blood with each beat.

You might recall from the self-assessment in chapter 1 that your resting heart rate is the number of heartbeats per minute when you are relatively inactive. A person who does regular physical activity might have a resting heart rate of 55 to 60 beats per minute, while a person who does not exercise regularly might have a resting heart rate of 70 or more beats per minute. A very fit person's heart beats approximately 9.5 million times less each year than that of the average person. As you can see in table 7.1, a fit person's heart works more efficiently by pumping more blood with fewer beats.

Blood

Although your body needs a certain amount of fat, excessive amounts trigger formation of fatty deposits along artery walls. **Cholesterol,** a fatlike substance found in meats, dairy products, and egg yolks, can be dangerous because high levels can build in your body without you noticing.

Cholesterol is carried through the bloodstream by particles called **lipoproteins.** One kind, **low-density lipoprotein (LDL),** is often referred to as bad cholesterol because LDLs carry cholesterol that is most likely to stay in the body and contribute to atherosclerosis.

An LDL lower than 100 is considered optimal for good health. Another kind, **high-density lipoprotein (HDL),** is often referred to as good cholesterol; HDLs carry excess LDLs out of the bloodstream and into the liver for elimination from the body. Therefore, HDLs appear to help prevent atherosclerosis. An HDL above 60 is considered optimal for good health. For more information on HDL and LDL consult the Internet address listed in the Web icon.

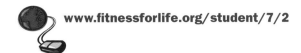

www.fitnessforlife.org/student/7/2

Regular physical activity helps improve your cardiovascular fitness by reducing LDL (bad cholesterol) levels and increasing HDL (good cholesterol) levels. Also, exercise can help prevent blood clots from forming by reducing the amount of **fibrin** in the blood. Fibrin is a substance involved in making your blood clot. High amounts of fibrin can contribute to the development of atherosclerosis.

Arteries

Each **artery** carries blood away from your heart to another part of your body. Blood is forced through your arteries by the beating of your heart. A strong heart and healthy lungs are not very helpful if your arteries are not clear and open. You know that fatty deposits on the inner walls of an artery lead to atherosclerosis. An extreme case of atherosclerosis can totally block the blood flow in an artery. Also, the hardened deposits allow blood clots to form, severely blocking blood flow. In either case, the heart muscle does not get enough oxygen and a heart attack occurs.

Regular physical activity has other cardiovascular benefits. Scientists have found that people who exercise regularly develop more branching of the arteries in the heart. In the drawing on page 106 you can see that the heart muscle has its own arteries (coronary arteries) that supply it with blood and oxygen. People who exercise regularly develop extra coronary arteries. The importance of a richer network of blood vessels can be shown in this example. After astronaut Ed White died in a fire in 1967 while training for a mission, an autopsy was performed. Doctors found that one of the major arteries in his heart was completely blocked due to atherosclerosis. Because of all the physical training astronauts do, scientists think White's body had developed an extra branching of arteries in his heart muscle. Therefore, he didn't die of a heart attack when a main artery was blocked. White had been able to continue a high level of physical fitness training without signs of heart trouble.

Table 7.1

Benefits of Physical Activity on the Cardiovascular and Respiratory Systems

Organ	Benefits
Heart	• Heart muscle gets stronger • Pumps more blood with each beat • Beats slower • Gets more rest • Works more efficiently
Blood vessels	• Healthy elastic arteries allow more blood flow • Less risk of atherosclerosis • Lower blood pressure • Less risk of a blood clot leading to heart attack • Development of extra blood vessels • Healthy veins with healthy valves
Blood	• Less bad cholesterol (LDL) and other fats in the blood • More good cholesterol (HDL) in the blood • Fewer substances in the blood that cause clots
Nerves of the heart	Regular exercise helps the nerves slow your heart rate at rest.
Lungs	• Lungs work more efficiently • Deliver more oxygen to the blood • Healthy lungs allow deeper and less frequent breathing
Cells	• Use oxygen efficiently • Get rid of more wastes • Use blood sugars and insulin more effectively to produce energy

Veins

Each **vein** carries blood filled with waste products from the muscle cells back to the heart. One-way valves in your veins keep the blood from flowing backward. Your muscles squeeze the veins to pump the blood back to your heart. Regular cardiovascular exercise helps make your muscles squeeze your veins efficiently. A lack of physical activity can cause the valves, especially those in the legs, to stop working efficiently, thereby reducing circulation in your legs.

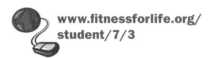
www.fitnessforlife.org/student/7/3

Nerves of Your Heart

Your heart muscle is not like your arm and leg muscles. When your arm and leg muscles contract, nerves in the muscles are responding to a message sent by the conscious part of your brain. In contrast, your heart is not controlled voluntarily; it beats regularly without you telling it to do so. Your heart rate is controlled by a part of the heart called a pacemaker. It sends out an electrical current telling the heart to beat regularly. People who do regular cardiovascular exercise often develop a slower heart rate because the heart pumps more blood with each beat and so it can beat less often. As a result your heart works more efficiently because each heartbeat supplies

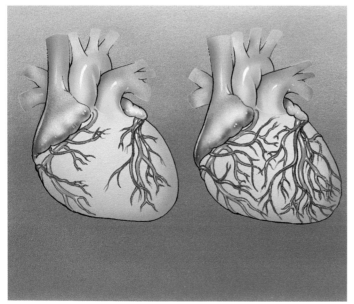
The richer network of blood vessels on the heart to the right is due to regular exercise.

FITNESS Technology

In chapter 1 you learned to count your heart rate using your wrist or neck pulse. Later in this chapter you will learn how to determine whether your heart rate is elevated enough to improve your cardiovascular fitness. A high-tech method is available to help you count your heart rate *during* your activity. The device is sometimes called a heart rate watch because you wear a heart rate monitor that looks like a wrist watch. You wear a band around your chest that senses the electrical stimulation from the heart's nervous system. A transmitter in the chest band sends a signal to a receiver in the watch on your wrist. The receiver picks up the signal and displays your heart rate. You can set a heart rate watch to tell you whether you are exercising in the heart rate target zone. You can also set it to keep track of how many minutes you stay in the target zone. If your school has heart rate watches you may want to use one to monitor your cardiovascular fitness activities.

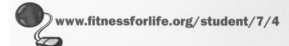
www.fitnessforlife.org/student/7/4

more blood and oxygen to your body than if you did not exercise. In addition, a person with a slower heart rate can function more effectively during an emergency or during vigorous physical activity.

Muscle Cells

For you to be able to do physical activity for a long time without getting tired, your muscle cells must function efficiently and effectively. Regular physical activity helps cells use oxygen and get rid of waste materials effectively. Physical activity also helps the muscle cells use blood sugar, with the aid of the hormone insulin, to produce energy. This function is important to good cardiovascular health.

Cardiovascular Assessment

You might be curious about your cardiovascular fitness—how good is it? Special tests can assess your cardiovascular fitness. The maximal oxygen uptake test is considered the best test of cardiovascular fitness. It is done in a laboratory using special equipment, including a gas meter and a treadmill or a stationary bicycle (see photo on page 107). Another type of lab test of cardiovascular fitness is the graded exercise test, sometimes called the exercise stress test. This test also requires a treadmill or stationary bicycle and a special heart rate monitor.

www.fitnessforlife.org/student/7/5

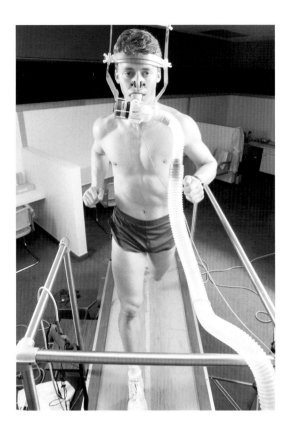

FIT FACTS

Because you may get different ratings on different tests of cardiovascular fitness, consider the strengths and weaknesses of each test when making decisions about which score is most indicative of your fitness.

How Much Cardiovascular Fitness Is Enough?

To get the health and wellness benefits associated with cardiovascular fitness, you should achieve the good fitness zone in the rating charts that accompany each self-assessment in this book. It is important to know that benefits are associated with moving out of the low fitness zone. Risk of hypokinetic diseases is greatest for those in the low fitness zone. Because cardiovascular fitness is a requirement for high-level performance in many sports, if you aspire to be an athlete you may want to train harder than most people to achieve the high performance zone. Achieving this level is not necessary to get most of the health and wellness benefits, and it may be difficult for some people.

Self-Assessment

The tests just described are often quite expensive because of the need for special equipment and fitness experts. For this reason several self-assessments have been developed to allow you to conveniently assess your own cardiovascular fitness with a minimum of equipment and expense. You will get an opportunity to try several self-assessments in this class.

Interpreting Self-Assessment Results

It is wise to do more than one self-assessment for cardiovascular fitness. Self-assessments are not as accurate as laboratory tests of fitness. However, they do give a good estimate of your fitness level. Each assessment has its own strengths and weaknesses. For example, the results of the PACER (chapter 8) and one-mile run (this chapter) are influenced by your motivation; if you don't try very hard, you won't get an accurate score. The walking test (chapter 6) is a good indicator of fitness for most people but is not best for assessing high-level fitness. The step test (this chapter) uses heart rate; therefore, motivation does not influence the results as much as in some other assessments. But results on the step test can be distorted if you have done other exercise that might elevate the heart rate before doing the assessment. The test also can be influenced by emotional factors that cause the heart rate to be higher than normal. Finally, your results may vary depending on the time of day the assessment is done.

Lesson Review

1. What are some benefits of cardiovascular fitness to health and wellness?
2. What is the relationship between physical activity and cardiovascular fitness?
3. What are some methods for assessing cardiovascular fitness and how are they performed?
4. How much cardiovascular fitness is enough?

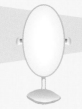

Self-Assessment

Cardiovascular Fitness—Step Test and One-Mile Run

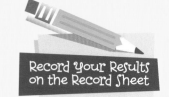

Record Your Results on the Record Sheet

As you learned in the previous lesson, several tests of cardiovascular fitness can be done in physical-fitness laboratories by trained technicians. But if you want a quicker, easier, and less expensive test, try the step test or the one-mile run. You might do either of these assessments to see how fit you are. After you have done regular exercise over a period of time, test yourself again to see how much you have improved.

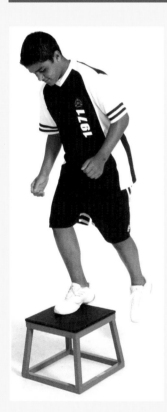
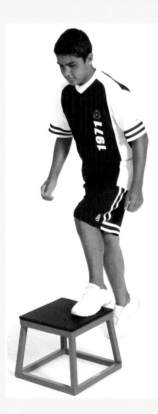

Step Test

1. Use a 12-inch-high bench. Step up with your right foot. Step up with your left foot.
2. Step down with your right foot. Step down with your left foot. Repeat this 4-count (up, up, down, down). Step 24 times each minute for 3 minutes.

Note: The height of the bench and the rate of stepping are both very important to getting an accurate test result. You should sit calmly for several minutes before the test to assure that your resting heart rate is normal.

3. Immediately after stepping for 3 minutes, sit and use the procedure you learned in the self-assessment in chapter 1 to count your own pulse. Begin counting within 5 seconds. Count for 1 minute.
4. Record your results on your worksheet. Check your cardiovascular rating in table 7.2 and write it on your record sheet.

Table 7.2

Rating Chart: Step Test (Beats per Minute)

	13 YEARS AND YOUNGER		14 TO 16 YEARS OLD		17 YEARS AND OLDER	
	Males	Females	Males	Females	Males	Females
High performance	90 or less	100 or less	85 or less	95 or less	80 or less	90 or less
Good fitness	91-98	101-110	86-95	96-105	81-90	91-100
Marginal fitness	99-120	111-130	96-115	106-125	91-110	101-120
Low fitness	above 120	above 130	above 115	above 125	above 110	above 120

Those who cannot step for 3 minutes receive a low fitness rating.

108

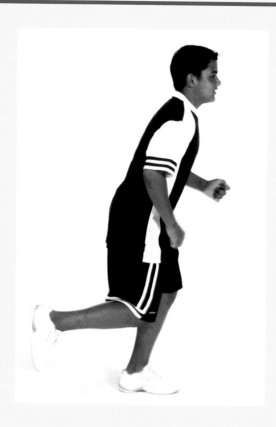

One-Mile Run

The one-mile run is an alternative test of cardiovascular fitness. Remember that this test is for your own information; it is not a race. Your goal is a good fitness rating. Once you achieve this rating, a faster time does not necessarily improve your health. However, it might help you perform better in a sport or other activity.

1. Run or jog for 1 mile in the shortest possible time. Try to set a pace that you can keep up for the full mile. A steady pace is best. If you start too fast and then have to slow down at the end, you will probably not be able to run for the entire distance.
2. Your score is the amount of time it takes you to run the mile. Record this score on your record sheet.
3. Find your rating in table 7.3 and write it on your record sheet.

Note: The one-mile run can be included in your *FITNESSGRAM* report if you choose.

Table 7.3

Rating Chart: One-Mile Run (Minutes:Seconds)

	13 YEARS AND YOUNGER		14 YEARS OLD		15 YEARS OLD		16 YEARS AND OLDER	
	Males	Females	Males	Females	Males	Females	Males	Females
High performance	7:30 or less	9:00 or less	7:00 or less	8:30 or less	7:00 or less	8:00 or less	7:00 or less	8:00 or less
Good fitness	7:31-9:00	9:01-10:30	7:01-8:30	8:31-10:00	7:01-8:00	8:01-9:30	7:01-7:45	8:01-9:00
Marginal fitness	9:01-10:00	10:31-11:30	8:31-9:30	10:01-11:00	8:01-9:00	9:31-10:30	7:46-8:30	9:01-10:00
Low fitness	above 10:00	above 11:30	above 9:30	above 11:00	above 9:00	above 10:30	above 8:30	above 10:00

Building Cardiovascular Fitness

Lesson Objectives

After reading this lesson, you should be able to

1. Explain the difference between aerobic activity and anaerobic activity.
2. Describe the FIT formula for developing cardiovascular fitness.
3. Explain how to determine a threshold of training and a target zone for building cardiovascular fitness using two different heart rate methods.

Lesson Vocabulary

active aerobic activity (p. 110), aerobic activity (p. 110), anaerobic activity (p. 111)

www.fitnessforlife.org/student/7/6

You now know that physical activity is important to your cardiovascular fitness. But how much physical activity do you have to do to improve your cardiovascular fitness? In this lesson you will learn about the best types of activity for building cardiovascular fitness. You will also learn to determine how much physical activity you need to build cardiovascular fitness.

Physical Activity and Cardiovascular Fitness

In chapter 6 you learned that aerobic physical activities of moderate intensity can provide many health benefits. The term *aerobic* means "with oxygen." **Aerobic activity** is activity that is steady enough to allow the heart to supply all the oxygen your muscles need. Moderate lifestyle physical activities are considered to be aerobic because you can do them for long periods without stopping, but they may not be intense enough to produce cardiovascular fitness. **Active aerobic activity** (or active aerobics) is a more vigorous type of aerobic activity that elevates the heart rate high enough to build cardiovascular fitness. Vigorous physical activity such as active aerobics can provide health benefits similar to lifestyle physical activity and have the added advantage

of helping you improve your cardiovascular fitness. In this chapter active aerobics will refer to physical activities that are more vigorous than lifestyle activities and that elevate the heart rate above the cardiovascular heart rate threshold of training. Later in this chapter you will learn more about the threshold of training and target zone for building cardiovascular fitness using active aerobics. In chapter 8, you will learn more about active aerobics as well as about sports and active recreation. All of these activities can build cardiovascular fitness.

How Much Cardiovascular Activity Is Enough?

In the previous chapter you learned that every American, including teens, should accumulate 30 minutes or more of moderate intensity physical activity on most, preferably all, days of the week. As you learned in chapter 6, moderate or lifestyle activity is as intense as moderate walking but can include activities such as working in the yard or riding a bicycle at a leisurely pace. This amount of activity is the minimum each person should do to get health and wellness benefits. But experts also indicate that teens should do vigorous physical activity such as active aerobics. Vigorous activity that increases

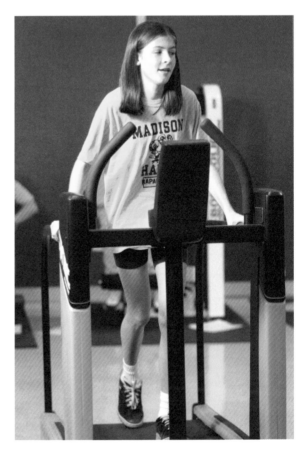

Exercise equipment such as the treadmill shown in the photo can help you keep active and build your cardiovascular fitness.

your heart rate above a threshold level is important to building good levels of cardiovascular fitness and building extra health benefits in addition to those resulting from lifestyle physical activity. Table 7.4 describes the threshold of training.

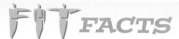

A health goal for the nation is to increase the percentage of teens who do vigorous physical activity at least three days a week to 85 percent. Currently 65 percent of teens do vigorous activity at least three days a week.

The FIT Formula for Building Cardiovascular Fitness

National guidelines suggest that teenagers should do regular vigorous physical activity. The guidelines state that teenagers should engage in three or more sessions per week of activities that last 20 or more minutes at a time and that require moderate to vigorous levels of exertion. To achieve cardiovascular fitness, your heart rate must be

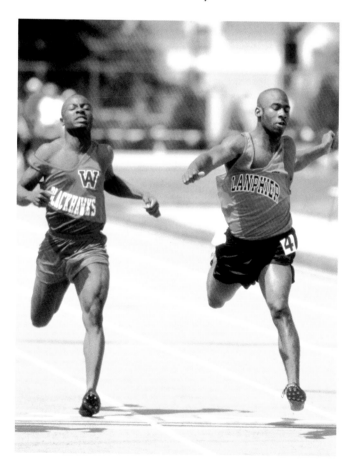

Anaerobic activity is so intense that you cannot sustain it for a long time.

Table 7.4

Physical Activity Threshold and Target Zone Threshold of Training

	Threshold of training	Target zone
Frequency	3 days/week	3-6 days/week
Intensity	50% HRR 65% maxHR	50-85% HRR 65-90% maxHR
Time	20 continuous min	20-60 continuous min

Note: The values in this table are for those with good cardiovascular fitness. Those with low fitness should use 40% of heart rate range or 55% for the maximal heart rate to calculate threshold values. See activity 2 in this chapter.

elevated above the threshold of training heart rate and into the target fitness zone. At a minimum you must be active three times a week for 20 minutes each time. For best results you should be active five or six days a week for up to 60 minutes each day. Experts have learned that you need one or two days of rest from this higher intensity physical activity. If you exercise more often, you risk getting injured. More details concerning the FIT formula for cardiovascular fitness are shown in table 7.4.

Counting Heart Rate to Determine Intensity

As noted earlier, vigorous active aerobic activities that elevate the heart rate are best for building cardiovascular fitness. In chapter 1 you learned to use your pulse to count heart rate at rest and after exercise. Table 7.4 tells you how high your heart rate should be elevated to produce cardiovascular fitness. You can determine the intensity of exercise necessary to build fitness using two different heart rate methods. The first is called the heart rate range (HRR) method. This formula uses the range between your resting and maximal heart rate for calculation. The second method is called the percent of maximal heart rate (% maxHR) method. You will get a chance to calculate your threshold heart rate and your exercise heart rate target zone using both of these methods when you do the activity at the end of this chapter. Heart rate counting is especially effective in producing cardiovascular fitness improvements such as those needed for participation in varsity sports or other activities requiring fitness in the good and high performance zones.

Anaerobic Physical Activity

The sprinters in the picture are doing **anaerobic activity.** Anaerobic activity is activity that is so intense that your body cannot supply adequate oxygen to sustain it for long periods of time. For this reason, it is frequently done in short bursts. Anaerobic activities include sprinting, swimming very fast, and bursts of activity in sports

Taking Charge: Learning to Self-Monitor

An activity log is a written account of the physical activities that you participate in during a specified time. It's a way to keep track of what you do so that you can tell whether you are meeting your activity goals.

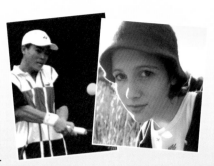

Mark enjoyed playing tennis on the weekends. He would start out full of energy but lacked the endurance to play well for a complete match. His instructor suggested that he do some daily activities to improve his endurance. For several weeks Mark reported that he faithfully engaged in the activities. But Mark's instructor was a little skeptical based on his level of improvement. Finally, she suggested that Mark keep a log of all the times he actually did the activities. "Boy, was I surprised. I rarely spent as much time as I thought on each activity. I really thought I was doing well until I actually saw the results written down."

Erica's situation was different. She had knee surgery and was ordered to limit the kinds and amount of activity she engaged in and follow a schedule of rehabilitation exercises. She was also supposed to elevate her leg whenever possible. Erica's leg was often swollen and sore at the end of the day. Her physical therapist suggested that she keep a daily log. Erica discovered that she spent much more time on her feet than she realized. She knew that she had to curtail more activities for her knee to heal yet still continue to do her rehabilitation exercises.

For Discussion

How did the logs help both Mark and Erica? What are some other ways in which a log could help people? What are some good suggestions that can help people keep up with their activity logs? Set a one-week physical activity goal for yourself. Use a weekly log to keep track of how well you meet your goal (available from your teacher). Consider the guidelines on page 113.

---

such as football. You need frequent rests between bursts of anaerobic activity to catch your breath. People who do frequent anaerobic exercise build anaerobic fitness that allows them to recover more quickly from anaerobic bursts. Anaerobic fitness is important to being a good sports performer, but anaerobic activities are not included in the Physical Activity Pyramid as a type of activity that provides significant health and wellness benefits.

www.fitnessforlife.org/student/7/7

If you are interested in doing anaerobic activity, you should perform it three to six days a week. The intensity of your activity should be at the upper level of the target zone because your exercise bouts are short. Keep your heart rate high for 10 to 40 seconds, then walk or jog slowly. This slow pace should last three times the length of the exercise. Alternate fast and slow exercise bouts. The total exercise time should be at least 15 minutes. Consult your teacher, coach, or the Web site listed above for more information on this type of activity.

Lesson Review

1. What is the difference between aerobic activity and anaerobic activity?
2. What is the FIT formula for developing cardiovascular fitness?
3. How do you determine a threshold of training and a target zone for building cardiovascular fitness? Use two different heart rate methods.

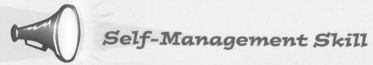

Self-Management Skill

Learning to Self-Monitor

One of the truths of human nature is that adults tend to underestimate how much they eat and overestimate how much physical activity they get. We make other errors in estimating what we do. For example, people often underestimate how much television they watch and how much money they spend on non-essential items. Self-monitoring is another name for keeping track of what you do. We all self-monitor our behavior in informal ways, but sometimes it is necessary to make formal assessments if we want accuracy. You can self-monitor current behaviors to help you set goals and plan. You can also use self-monitoring to help you determine whether you are meeting your goals and fulfilling your plans. Self-monitoring of physical activity is sometimes referred to as record keeping or keeping activity logs. Follow these guidelines to effectively monitor your physical activity:

▶ **Keep a written log.** Make a formal record of the physical activities you perform by using the activity log provided by your instructor or a computer program such as *ACTIVITYGRAM* (see Fitness Technology in chapter 4, page 65).

▶ **Record information as frequently as possible.** The longer you wait before you write down what you do, the more likely you are to make an error. Write things down as soon after you do them as possible.

▶ **Start by self-monitoring your current activity patterns.** Use the activity log or *ACTIVITYGRAM* computer program to determine your current activity level. To get an accurate picture of your true activity level you should monitor for at least three days, at least one of which should be a weekend day. For most people, activity patterns are different on weekends than on weekdays.

▶ **Use your current activity patterns to help you to determine your future goals and plans.** People who are already active can set higher goals than those who are less active (just beginning).

▶ **Determine how much activity you do in each area of the Physical Activity Pyramid.** For each of the different types of activity in the pyramid, you can determine the frequency, intensity, and time for each.

▶ **Write down your goals and plans and then keep records to see whether you fulfill them.** In chapter 5 you learned to set goals and develop plans for different types of activity. Putting your goals and plans in writing can help you self-monitor. Keep records to see whether you did what you planned to do. Keep a diary or an activity chart. A sample of a written plan is included in chapter 18, page 309. Also you can ask your teacher for a record-keeping worksheet.

▶ **Consider using an activity monitor to monitor your activity.** Pedometers and heart rate watches are examples of activity monitors. You learned about pedometers in chapter 6 and about heart rate monitors earlier in this chapter.

▶ **Use these guidelines to self-monitor other behaviors such as eating patterns.**

113

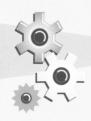

Activity 2

Cardiovascular Fitness: How Much Activity Is Enough?

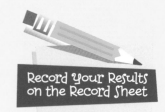

Record your Results on the Record Sheet

PART 1: Calculating Target Heart Rate Zone

In chapter 1 you learned how to count your radial and carotid pulse at rest and after exercise. In this activity you will learn how to use heart rate counting to determine whether you are doing enough physical activity to build cardiovascular fitness. As you learned earlier in this chapter, if you have a heart rate watch you can use it to count your heart rate.

To build cardiovascular fitness you must elevate the heart rate above the threshold of training and into the target zone (see table 7.4 on page 111). Two methods exist to determine your target heart rate zone. They are explained next. Use your record sheet to calculate your target heart rate zone using both methods.

 www.fitnessforlife.org/student/7/8

Finding Your Maximal Heart Rate

For both methods of determining your target heart rate zone you will need to know your maximal heart rate, the highest your heart rate ever gets. A formula can be used to estimate your maximal heart rate:

Maximal heart rate = 208 – (.70 × your age)

For a 16-year-old the estimated maximal heart rate would be 208 – (.70 × 16) or 208 – 11 = 197. This formula was recently developed by researchers to replace a formula that made estimates that were too high for young people. You can calculate your own maximal heart rate using the formula or using table 7.5.

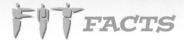 FACTS

Small animals have very high heart rates. For example, a hummingbird has a heart rate near 500 beats per minute. Larger animals have lower heart rates. For example, elephants typically have heart rates well below 50 beats per minute. Humans typically have resting heart rates near 60 or 80 beats per minute and maximal heart rates near 200 beats per minute. Older people typically have lower maximal heart rates than young people.

Table 7.5

Estimated Maximal Heart Rates

Your age	12	13	14	15	16	17	18	19
MaxHR	200	199	198	197	197	196	195	195

Table 7.6

Calculating Heart Rate Target Zone (HRR Method)

Threshold HR	Step 1	197	(maxHR)*
	Step 2	– 67	(resting HR)
		130	(HRR)
	Step 3	× .50	(threshold %)
		65	
		+ 67	(resting HR)
		132	(threshold HR)
Target ceiling rate	Step 1	197	(maxHR)*
	Step 2	– 67	(resting HR)
		130	(HRR)
	Step 3	× .85	(target ceiling %)
		111	
		+ 67	(resting HR)
		178	(target ceiling rate)
Target HR zone	132-178 beats/min		

*Example for a 16-year-old with a resting HR of 67.

Heart Rate Range Method

This method is considered the most accurate, but it is a bit more difficult to calculate. To use this method you must know both your maximal and your resting heart rates. Table 7.6 provides an example of this calculation for a 16-year-old person.

1. Begin by estimating your maximal heart rate using the information provided earlier. The maximal heart rate in the example is 197.
2. Next, determine your heart rate range by subtracting your resting heart rate from your maximal heart rate. The resting heart rate in the example is 67 and the heart rate range is 130.
3. To calculate your threshold heart rate, multiply your heart rate range by 50 percent (0.5). Then add your resting heart rate. In the example the threshold would be 132.
4. Calculate your target ceiling rate by repeating steps 1 through 3, but in step 3 multiply by 85 percent, not 50 percent. In the example the target ceiling heart rate is 178.
5. The target heart zone for the 16-year-old person in this example is 132 to 178.

Table 7.7

Calculating Heart Rate Target Zone (% maxHR Method)

Threshold HR	Step 1	197	(maxHR)*
	Step 2	× .65	(threshold %)
		128	(threshold HR)
Target ceiling rate	Step 1	197	(maxHR)*
	Step 2	× .90	(target ceiling %)
		177	(target ceiling rate)
Target HR zone	128-177 beats/min		

*Example for a 16-year-old with a resting HR of 67.

Percent of Maximal Heart Rate Method

This method is not quite as accurate as the heart rate range method but it is easier to calculate. In this method you do not use your resting heart rate.

1. Estimate your maximal heart rate. The maximal heart rate in the example is 197.
2. To find your threshold heart rate, multiply this number by 65 percent (0.65). For the example in table 7.7, the threshold would be 128.
3. To calculate your target ceiling rate, repeat steps 1 and 2, but in step 2 multiply by 90 percent. For the example in table 7.7, the ceiling rate would be 177.
4. The target heart rate zone for the 16-year-old person in this example is 128 to 177. The numbers are slightly lower than for the HRR method.

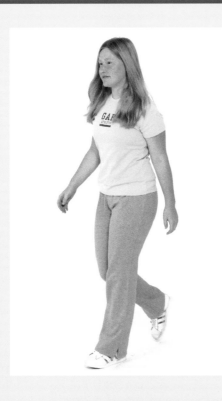

PART 2: Walking and Jogging

When using the heart rate counting method for determining how much activity you need, it is important to be able to continue to exercise in your target heart rate zone. In this part of the activity you will walk and jog in your target heart rate zone.

Walking

1. Walk briskly for 5 minutes.
2. At the end of your walk, immediately count your one-minute heart rate. Record your heart rate on your record sheet.
3. Determine whether your heart rate reached your heart rate threshold of training (lower limit of your target heart rate zone). You can use the zone you calculated with either method discussed earlier.
4. Check to see that your heart rate did not exceed your target ceiling heart rate (the upper limit of your target heart rate zone).

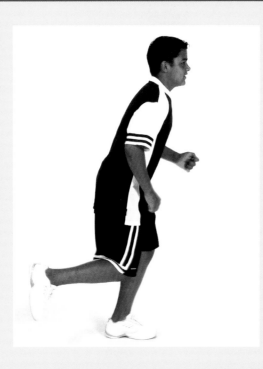

Jogging

1. Jog at a steady pace for 5 minutes.
2. At the end of your jog, immediately count your one-minute heart rate. Record your heart rate on your record sheet.
3. Determine whether your heart rate reached your heart rate threshold of training (lower limit of your target heart rate zone). You can use the zone you calculated with either method discussed earlier.
4. Check to see that your heart rate did not exceed your target ceiling heart rate (the upper limit of your target heart rate zone).

Additional Activity

Use the remainder of the class performing an activity of your choice. Choose an activity that keeps your heart rate above the threshold heart rate and in the target zone. Try to get 20 minutes of total activity above the threshold, including the 5-minute jog that you performed. Count your heart rate at least twice in this part of the activity to see whether you are in your target heart rate zone.

116

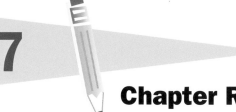

7 Chapter Review

Reviewing Concepts and Vocabulary

Number your paper from 1 to 5. Next to each number, write the word (or words) that correctly completes the sentence.

1. Vessels that carry blood to the heart are called _____.
2. Walking, jogging, and bicycling are examples of _____ activity.
3. The body system that includes your heart, blood vessels, and blood is the _____.
4. Carriers of cholesterol in the blood are called _____.
5. The body system that includes your lungs and air passages is the _____.

Number your paper from 6 to 10. Next to each number, choose the letter of the best answer.

Column I	Column II
6. aerobic activity	a. fatlike substance in the blood
7. cholesterol	b. heart can supply necessary oxygen to muscles
8. high-density lipoprotein	c. bad cholesterol
9. low-density lipoprotein	d. heart cannot supply necessary oxygen to muscles
10. anaerobic activity	e. carries cholesterol out of the bloodstream

Number your paper from 11 to 15. Write a short answer for each statement or question.

11. Describe the two different methods of determining your heart rate target zone.
12. Why is it important to monitor your heart rate to make sure that it is in the target heart rate zone?
13. Explain how cardiovascular fitness helps your cardiovascular system work more efficiently and helps prevent cardiovascular diseases.
14. Explain why cholesterol can be dangerous to your health.
15. Why should you do more than one self-assessment for determining cardiovascular fitness?

Thinking Critically

Write a paragraph to answer the following question.

You decide that you need to develop a program to improve your cardiovascular fitness. What are some lifelong changes that you should incorporate into your program? Explain.

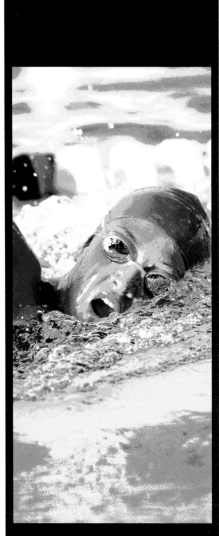

Project

Investigate the heart rates of people of different fitness levels. Check the pulse rates of athletes who do activities requiring a lot of cardiovascular fitness such as cross-country running and distance swimming. Compare these heart rates to heart rates of nonathletes.

8

Active Aerobics and Recreation

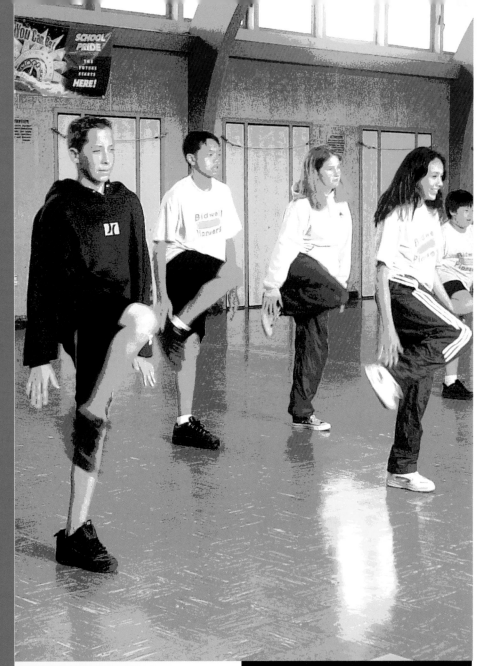

Activity 1

STEP AEROBICS

If you performed the aerobic dance routine in chapter 7, you have an idea of how you can make physical activity fun by using various foot and arm movements. Step aerobics uses arm and leg movements similar to those in aerobic dance, but in step aerobics you use a step, or an elevated platform, to create interesting additional movements. Stepping up and down on the step during a step aerobics routine can increase the cardiovascular intensity of the exercise without causing stress to the joints. Also, stepping helps increase muscular endurance of the legs. The height of the step can be adjusted to alter exercise intensity.

Active Aerobics

Lesson Objectives

After reading this lesson, you should be able to

1. Explain the difference between lifestyle physical activity and active aerobics.
2. Describe some of the benefits and risks of active aerobic activities.
3. Describe several types of active aerobic activity.

Lesson Vocabulary

active aerobics (p. 119), aerobics (p. 120), circuit training (p. 120)

 www.fitnessforlife.org/student/8/1

Two types of physical activity lie at the second level of the physical activity pyramid: active aerobics and active sports and recreation. Activities at this level are more vigorous than lifestyle activities (level 1 of the Physical Activity Pyramid) and are especially good for building cardiovascular fitness and providing the health benefits of physical activity described in chapter 3. In this lesson you will learn more about the many different types of active aerobics.

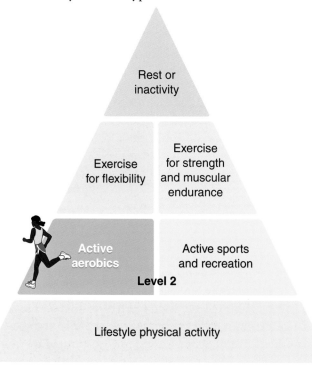

The Popularity of Active Aerobic Activity

Most activities in the Physical Activity Pyramid (including lifestyle activities) can be considered aerobic. But only those that are vigorous enough to elevate the heart rate above the heart rate threshold and into the target zone are considered **active aerobics.** Aerobic activities are among the most popular and the most beneficial of all activities in the Physical Activity Pyramid. For example, jogging or running, aerobic dance, cycling, and swimming are all among the most popular activities. Reasons for the popularity include:

- ▶ They often do not require high levels of skill.
- ▶ They frequently are not competitive.
- ▶ They often can be done at home or near home.
- ▶ They often do not require a partner or a group.

In general, active aerobic activities are safe compared to other activities such as sports and recreational activities. However, they can result in injury if overdone. Jogging or running is one of the top five activities in terms of injuries to participants. People who do a lot of high-impact and step aerobics also are often injured. Unlike sports injuries that are often sprains and muscle strains, joggers and aerobic dancers typically get overuse injuries such as heel bruises, sore shins, stress fractures in the legs and feet, and sometimes knee or back injuries. Most of these injuries can be prevented simply by not overexercising. People most prone to injury are those who train every day and who participate in several exercise sessions a day. Long distance runners and aerobic dance instructors have a higher than normal injury rate. Taking at least one day a week to rest is generally a good idea for injury prevention.

Types of Active Aerobics

Many types of active aerobics exist. Some of the most popular will be described here. Some activities could be classified in more than one of the sections of the Physical Activity Pyramid. For example, swimming is an active aerobic activity but is also a sport and a type of active recreation. In this book it will be classified as an active aerobic activity. Many activities are described in this chapter and in the one that follows. Each activity will be described only once, even though it could fit in several places.

Aerobic Dance

Aerobic dance involves the continuous performance of various dance steps to music. Unlike various forms of social dance, performers typically dance by themselves, often following a leader or a video. This activity first became popular in the 1970s and remains one of the most popular forms of aerobic exercise. Various forms of aerobic dance include low impact, high impact, and step aerobics. Low impact is typically done with one foot staying on the ground at all times. This form is best for beginners because it has fewer injuries than other forms. High impact is typically more vigorous and involves jumping. Step aerobics involves dance steps done on a step or box. Some types of aerobic dance use light weights, rubber bands, and other types of exercise equipment.

Aerobic Exercise Machines

Types of aerobic exercise machines include treadmills, stair steppers, exercise bicycles, rowing machines, and ski machines. You can purchase these machines for use in your own home or you can find them in health clubs and schools. They can be effective if used properly, but some people do not find exercise on machines as enjoyable as activities that allow them to move more freely. For example, actual skiing may be more enjoyable than using a ski machine. On the other hand, exercise machines are often convenient and efficient.

Bicycling

Bicycling could be classified as a sport because some compete in it or as a recreational activity because some do it for fun. It is included here because it is often done continuously at a consistent rate of speed that elevates the heart rate. If done relatively slowly it can also be considered as a form of lifestyle physical activity. Some forms of cycling such as BMX are considered to be extreme sports (see chapter 9).

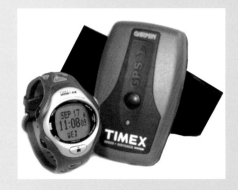

FITNESS Technology

GPS (global positioning systems) technology provides a system that communicates information. A satellite sends signals to a receiver, which sends the signal to a computer that analyzes the information. Originally GPS was developed by the government to help in national defense, but the technology is now available for consumer use. GPS has been used in automobiles to help drivers find their way, and now it can also help bikers and joggers. The system for bikers and joggers includes a GPS receiver that is strapped on the upper arm and a watch that is worn on the wrist. A satellite sends a signal to the receiver, which sends it on to the watch. The watch provides information about how fast you are moving (speed), the distance you have traveled, and the average pace for your total workout. It is extremely accurate.

Cooper's Aerobics

Dr. Ken Cooper, the founder of the Cooper Institute in Dallas, Texas, popularized the term **aerobics.** He developed a system of points that can be earned for doing active aerobic activities. The goal of those who do this program is to earn at least 30 aerobics points each week.

 www.fitnessforlife.org/student/8/2

Circuit Training

Circuit training refers to performing several different exercises one after the other. The performer does one exercise for a period of time and then moves on to the next with only a brief time between exercises. The goal is to keep the heart rate in the target zone. Circuit training can use exercise machines, small equipment such as jump ropes or rubber bands, free weights, or no equipment at all (for example, calisthenics). Sometimes people use music to determine how much time is spent on each exercise. Breaks in the music signal that it is time to move to the next exercise.

Dance

Dance is one of the oldest art forms and has been a means of expression for many cultures. Some forms of dance are not only enjoyable but also excellent forms of active aerobic exercise. Modern, ballet, folk, and square dance are among the more traditional dance activities. Another form of dance is social dance. It includes more traditional types such the waltz, country dancing, Latin dancing, and newer dance forms including hip-hop and line dance. All can be good forms of active aerobics if you do them vigorously enough to elevate your heart rate.

Martial Arts Exercise

Judo and karate are just two of the many martial arts. Martial arts can build various parts of fitness, but they are not always good at building cardiovascular fitness because they may not involve enough continuous activity to keep the heart rate elevated. Recently some forms of martial arts have been combined with aerobic dance to create martial arts exercise such as TaeBo and cardio-karate. This form of exercise can build cardiovascular fitness but may not be as effective in learning self-defense as other more traditional techniques.

Rope Jumping

Jumping rope has been used by boxers and other athletes as a method of training. Because it requires moving both the arm and legs as well as the entire body, it can be quite vigorous. For this reason people sometimes alternate jumping rope with other forms of exercise such as calisthenics. You can use many different jump rope steps. Advantages of jumping rope are that it is inexpensive and you can easily do it at home or in the neighborhood. Also, you can easily transport the equipment when you are away from home. One limitation is that not all people find it enjoyable.

Swimming

Swimming is a sport and a form of recreation. It is included here because it is one of the most popular fitness activities among adults and it can be good for improving cardiovascular for almost all people. Like water aerobics, it is good for people who are overweight, elderly, or suffering from joint problems. For swimming to be effective aerobic exercise, your heart rate must be elevated and you must swim continuously for many minutes. Many people who say they swim do not meet either of these standards.

Water Aerobics

Water aerobics, sometimes called aqua-dynamics, involves doing calisthenics or dance steps in a swimming pool. This form of aerobic exercise is especially good for people who are overweight, elderly, or suffering from arthritis or other joint problems. The water prevents the exercises from causing stress on the joints. Water also can offer resistance and increase the intensity of exercise for the able-bodied exerciser.

Finding the Best Type of Active Aerobics for You

In this class you will get the opportunity to try out many types of active aerobics. Examples include aerobic dance, step aerobics, line dance, jogging, exercise circuits, and jumping rope. It is important that you try a variety of activities so that you can discover the ones you like best. It is also important to try an activity more than once before you decide whether to do that activity in the future. If you are going to stick with an activity over the long term, it must be enjoyable. To help you enjoy an activity, you should consider getting good instruction, wearing appropriate activity clothing, getting good equipment if necessary, and finding others with whom you can participate.

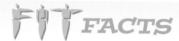

More teen boys (72 percent) are vigorously active at least three times a week than teen girls (57 percent). High school girls are especially likely to become less active as they grow older. Health experts are interested in finding ways to help teen girls to be more physically active.

Lesson Review

1. What are active aerobics and how do they differ from lifestyle activities?
2. What are some of the benefits and risks of active aerobic activities?
3. What are some types of active aerobic activity?

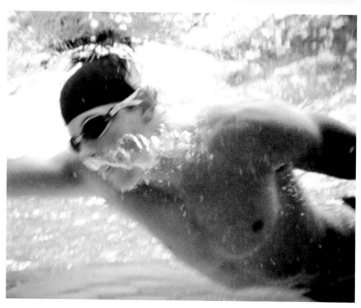

Swimming is a good form of active aerobics.

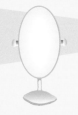

Self-Assessment

FITNESSGRAM 3—Cardiovascular Fitness, Flexibility, and Strength

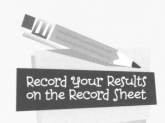

Record Your Results on the Record Sheet

In chapter 2 you performed two *FITNESSGRAM* assessments to measure strength and muscular endurance. In this assessment you will perform two more *FITNESSGRAM* tests to measure cardiovascular fitness and the strength and flexibility of your back and trunk muscles.

Table 8.1

Rating Chart: Trunk Lift

Rating	Inches
High performance	11-12
Good fitness	9-10
Marginal fitness	7-8
Low fitness	<6

Adapted with permission from *FITNESSGRAM*.

Trunk Lift (Upper Back)

1. Lie facedown with your arms to your sides and your hands under your thighs.

2. Lift the upper part of your body very slowly so that your chin, chest, and shoulders come off the floor. Lift your trunk as high as possible to a maximum of 12 inches. Hold this position for 3 seconds while a partner measures the distance your chin lifts off the floor. Hold the ruler at least 1 inch in front of your chin. Look straight ahead so that your chin is not tipped upward abnormally.

⚠ **Caution:** Do not place the ruler directly under your chin in case you have to lower your trunk unexpectedly.

3. Do the trunk lift 2 times and record the number of inches you can lift and hold your chin. Do not record scores above 12 inches. Use table 8.1 to determine your fitness rating. Record your results.

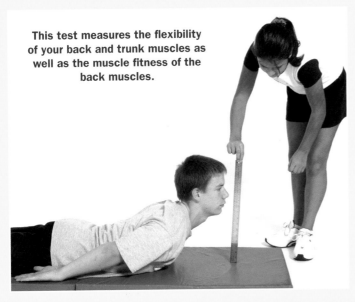

This test measures the flexibility of your back and trunk muscles as well as the muscle fitness of the back muscles.

The PACER

PACER stands for Progressive Aerobic Cardiovascular Endurance Run and is a test of cardiovascular fitness. You will need a tape recorder and a special audiotape to perform the test. Because the test requires this special equipment, it may not be as easy to do as other cardiovascular assessments you will do later. However, by taking this test you can see whether you meet the national health-related cardiovascular fitness standard. The objective of the test is to run back and forth across a 20-meter distance as many times as you can.

1. When you hear the beep, run across the 20-meter area and touch the line before the tape beeps again. Turn around.
2. At the sound of the next beep, run back to the other side. (You must wait for the beep before running in the opposite direction.) The beeps will come faster and faster, causing you to run faster and faster. The test is finished when you twice fail to reach the opposite side before the beep.
3. Your score is the number of times you can run the 20-meter distance before your test is finished. Record this number on your record sheet. Then find your fitness rating on table 8.2.

Table 8.2

Rating Chart: PACER (Scores Are Laps Completed)

	13 YEARS AND YOUNGER		14 YEARS OLD		15 YEARS OLD		16 YEARS OLD		17 YEARS AND OLDER	
	Males	Females	Males	Females	Males	Females	Males	Females	Males	Females
High performance	55-74	31-42	61-80	33-44	65-85	38-50	70-90	43-56	74-94	50-61
Good fitness	35-54	15-30	41-60	18-32	46-64	23-37	52-69	28-42	57-73	34-49
Marginal fitness	30-34	13-14	36-40	16-17	41-45	21-22	47-51	25-27	52-56	30-33
Low fitness	<29	<12	<35	<15	<40	<20	<46	<24	<51	<29

Adapted with permission from *FITNESSGRAM*.

Lesson 8.2

Active Recreation

Lesson Objectives

After reading this lesson, you should be able to

1. Define recreational activity and leisure time.
2. Describe several types of active recreation including their benefits and risks.
3. Describe some safety considerations for active recreation and active aerobics.
4. Define social support and describe how it can help you to be physically active.

Lesson Vocabulary

active recreation (p. 124), leisure time (p. 124), recreational activity (p. 124)

www.fitnessforlife.org/student/8/3

We would all like to have more **leisure time.** It is time free from work, or in the case of teens, free from commitments such as school, homework, and jobs. Leisure is more than free time. It is an attitude that refers to being free from doing things you have to do. The word recreation refers to re-creating or refreshing yourself. Accordingly a **recreational activity** is an activity that you do during your leisure or free time to refresh or re-create yourself. Recreational activities are done for fun and enjoyment. They need not be vigorous or purposeful. They can include watching TV, reading a book, playing chess, and many other relatively inactive pursuits. Some activities such as fishing, some forms of boating, and camping can be considered lifestyle activities.

www.fitnessforlife.org/student/8/4

Types of Active Recreation

Active recreation includes activities that are fun and typically non-competitive. The main purpose of doing

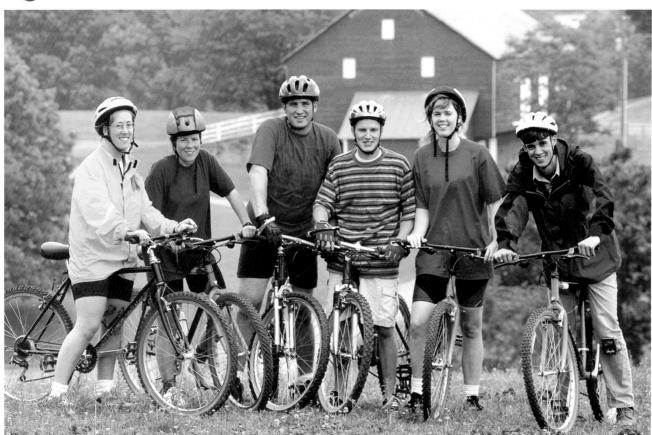

Biking is an aerobic activity that is also a form of active recreation. Many communities have cycle clubs that involve members of all ages in riding for fun and fitness. Ask at your local cycle shop—they will likely have information on how to get involved.

the activity may not be to build fitness, but if the activity is continuous and vigorous, it can be good for this purpose. Recreational activities that are vigorous enough to elevate the heart rate in the cardiovascular target zone are considered to be active recreation. Many types of active recreation are done outdoors because participants feel that the beauty of the outdoor setting and the fresh air help them become refreshed. Examples of active recreation include:

▶ **Backpacking and hiking.** Hiking is a particularly enjoyable activity because it is an outdoor activity that can be done independently or in groups. Most county, state, and national parks have a wide variety of scenic trails for hikers of all levels of experience. Hiking usually involves a one-day trip. Backpacking is often a several-day venture that requires carrying food, shelter, and other supplies on your back.

▶ **Boating, canoeing, kayaking, and rowing.** Various types of boating are done outdoors on water, free from the hassles of normal daily life. When done vigorously they can also be good for building fitness and promoting good health. Kayaking and rowing can be especially vigorous and require considerable skill to perform well and safely. Even when not done vigorously, boating activities can be relaxing and refreshing.

▶ **Orienteering.** Orienteering combines walking, jogging, and map-reading skills. It is usually done in a rural area and might include hiking through rugged terrain. One participant departs from a starting point

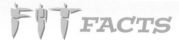

every few minutes so that he or she cannot follow the person ahead. Each participant has a compass and a map that describes a course from 1 to 10 miles. The compass is used to help locate several checkpoints that are marked by flags or other identification. At each checkpoint the participant marks a card to indicate that the checkpoint has been located. In some cases the activity can be competitive if the goal is to cover the course in as little time as possible.

▶ **Skating.** Types of skating include inline skating, roller skating, and ice skating. Inline skating is one of the fastest growing participation activities. It was originally developed as a method of training for skiers in the summer. It has become popular, and now many nonskiers do inline skating. Inline hockey and other inline sports have now developed. One study by a sports medicine group found that inline skating was the most risky of the many participation activities studied, possibly because people fail to use safety equipment or they try advanced skills too soon. Because of the risk in this activity the safety guidelines described here are

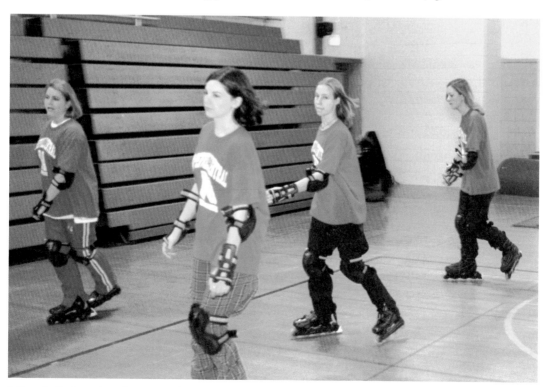

Inline skating can be a fun way to keep active.

Safety Tips for Active Aerobics and Recreation

Wear Proper Safety Equipment

For example, bikers and skaters should wear helmets. Skaters should wear hand and knee pads. Dress appropriately for the weather. Choose warm clothes for winter activities and clothing that allows you to stay cool in the heat.

Use Safe Equipment

Bikes should have lights and reflectors. Backpacking equipment should fit your body size, and loads should not be too heavy. Skis and other equipment should be in good repair, be of the correct size, and have proper safety releases. Boaters should wear life preservers. Rock climbers should have appropriate safety equipment. As described in chapter 2, it is important to drink water regularly when doing vigorous activity, especially in the heat.

Get Proper Instruction

Whether it is skiing, inline skating, boating, rock climbing, or some other activity, it is important to get proper instruction before participation. Many injuries and accidents occur because people are not performing activities properly.

Perform Within the Limits of Your Current Skills

Many injuries occur because people attempt to perform beyond the limits of their current skills. For example, beginning skiers should not attempt to ski advanced slopes until they acquire more skill. For all activities, start with simple skills and gradually attempt more difficult skills as your abilities improve.

Plan Ahead

Planning is very important. If you are going on a hike, make sure you have a map and that you know where you are going. Carry an emergency phone. If you are going skiing, make sure that the trail is open and don't ski in restricted areas. When backpacking, carry enough food and water to supply you if you get lost. When planning trips to unfamiliar areas it is important to stay with a group.

---

especially important. Roller skating is a more traditional activity that uses skates with four wheels as opposed to one line of several wheels. Ice skating has been around for a long time and is now performed by people of all ages. Ice skating is very popular in colder climates. Figure skating, speedskating, and hockey are Olympic sports, so this activity could easily be included in the next chapter on sports.

▶ **Skateboarding.** Skateboarding is a recreational activity that is popular among teens. Like inline skating it is a risky activity, so proper safety equipment is essential, as is proper instruction. Serious skateboarding is now considered an extreme sport, and for this reason it could be included in the next chapter on sports. Finding a proper place to perform skateboarding is very important. Many cities have planned skate parks to provide safe places to skate because many skate hangouts are unsafe and sometimes are in locations where skating is prohibited.

▶ **Rock climbing.** Many schools now teach rock climbing on climbing walls. Learning on a climbing wall is a good idea because you can get proper

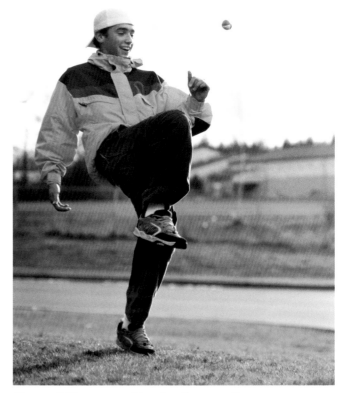

Many activities are considered active recreation.

Taking Charge: Finding Social Support

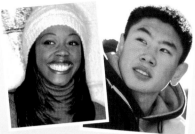

Social support is when members of your family, your friends, teachers, and members of the community encourage your physical activities or participate with you. You are more likely to begin or continue an activity if the people you associate with also do it.

Shannon's family has always enjoyed riding bikes. As a toddler, she would ride in the child's seat behind her mother. Every evening the family would ride through the neighborhood. By the time she was in school, Shannon had her own two-wheeler. Now as a teenager, Shannon still loves to ride. Because of school activities, she can't always ride with her family. Shannon wants to continue riding, but she doesn't want to do it alone.

Jim's family never has been very active. Most of his friends tend to watch television, play video games, or just hang out rather than do anything active. Sometimes, Jim watches while a group of his classmates plays a quick game of volleyball after school. They often invite him to join the game. He has been tempted to join, but he has hesitated because he is not friends with any of the players. He has enjoyed the activities he has tried in the past, although he never continued them for very long.

Both Shannon and Jim need social support. Shannon needs it to continue an activity she already enjoys. Jim needs it to begin an activity and then to continue to reinforce participation in it.

For Discussion

Whom might Shannon ask to go riding with her? What could Jim do to become involved in physical activity? What groups of people provide the social support a person receives? Fill out the questionnaire provided by your teacher to find out what social support you have. Consider the guidelines on page 128.

instruction and can have proper spotting (protection against falling). More advanced climbers will have special safety ropes and equipment and the skill to use them. Beginners and intermediate climbers should always climb with the assistance of an expert. When done properly, rock climbing is a relatively safe activity.

▶ **Bouldering.** It is a safe alternative to rock climbing that can be done in the natural environment with minimal gear.

▶ **Skiing.** Kinds of skiing include cross-country (Nordic), downhill, snowboarding, and ski jumping. Cross-country skiing is typically done at a steady pace over relatively long distances. For this reason it could be considered an active aerobic activity. Downhill skiing typically involves faster skiing, sometimes over moguls and jumps. Snowboarding is like skateboarding on snow and has become extremely popular. It has joined the other forms of skiing as an Olympic sport and can also be considered an extreme sport. All types of skiing could be considered sports, but they are classified here because so many people do them just for fun and recreation.

Safety Considerations for Active Recreation

In general active recreation activities are safe, but some activities are more risky than others. For example, skating is the most risky of all forms of physical activity. Inline skating is especially risky. Skateboarding, downhill skiing, and rock climbing are others that are relatively risky. Some general information concerning safety for all activities at level 2 of the Physical Activity Pyramid are listed in the box on page 126.

Lesson Review

1. What are the definitions of recreational activity and leisure time?
2. What are some types of active recreation? What are their benefits and risks?
3. What are some safety considerations for active recreation and active aerobics?
4. What is meant by social support? Describe how it can help you to be physically active.

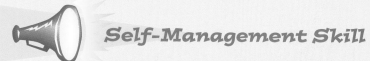

Self-Management Skill

Finding Social Support

Experts indicate that people who find the support of others are more likely to participate in regular physical activity, especially over a lifetime. Social support is also helpful to people who are interested in losing weight, building muscle fitness, and improving their eating habits. Consider these guidelines to help you get the support of others for your physical activity:

▶ **Do a self-assessment of your current level of social support.** Ask your teacher about the social support worksheet that can help you do this assessment.

▶ **Use the self-assessment to determine areas in which you can improve your social support.**

▶ **Find friends who have interests in the activities that interest you,** or encourage your current friends to support you or join you in your participation.

▶ **Join a club or a team.** If no club or team exists, talk to a teacher, family members, or a community recreation leader about starting one.

▶ **Discuss your interests with family and teachers.** Ask them for their support. Ask them to help you in learning the activity.

▶ **Get lessons if possible.** In addition to formal lessons, teachers and others can support you by helping you learn to perform an activity properly.

▶ **Encourage other family members to try the activity.**

▶ **Get proper equipment.** Ask for equipment for birthdays or for other special occasions.

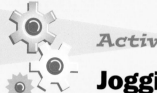

Activity 2

Jogging: Biomechanical Principles and Guidelines

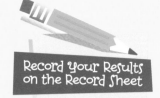

Record Your Results on the Record Sheet

If you are looking for an excellent cardiovascular activity requiring little skill and no equipment except a good pair of running shoes and proper clothing, jogging might be for you. More than 6 million people in the United States are joggers. Many more could learn to enjoy this activity if they knew how to jog properly. If you plan to start jogging, be sure to consider these biomechanical principles and guidelines:

▶ **Use a foot action appropriate for jogging.** The foot action for jogging is not the same as for fast running. In fast running, your weight is mainly on the front of your foot. In jogging, you land on your heel or on the entire foot. Then you rock forward and push off with the ball of the foot, followed by the toes. Improper jogging technique can cause injuries such as sore shins, sore calves, or even a sore back.

▶ **Swing your legs and feet straight forward.** Do not let your feet turn out to the sides. Feet and legs out of alignment cause unnecessary strain on your joints and muscles. When jogging, step farther than your normal walking step.

▶ **Swing your arms straight forward and backward.** Do not swing them across your body. Keep your arms bent at the elbows, and keep your hands relaxed. Try to keep your shoulders relaxed. If you jog with a floppy jaw, your upper body will relax more.

▶ **Keep your trunk fairly erect.** When jogging, do not lean forward as you would when starting to run fast.

▶ **Learn your own best pace.** Learn how fast or slow you should jog to raise your heart rate to the appropriate level. A correct jogging pace is different for each person. Find your own pace; do not try to jog at someone else's pace, especially if it is faster than your own best pace.

▶ **Avoid running on hard surfaces.** If possible, jog on running tracks, grassy places, or dirt paths. These surfaces have more give than concrete sidewalks and put less stress on your feet and legs. If you jog indoors, try to jog on a wooden floor rather than on concrete.

▶ **Breathe easily.** If you are jogging with a friend, you should be able to carry on a conversation as you jog. If you are jogging alone, you should be able to breathe comfortably. If you are panting or gasping for breath, you are jogging too fast.

Jogging Practice

Work with a partner to practice the jogging techniques discussed above. Jog about 100 yards while your partner stands behind you and checks your technique. Have your partner check your feet and legs and answer these questions:

1. Does your heel or whole foot hit the ground first?
2. Do you push off with the ball of your foot?
3. Do your legs and feet swing and land straight ahead?
4. Is your jogging stride longer than your walking stride?

Now do a second 100-yard jog. Have your partner look at you from a side view, checking your arms and body, and answer these questions:

1. Are your elbows bent properly (90 degrees) with your hands relaxed?
2. Do your arms swing straight forward and backward?
3. Are your head and chest up?
4. Is your body leaning only slightly?

Discuss your assessment with your partner. Then have your partner jog twice while you evaluate his or her technique. Try to correct your technique and have your partner check you again. Do the same for your partner. Both you and your partner may jog more than twice if necessary.

Table 8.3

Target Heart Rates (in Beats per Minute)

Resting HR	Beginner (low fit)	Regularly active (good fitness)
<50	127-143	143-182
51-70	132-147	147-183
71+	140-153	153-185

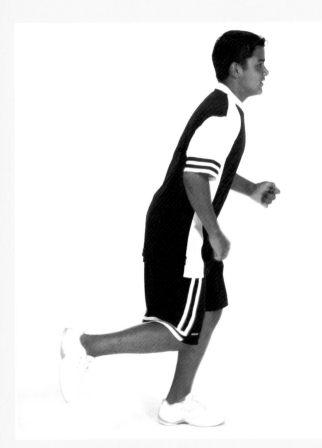

Beginner's Jogging Workout

This workout helps you learn about how fast to jog to get a fitness benefit (by reaching your target heart rate). You learned about target heart rate in chapter 7. Try this workout after you have practiced your jogging technique.

1. Begin your workout by taking your resting heart rate using the procedure you learned in the self-assessment in chapter 1.

2. Determine your target heart rate using the method described on page 115 or use your resting heart rate and table 8.3 to determine the appropriate target heart rate for your workout. If you are a beginner or if you are low or marginal in cardiovascular fitness, use the target zone in the first column. If you have been exercising regularly and you are in the good fitness or high performance fitness levels, use the second column.

3. Jog for 5 minutes trying to get your heart to the target level. Use your watch to keep track of how long you run. How long you run is more important than how far. By using time instead of distance, you can jog anywhere. Set your own course. Try to jog half the time away from your starting point and the other half returning to your starting point. If you are not somewhere near your starting point at the end of 5 minutes, walk back to it.

4. At the end of 5 minutes, count your heart rate to get your one-minute exercise heart rate. Record this score on your record sheet. Determine whether your exercise heart rate was in your target heart rate zone.

5. Jog for 5 minutes again. If your exercise heart rate was lower than your target heart rate on the first jog, then jog faster this time. If your exercise heart rate was higher than your target rate on the first jog, then jog slower this time. If your exercise heart rate was in the target zone on the first jog, then jog at the same speed this time. After the second run, count your exercise heart rate again. Record your score on the record sheet.

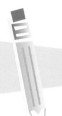

8 Chapter Review

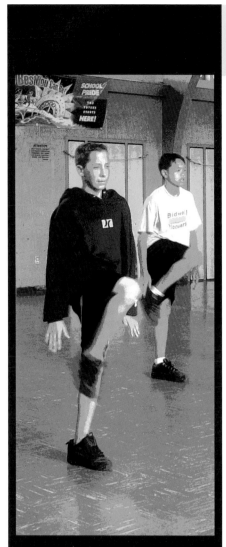

Reviewing Concepts and Vocabulary

Number your paper from 1 to 4. Next to each number, write the word (or words) that correctly completes the sentence.

1. The word _____ means "with oxygen."
2. Free time or time free from work is called _____.
3. TaeBo is a type of _____ exercise.
4. Jogging, swimming, and skating are examples of _____.

Number your paper from 5 to 9. Next to each number, choose the letter of the best answer.

Column I	Column II
5. water aerobics	a. aqua-dynamics
6. orienteering	b. several exercise stations
7. inline skating	c. done for fun during free time
8. recreational activity	d. uses map-reading skills
9. circuit training	e. has relatively high injury risk

Number your paper from 10 to 15. On your paper, write a short answer for each statement or question.

10. What are some good safety tips for performing active aerobics and active recreation?
11. Why is it important to include in your activity plan choices from the active aerobics and active recreation part of the Physical Activity Pyramid?
12. Why is aerobic activity among the most beneficial types of activity?
13. Why might team sports not be good as an only choice for your lifetime activity plan?
14. Why is good equipment important to safe physical activity?
15. Why are active aerobics among the most popular physical activities among adults?

Thinking Critically

Write a paragraph to answer the following question.

What are some active aerobic and active recreational activities you might include in your lifetime activity program? Explain why you made each choice.

9

Active Sports and Skill-Related Physical Fitness

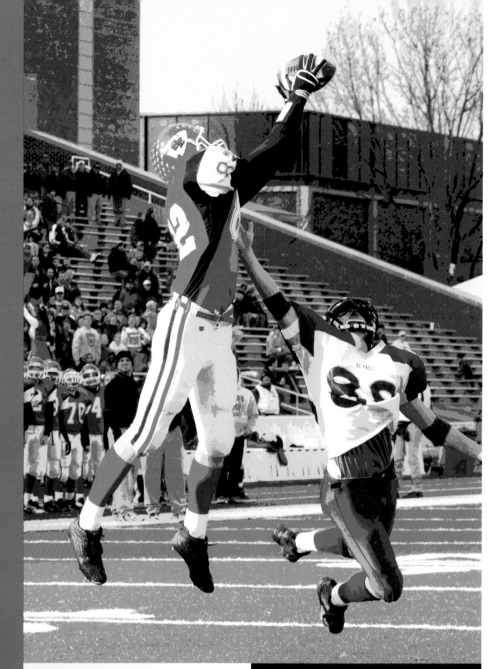

In this chapter...

Activity 1
Orienteering

Lesson 9.1
Skills and Skill-Related Physical Fitness

Self-Assessment
Assessing Skill-Related Physical Fitness

Lesson 9.2
Active Sports

Taking Charge
Building Performance Skills

Self-Management Skill
Building Performance Skills

Activity 2
The Sports Stars Program

Activity 1

ORIENTEERING

In chapter 8 you learned about orienteering. It combines walking, jogging, and map-reading skills. It is usually done in a rural area, but in recent years urban orienteering has become more popular. Each participant has a compass and a map that describes a course. The compass is used to help locate several checkpoints marked by flags or other identification. At each checkpoint the participant marks a card to indicate that the checkpoint has been located. In some cases the activity can be competitive if the goal is to cover the course in as little time as possible.

Skills and Skill-Related Physical Fitness

Lesson Objectives

After reading this lesson, you should be able to

1. Define physical skills and give examples.
2. Explain how skill-related fitness abilities differ from physical skills.
3. Identify and explain factors that affect skill-related fitness and skills.
4. Discuss the importance of assessing personal skill-related fitness.

Lesson Vocabulary

skill (p. 133), skill-related physical fitness (p. 133)

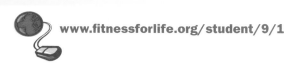

www.fitnessforlife.org/student/9/1

You already know that physical fitness is divided into two categories: health-related physical fitness and **skill-related physical fitness.** Health-related physical fitness is considered the most important because you need it to maintain good health and wellness. Skill-related physical fitness is less related to good health and more related to your ability to learn sports and other kinds of physical **skill.**

Learning about your own skill-related fitness will help you determine which sports and lifetime activities will be easiest for you to learn and enjoy. Because people differ in their levels of each part of skill-related fitness, different people will find success in different activities. In this lesson you will learn how to assess your own levels of skill-related fitness so that you can choose activities that match your abilities, work to improve your abilities, and find activities you can enjoy for a lifetime.

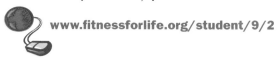

www.fitnessforlife.org/student/9/2

Factors That Affect Skill-Related Fitness

You learned in chapter 1 that skill-related physical fitness is a group of basic abilities that helps you perform well in sports and activities requiring certain physical skills. These abilities include agility, balance, coordination, power, speed, and reaction time.

Notice that skill-related fitness abilities and physical skills are not the same thing. Physical skills are specific physical tasks that people perform, such as the sport skills of catching, throwing, swimming, and batting, and other skills such as dancing. Skill-related fitness abilities help you learn particular skills. For example, if you have good skill-related fitness abilities in speed and power, you will be able to learn football running skills easily; if you have good balance, you will be able to learn gymnastics skills more easily.

Several factors affect your skill-related fitness and your skills, including heredity, practice, and the principle of specificity. The diagram below shows how these factors are related.

Heredity

Heredity influences skill-related fitness abilities. For example, some people are able to run fast or react quickly because they inherited these traits from their parents. A person who did not inherit a tendency to excel in these areas may have more difficulty performing skills that require those abilities. Improving your skills is always possible, and often extra practice and desire make up for lack of inherited ability.

Practice

Anyone can learn the skills required for sports, games, and other lifetime activities. Practice—repeating a skill over and over—is the key. If you repeat a skill such as a tennis serve and do it correctly, you will become better at that skill. You probably will learn the skill faster if you have good skill-related fitness in an area such as coordination. While everyone cannot become an Olympic athlete, with practice everyone can learn the basic skills necessary to enjoy some sports and to perform physical tasks efficiently. Learning about your own skill-related abilities can help you choose a sport or activity in which you are more likely to succeed.

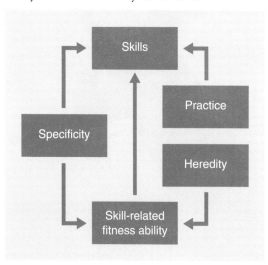

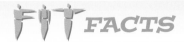

Principle of Specificity

The principle of specificity applies to all parts of skill-related fitness and to physical skills. Just because you excel in one part of skill-related fitness does not mean you will excel in another part. This is often the case even when abilities seem closely related, such as reaction time and speed. For example, you might have great speed, which helps you run fast, but lack good reaction time, which prevents you from getting a good start. Apply the principle of specificity to choose a sport or activity that requires the specific skill-related fitness abilities you perform best.

The principle of specificity also tells you that once you choose an activity or sport that you would like to learn, it is best to practice the specific skills of that activity. With practice you may be able to make some improvement in skill-related fitness, but it is best to use practice time on the specific skills of the activities in which you want to improve.

Assessing Skill-Related Fitness

A good first step for a person interested in learning a lifetime sport or physical activity is to assess skill-related fitness abilities. Assessing each of the abilities can help

you identify those that will help you succeed in a particular activity. Perform the skill-related fitness assessments in this chapter. As you perform these assessments you should be aware that skill-related fitness has many subparts. For example, coordination is a skill-related ability that includes eye-hand coordination—the ability to use the hands and eyes together as in hitting a ball—and eye-foot coordination—the ability to use the eyes and feet together as in kicking a ball.

Once you have assessed your skill-related fitness abilities, you can develop a profile of your results that will help you in selecting lifetime activities and sports. In this lesson you will learn how to use a profile to select lifetime activities and make plans for becoming proficient in those activities.

Developing a Skill-Related Fitness Profile

One student, Sue, did all of the skill-related physical fitness assessments in this chapter. You can see the profile she developed for her skill-related fitness in table 9.1. Sue's profile helped her identify her strengths and weaknesses. She used her profile to develop her fitness program.

You can see that Sue has better abilities in some parts of fitness than in others. One way she can use her profile is to see how she can improve her skill-related fitness in areas in which she didn't do so well. She can use table 9.2 to identify activities that provide the most benefits for each part of skill-related fitness.

The second way Sue can use her profile is to find physical activity that is suited to her abilities. Activities that give the most benefits in a specific part of skill-related fitness will also require the greatest amount of fitness in that part. Sue did not do well in power, so she decided to take karate lessons to help her improve. She also didn't do well in speed and reaction time but realized that, because of heredity, she probably would not be a really fast person with good reaction time. Still, she thought that karate might help these abilities some. She also decided not to worry if she wasn't as able as other people in these parts of fitness. Sue used table 9.2 to help her determine which activities helped to build specific parts of skill-related fitness.

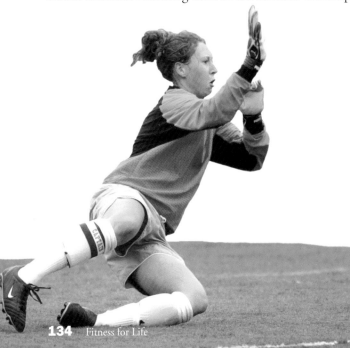

Table 9.1

Sue's Skill-Related Fitness Profile

Fitness part	SKILL-RELATED PERFORMANCE RATING			
	Low	Marginal	Good	High
Agility				X
Balance		X		
Coordination			X	
Power		X		
Speed		X		
Reaction time	X			

Table 9.2

Skill-Related Benefits of Sports and Other Activities

Activity	Balance	Coordination	Reaction time	Agility	Power	Speed
Badminton	Fair	Excellent	Good	Good	Fair	Good
Baseball	Good	Excellent	Excellent	Good	Excellent	Good
Basketball	Good	Excellent	Excellent	Excellent	Excellent	Good
Bicycling	Excellent	Fair	Fair	Fair	Poor	Fair
Bowling	Good	Excellent	Poor	Fair	Poor	Fair
Circuit training	Fair	Fair	Poor	Fair	Good	Fair
Dance, aerobic or social	Fair	Good	Fair	Good	Poor	Poor
Dance, ballet or modern	Excellent	Excellent	Fair	Excellent	Good	Poor
Fitness calisthenics	Fair	Fair	Poor	Good	Fair	Poor
Extreme sports	Good	Good	Excellent	Excellent	Fair	Good
Football	Good	Good	Excellent	Excellent	Good	Excellent
Golf (walking)	Fair	Excellent	Poor	Fair	Good	Poor
Gymnastics	Excellent	Excellent	Good	Excellent	Excellent	Fair
Interval training	Fair	Fair	Poor	Poor	Poor	Fair
Jogging or walking	Poor	Poor	Poor	Poor	Poor	Poor
Martial arts	Good	Excellent	Excellent	Excellent	Excellent	Excellent
Racquetball or handball	Fair	Excellent	Good	Excellent	Fair	Good
Rope jumping	Fair	Good	Fair	Good	Fair	Poor
Skating, ice or roller	Excellent	Good	Fair	Good	Fair	Good
Skiing, cross-country	Fair	Excellent	Poor	Good	Excellent	Fair
Skiing, downhill	Excellent	Excellent	Good	Excellent	Good	Poor
Soccer	Fair	Excellent	Good	Excellent	Good	Good
Softball (fastpitch)	Fair	Excellent	Excellent	Good	Good	Good
Swimming (laps)	Poor	Good	Poor	Good	Fair	Poor
Tennis	Fair	Excellent	Good	Good	Good	Good
Volleyball	Fair	Excellent	Good	Good	Fair	Fair
Weight training	Fair	Fair	Poor	Poor	Good	Poor

135

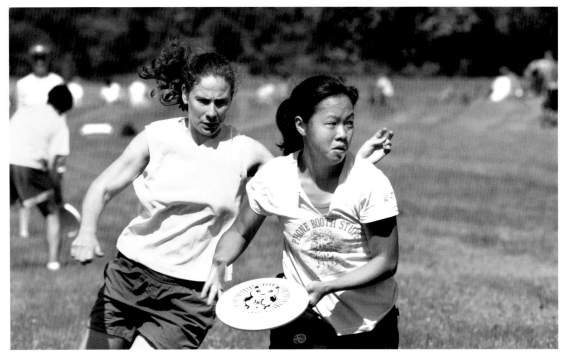

Playing ultimate requires good eye-hand coordination.

Sue also decided to use her profile to help her choose other activities that would be easier to learn. She scored well in coordination. Because bowling is excellent for building coordination, it is also an activity in which a person with good coordination is likely to succeed.

Sue selected bicycling as another activity she would include in her activity program because it did not require high levels of skill-related fitness, did not require her to learn new skills, but did have a lot of health benefits.

You can develop your own skill-related fitness profile similar to the one Sue developed (see table 9.1). Use your profile to determine which activities might help you improve where you need it and which activities will be the ones you can most easily learn.

FITNESS Technology

Many new technological advances have helped people to become more successful in sports, even those who are not highly skilled. One of the most noteworthy is the development of sports equipment made from lightweight metals such as titanium, magnesium, and aluminum. Because these metals are light in weight, equipment such as tennis rackets, golf clubs, and baseball bats can be made larger without being excessively heavy.

Oversized tennis rackets have a larger sweet spot, and for this reason even beginners are more likely to hit the ball well than with a smaller racket. Large golf clubs allow beginning golfers to hit the ball straighter and farther. Lightweight metals are also quite strong, so equipment made with them is less likely to break. For example, baseball and softball bats are less likely to break than wooden bats. Schools often use them so that they don't have to spend so much money to replace wooden bats. One negative aspect of using new, lightweight metal bats is that they allow the ball to be hit harder. Some experts think that they are especially dangerous for pitchers, who are more likely to be injured if struck by a ball hit with these bats.

 www.fitnessforlife.org/student/9/3

Lesson Review

1. What are some examples of physical skills?
2. How do skill-related fitness abilities differ from physical skills?
3. What are three factors that affect skill-related fitness and skills?
4. Why is assessing personal skill-related fitness important?

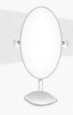

Self-Assessment

Assessing Skill-Related Physical Fitness

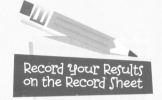
Record Your Results on the Record Sheet

Use these stunts to assess your skill-related fitness abilities. Keep these points in mind, especially if you score low:

▶ You can improve all parts of your skill-related fitness, but it is often harder to improve on skill-related fitness abilities than on health-related fitness abilities.

▶ With practice you can improve your skills even if you are low in a skill-related fitness ability.

▶ Many activities do not require high levels of these abilities.

▶ You do not need to excel in an activity or sport to enjoy it.

▶ Many subparts of skill-related fitness are not included in these stunts. You may excel in some of these other subparts. Ask your teacher to help you find stunts to test more specific abilities not measured by these stunts.

PART 1: Side Shuttle (Agility)

Use masking tape or other materials to make five parallel lines on the floor, each 3 feet apart. Have a partner count while you do the side shuttle. Then count while your partner does it.

1. Stand with the first line to your right. When your partner says "go," slide to the right until your right foot steps over the last line. Then slide to the left until your left foot steps over the first line.

 Caution: Do not cross your feet.

2. Repeat the exercise, moving from side to side as many times as possible in 10 seconds. Only one foot must cross the outside lines.

3. When your partner says "stop," freeze in place until your partner counts your score. Score 1 point for each line you crossed in 10 seconds. Subtract 1 point for each time you crossed your feet.

4. Do the side shuttle twice. Record the better of your two scores on your record sheet.

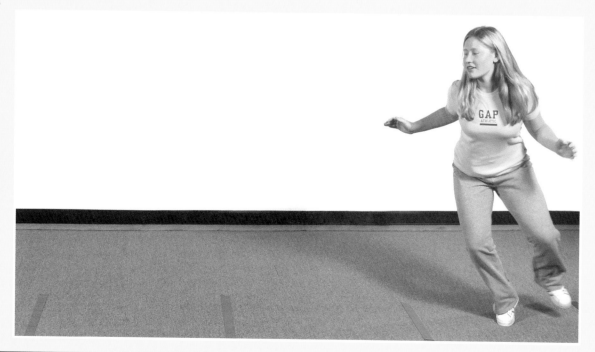

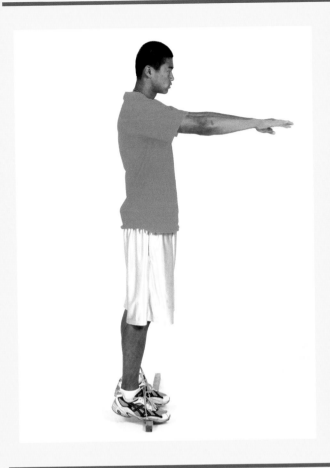

PART 2: Stick Balance (Balance)

You may take one practice try before doing each stunt for a score.

Stunt 1

1. Place the balls of both feet across a stick so that your heels are on the floor.
2. Lift your heels off the floor and maintain your balance on the stick for 15 seconds. Hold your arms out in front of you for balance. Do not allow your heels to touch the floor or your feet to move on the stick once you begin.

Hint: Focus your eyes on a stationary object in front of you.

3. Try the stunt twice. Give yourself 2 points if you are successful on the first try, 1 point if you failed on the first try but succeeded on the second, and 3 points if you were successful on both tries. Try stunt 2 even if you did not do well on stunt 1.

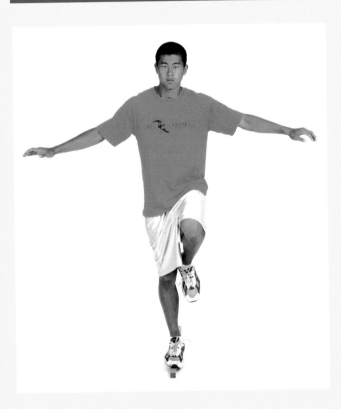

Stunt 2

1. Stand on a stick with either foot. Your foot should run the length of the stick.
2. Lift your other foot off the floor. First, balance for 10 seconds with your foot flat. Then rise up on to your ball of foot (heel off the stick) and continue balancing for 10 seconds.

Hint: Balance on your dominant leg—the one you balance on when you kick a ball.

3. Try the stunt twice. Give yourself 1 point if you balanced flat-footed for 10 seconds, and another point if you balanced on the ball of your foot for 10 seconds. Give yourself another point if you successfully balanced both flat-footed and standing on your toes. Your maximum score is 3 points.

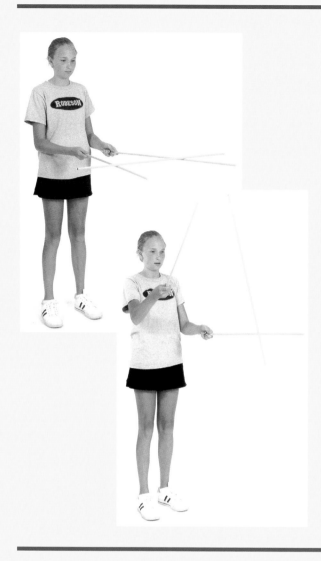

PART 3: Wand Juggling (Coordination)

1. Take three practice tries before doing this stunt for a score. Hold a stick in each hand. Have a partner place a third stick across your sticks.

2. Toss the third stick in the air so that it makes a half turn. Catch it with the sticks you are holding. The tossed stick should not hit your hands.

3. Do this stunt 5 times tossing the stick to the right, and then do it 5 times tossing the stick to the left. Score 1 point for each successful catch.

Hint: Absorb the shock of the catch by giving with the held sticks, as you might do when catching an egg or something breakable.

PART 4: Standing Long Jump (Power)

Use masking tape or other materials to make a line on the floor.

1. Stand with both feet behind the line on the floor. Swing your arms forward, and jump as far forward as possible. Keep both feet together. Do not run or hop before jumping.

2. Have a partner measure the distance from the line to the nearest point where any part of your body touched the floor when you landed.

3. Do this stunt twice. Record the better of your two scores on your record sheet.

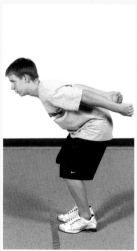
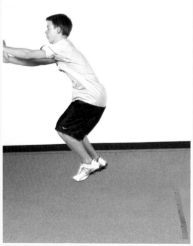
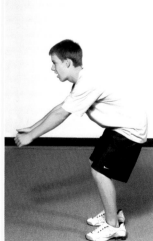

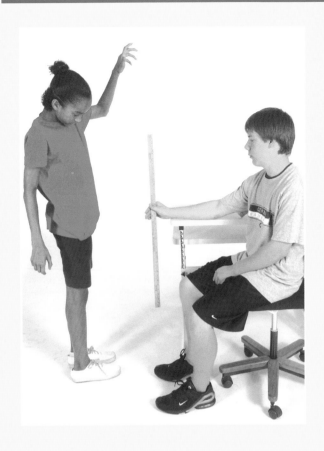

PART 5: Yardstick Drop (Reaction Time)

1. You will need a partner for this stunt. Have your partner hold the top of a yardstick with his or her thumb and index finger between the 1-inch mark and the end of the yardstick.
2. Position your thumb and fingers at the 24-inch mark on the yardstick. They should not touch the yardstick. Your arm should rest on the edge of a table with only your fingers over the edge.
3. When your partner drops the stick without warning, catch it as quickly as possible between your thumb and fingers.

Hint: Focus on the stick, not your partner, and be very alert.

Try this stunt 3 times. Your score is the number on the yardstick at the place where you caught it. Record your scores. Your partner should be careful not to drop the yardstick after the same waiting period each time. You should not be able to guess when the yardstick will drop. To get your rating, use the middle score (between your lowest and highest score).

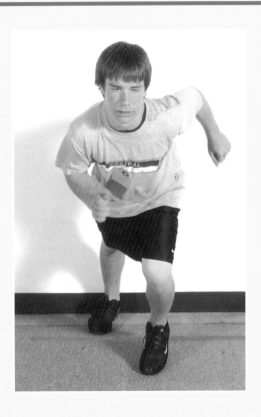

PART 6: Short Sprint (Speed)

Use masking tape or other materials to make lines 2 yards apart beginning 10 yards from the starting line for a total distance of 26 yards. Work with a partner who will time you and blow a whistle to signal you to stop.

Try this once for practice without being timed; then try it for a score. Record your score on your record sheet.

1. Stand 2 or 3 steps behind the starting line.
2. When your partner says "go," run as far and as fast as you can. Your partner will start a stopwatch when you cross the starting line. Then your partner will blow the whistle 3 seconds later. When the whistle blows, do not try to stop immediately, but begin to slow down.
3. Your partner should mark where you were when the 3-second whistle blew. Measure the distance to the nearest yard line. Your score is the distance you covered in the 3 seconds after crossing the starting line.

Scoring and Rating

Record your individual scores on your record sheet. Then follow the instructions for each stunt to find your fitness rating in tables 9.3 and 9.4.

Table 9.3

Rating Chart: Agility, Balance, and Coordination

	SIDE SHUTTLE (LINES CROSSED)		STICK BALANCE	WAND JUGGLING
	Males	Females	Males and females	Males and females
Excellent	31+	28+	6	9-10
Good	26-30	24-27	5	7-8
Fair	19-25	15-23	3-4	4-6
Poor	<18	<14	<3	<4

Table 9.4

Rating Chart: Power, Reaction Time, and Speed

	STANDING LONG JUMP (INCHES)		YARDSTICK DROP (INCHES)	SHORT SPRINT (YARDS RUN)	
	Males	Females	Males and females	Males	Females
Excellent	87+	74+	21+	24+	22+
Good	80-86	66-73	19-21	21-23	19-21
Fair	70-79	58-65	14-18	16-20	15-18
Poor	<69	<57	<13	<15	<14

Note: The rating categories used for health-related physical fitness are not used for skill-related physical fitness. The categories for skill-related physical fitness describe levels of performance ability, not health or wellness.

Active Sports

Lesson Objectives

After reading this lesson, you should be able to

1. Identify four categories of sports.
2. Explain why fitness is important to sports participants.
3. Identify categories of sports for which participants must be especially fit.
4. Discuss guidelines for choosing a sport.

Lesson Vocabulary

active sports (p. 142), lifetime sports (p. 144), sports (p. 142)

 www.fitnessforlife.org/student/9/4

You already know that regular physical activity contributes to good health and well-being. You also know that no single activity or set of exercises is best for everyone. An individual's choice of physical activities is based on such factors as age, skill-related fitness abilities, skills, interests, and personal fitness goals. In this lesson you will learn about the many kinds of sports and their benefits.

Sports of Different Intensities

As you will see, many different types of sports exist. **Sports** are physical activities that are competitive (have a winner and loser) and that have well-established rules. Some, such as golf and bowling, are relatively moderate in intensity. For this reason they are classified in the first level of the Physical Activity Pyramid with lifestyle activities that are also moderate. **Active sports** are included at the second level of the Physical Activity Pyramid because they are vigorous in nature. Active sports are considered at the same level of the pyramid (second level) as active aerobics because they elevate the heart rate above the threshold level and into the target zone for cardiovascular fitness. Active sports such as soccer, tennis, and basketball are not truly aerobic in nature because they involve frequent stops and starts. Short sprints or intense movements in these sports are typically anaerobic because these spurts are so vigorous that

they could not be continued for long periods without a rest. Experts still consider these sports to be similar to active aerobics if the rests between spurts of activity are brief and if the average heart rate during the activity stays above the threshold level. Some sports such as sprints in track and field are so intense for such a short period that they are totally or almost totally anaerobic. Examples include the 100-, 200- and 400-meter dashes. Training for sports typically involves both aerobic and anaerobic components. If you want to learn more about different types of anaerobic training consult the *Fitness for Life* Web site.

 www.fitnessforlife.org/student/9/5

The Health-Related Benefits of Active Sports

Active sports can be effective in building many parts of health-related physical fitness. Table 9.5 illustrates the health-related benefits of a wide variety of sports as well as some active recreation activities. You may also want to consult table 9.2 on page 135 for some of the skill-related benefits of a variety of sports. These two tables may be of value in helping you choose a sport for lifetime participation. As you read this lesson, think about which sports are best for you.

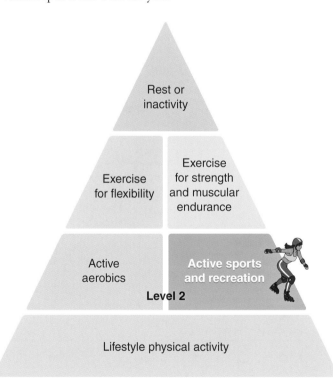

Table 9.5

Health-Related Benefits of Sports

Sport	Develops cardio-vascular fitness	Develops strength	Develops muscular endurance	Develops flexibility	Helps control body fat levels
INDIVIDUAL SPORTS					
Badminton +	Fair	Poor	Fair	Fair	Fair
Bowling +	Poor	Poor	Poor	Poor	Poor
Golf (walking) +	Fair	Poor	Poor	Poor	Poor
Gymnastics	Fair	Excellent	Excellent	Excellent	Fair
Rowing, crew	Excellent	Fair	Excellent	Poor	Excellent
Skiing, cross-country +*	Excellent	Fair	Good	Poor	Excellent
Skiing, downhill +*	Fair	Fair	Good	Poor	Fair
Snowboarding	Fair	Fair	Good	Fair	Fair
DUAL OR PARTNER SPORTS					
Handball/Racquetball +*	Good/Excellent	Poor	Good	Poor	Good/Excellent
Martial arts +*	Poor	Fair	Fair	Fair	Poor
Table tennis +*	Poor	Poor	Poor	Poor	Poor
TEAM SPORTS					
Baseball/Softball *	Poor	Poor	Poor	Poor	Poor
Basketball, half-court +*	Fair	Poor	Fair	Poor	Poor
Basketball, vigorous +*	Excellent	Poor	Good	Poor	Excellent
Football *	Fair	Good	Fair	Poor	Fair
Soccer *	Excellent	Fair	Good	Fair	Excellent
Volleyball +*	Fair	Fair	Poor	Poor	Fair
OUTDOOR, CHALLENGE, OR EXTREME SPORTS					
BMX cycling	Good	Good	Excellent	Fair	Good
Canoeing +	Fair	Poor	Fair	Poor	Fair
Horseback riding +	Poor	Poor	Poor	Poor	Poor
Mountain climbing +*	Good	Good	Good	Poor	Good
Sailing +	Poor	Poor	Poor	Poor	Poor
Surfing +*	Fair	Poor	Good	Fair	Fair
Waterskiing +*	Fair	Fair	Good	Poor	Fair

+ Lifetime sport.

* Fitness needed to prevent injury.

Sports of Many Kinds

There are so many different active sports that it is impossible to mention them all. Sports are generally grouped into several categories: team sports; dual sports; individual sports; and outdoor, challenge, or extreme sports. Other sports will not be considered here because they are not among the most popular or because they have little importance to the personal physical activity program of the typical person. Examples include motor sports (car racing), and racing (dogs and horses).

Team Sports

Team sports, such as the volleyball game in the photo below, are among the most popular for high school students and for adult spectators. Other examples are football, hockey, and soccer. These activities can be very good for building fitness for participants but do little for the fitness of spectators. Team sports are hard to do after the school years because they require other participants (teammates) as well as special equipment or facilities. Even though baseball and softball involve some vigorous activity, they are sometimes considered to be more like lifetime physical activities because their average intensity is low.

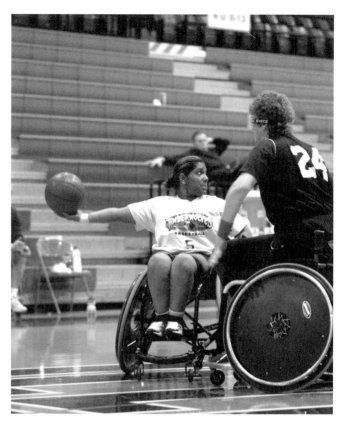

Basketball is one of the few team sports listed among the top 20 activities performed by adults.

No team sport is among the 10 most popular types of physical activities performed by adults 18 and over, but basketball is one of the few that is listed among the top 20 activities. The 10 most popular activities are primarily lifestyle physical activities and active aerobics. Because relatively few people who play team sports when they are young continue to pursue them for a lifetime, it will be important for you to find opportunities to continue if you want to play team sports as you grow older. Another way to stay active is to begin learning an individual sport, a dual sport, or an aerobic activity that you can enjoy later in life.

Dual or Partner Sports

Dual sports, sometimes called partner sports, are those you can do with one other person. Examples include tennis, badminton, fencing, and judo. Because they require fewer people than team sports, dual sports are often referred to as **lifetime sports.** Dual sports can be practiced individually, so you can get activity in these sports without a partner.

Tennis is often included in the top 10 participation activities, partly because it can be done with one other person and tennis courts are now available to most people. Some dual sports are not activities that large numbers of people do as adults. For example, wrestling is considered a dual sport but is not often done as a

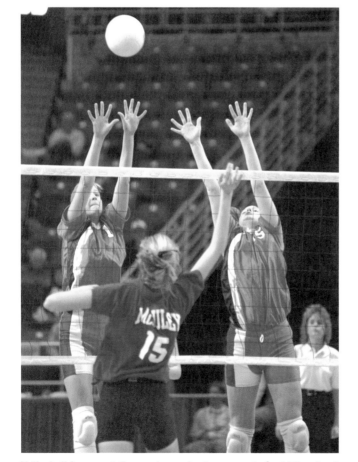

Volleyball is among the most popular team sports for high school students.

lifetime sport even though it does develop many important parts of health-related fitness. Dual sports that are not done by many adults are not considered lifetime sports.

Individual Sports

Individual sports are those that you can do by yourself. Golf, gymnastics, and bowling are truly individual sports because you do not have to have a partner or a team to perform them. Many of these types of sports are also lifetime sports because they are more likely to be done throughout life, although some such as gymnastics are not done by many later in life. Also gymnastics often requires a spotter. Skiing and skating are two forms of active recreation that are also sometimes classified as individual sports.

Outdoor, Challenge, or Extreme Sports

Many of the types of active recreation discussed in chapter 8 can also classified as sports. Active recreation activities such as those included in the previous chapter as well as sailing and water skiing are sometimes referred to as outdoor or challenge sports. Snowboarding, skateboarding, surfing, and BMX cycling are examples of activities sometimes referred to as extreme sports.

Fitness for Sports

Just as sports can contribute to good fitness, you also must stay fit to participate actively in sports. A weekend athlete is someone who neither exercises nor plays a sport on a regular basis. For example, some people snow ski only once or twice a year but otherwise do not exercise regularly. Nevertheless, they believe they are fit enough to ski. These people should exercise regularly for several weeks before skiing to get ready for it and to avoid injury.

Some individuals mistakenly assume that fitness is not necessary for certain sports, especially if the sports do little to build fitness. For example, softball is not particularly good for developing fitness, but it does

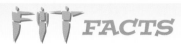

People who inherit a large number of fast-twitch muscle fibers are especially likely to be good at activities requiring sprinting and jumping, while those who inherit a large number of slow-twitch muscle fibers are likely to be good at activities requiring long, sustained performances such as distance running or swimming. You will learn more about fast- and slow-twitch muscle fibers in chapter 11.

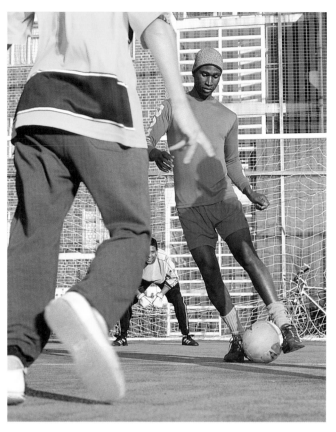

Fitness is necessary for weekend athletes as well as those who participate in sports on a regular basis.

require fitness if you are to perform well. A player must sprint between bases, slide into bases, and jump to catch the ball. Each action could result in an injury if the player is not physically fit.

Each sport could result in injury if you are not physically fit. Be fit before actively playing a sport that involves these factors:

- ▶ Physical contact (football, wrestling, ice hockey)
- ▶ Fast sprinting (baseball, softball, soccer)
- ▶ Sudden fast starts and stops (racquetball, track, basketball)
- ▶ Vigorous jumping (basketball, high jump, soccer)
- ▶ Danger of falling (skiing, skating, judo)
- ▶ Danger of overstretching muscles (tennis, football)

Choosing a Sport

If you decide that participation in a sport should be a part of your lifetime physical activity plan, follow these guidelines:

- ▶ **Consider your skill-related abilities.** In the previous lesson you learned how to match your abilities to different activities. Consider your abilities as you choose a sport, too.

Taking Charge: Building Performance Skills

To enjoy a physical activity, it is good to have skills needed for the sport or game. Skills such as kicking, throwing, hitting, and swimming can be learned by anyone with practice. It does take some people longer than others to learn skills, though.

Zack felt that he was never really good at sports. He tried several activities and found that he was not as good at any of them as were other people he knew. He even tried out for sport teams at school. Once he tried to make the soccer team and then he tried out for the swim team but did not make either one. His biggest problem was that he did not learn to play sports when he was young, and now he was behind others who played sports.

Zack wanted to learn a sport but was afraid that he would be unsuccessful again and that his friends might laugh at him. He did a self-assessment of his skill-related abilities and found that he did pretty well on most of the assessments. He found that he did best in coordination and agility, though his power was not especially high.

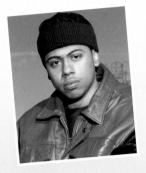

Before trying out for a team again, Zack thought it would be best to try to learn some skills of a sport that matched his abilities. Being over 6 feet tall and weighing 180 pounds seemed to be an advantage, though he wanted to get stronger. Still, he was not sure which sport would be best for him. He wanted to be on a team but he also wanted to learn something that would be fun and interesting.

For Discussion

What advice would you give Zack for choosing a sport? Once he chooses a sport, what steps could he take to improve his performance skills? Who could he talk to for help? Zack knew that he needed to practice but was not sure exactly what to practice. What practice advice would you give him? Fill out the questionnaire provided by your teacher to see how you might improve your performance skills. Consider the guidelines on pages 145 to 147.

▶ **Consider the health-related benefits of the sport.** Use the information from this lesson to help you choose a sport that will help you build important parts of fitness.

▶ **Consider a lifetime sport.** Sports that can be done throughout life are good choices because you are likely to stick with them.

▶ **Learn the skills of the sport.** Skill is important if you are going to do an activity on a regular basis. Set aside time to practice your sport skills.

▶ **Be fit for sports.** Remember, you need to be physically fit even for sports that do not build fitness.

▶ **Choose sports that you enjoy doing.** Sports can be fun. Sometimes it is pleasant and worthwhile to just get away from the pressures of life and do something that you enjoy.

Choosing Your Role

We know that sports offer opportunities for leadership. Coaches provide leadership, and so do team captains. Some roles in sports require more leadership than others. For example, quarterbacks call plays in football and catchers call pitches in softball and baseball. In recreational sports, such as intramurals or community programs, there is no coach. Someone must provide leadership to get a team organized and take care of details. Without this leadership there would be no team—and there would be no participation.

However, not all participants need to be leaders. Being a good team member, following the team leader, and playing an important role are all important to team success and enjoyment. Without good followers, no team can be successful. You may play a different role in different situations; you may lead in one instance and follow in another. This is good because it allows all people to play a variety of roles and to enjoy their involvement.

Lesson Review

1. What are four categories of sports? Give an example of each.
2. Why is fitness important to sports participants?
3. What are some categories of sports for which participants must be especially fit?
4. What are six guidelines for choosing a sport?

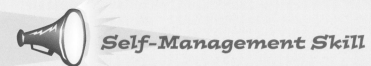

Self-Management Skill

Building Performance Skills

Many sports require practicing more than a few skills to become proficient. For example, basketball players must practice shooting, dribbling, passing, catching, and defensive skills. Follow these guidelines to improve your sport skills:

▶ **Get good instruction.** If you learn a skill incorrectly, it will be hard to improve, even with practice.

▶ **At first do not worry about details.** When you first learn a skill, concentrate on the skill as a whole. You can deal with the details after learning the main skill.

▶ **As you improve, concentrate on one detail at a time.** If you try to concentrate on too many details at once, you may develop what is called paralysis of analysis. This condition occurs when you analyze an activity and try to correct several problems all at once. For example, if you are learning the tennis serve it is not wise to try to work on your ball toss, your grip, your backswing, and your follow-through all at once. It is better to practice changes one at a time.

▶ **Keep practicing.** Many people do not like to practice skills; they just want to play the game. However, just playing the game does not provide practice for a particular skill. Also, when you play a game without having the proper skills, you often develop bad habits that hinder your success.

▶ **Avoid competing while learning a skill.** Although competition can be fun, competing while you are learning a skill is stressful and does not promote optimal learning.

▶ **Think positively.** Experts have shown that if you think negatively you are likely to perform poorly. If you think positively while you practice, you will learn faster and become more confident in your abilities.

▶ **Choose an activity that matches your skill-related fitness.** As mentioned earlier, your heredity may play a role in your success in sports. Use the information from your self-assessment of skill-related fitness earlier in this chapter to help you select a sport in which you are most likely to succeed.

Resolving Conflict in Sports

In a highly charged, competitive situation, conflicts sometimes arise. Too often emotions, rather than clear thinking, cause people to do things they would not normally do. For example, one player in a basketball game commits a hard foul, so the opponent commits a hard foul to get even. This type of conflict can damage relationships, cause hard feelings, and even lead to injury.

The most important step to resolving this type of conflict is controlling emotions. You can take steps such as calling a time-out to let tempers cool off and making a change in defensive assignments to prevent further incidents. During the time-out, reflection on the consequences of "getting even" can be helpful. For example, rough play can result in fouling out or ejection from the game. When incidents occur in games with friends, postgame negotiation and discussion can help. Negotiation might include the following:

▶ Reach an agreement on what the conflict is about, including describing the situation as a mutual problem to be solved, not a win–lose struggle.

▶ Communicate your cooperative intentions and let the other person know you want to resolve the conflict constructively.

▶ Take the other person's perspective on the problem.

▶ Determine how both people can gain from resolving the conflict.

▶ Use discussion, understanding, and negotiation to reach an agreement that satisfies both parties.

▶ Communicate to prevent future conflicts.

Controlling emotions takes practice, just as learning skills takes practice. Learning how to control competitive anxiety can also be useful (see page 299). Additional conflict recognition and resolution guidelines are on pages 191 and 315.

147

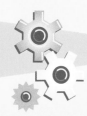

Activity 2

The Sports Stars Program

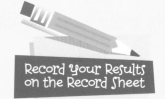
Record Your Results on the Record Sheet

The Sports Stars Program is designed to help you use sports in your physical activity program. The program is based on earning a certain number of stars, or points, each week as you participate in sports of your choice. If sports are your only form of exercise, you should earn 100 stars each week to build good health-related fitness, especially cardiovascular fitness. If you do other activities from the Physical Activity Pyramid, you can substitute them and earn fewer sports points. You may only have the opportunity to perform one day of the Sports Stars Program. If this is the case, choose a sport from table 9.6 and earn as many Sports Stars Points as time will allow. If you use the Sports Stars Program as your main source of exercise, follow these guidelines:

▶ Earn stars at least three days each week. Ideally, you should earn sports stars four to six days a week.

▶ Use table 9.6 to determine how many points you earn for participation in different sports for different lengths of time.

▶ If you have not been active on a regular basis before beginning the program, start gradually. Earn 50 points a week for the first two weeks, 75 points a week for the next two weeks, and then earn 100 points a week.

▶ You may select from a variety of activities in table 9.6. Some people will enjoy doing the same activities from day to day and week to week. Others will enjoy variety and may change activities as time passes.

▶ Try to earn at least half of your sports stars from active sports that elevate your heart rate into the target zone for cardiovascular fitness.

▶ Remember to warm up before and cool down after your workout.

▶ Keep records of your participation. You may make up your own chart for keeping records or use one supplied by your teacher.

148

Table 9.6

Number of Stars Earned in Sports

Sport	15 min	30 min	1 h	2 h	Comments
Archery	3/4	1-1/2	3	6	

Badminton
  doubles
  singles
	
	1
	3
		
		2
		6
			
			4
			12
				
				8
				24	

Baseball
  recreational
  school team
	
	1
	3
		
		2
		6
			
			4
			12
				
				8
				24
					
					Team practice

Basketball
  recreational
  school team
	
	3
	4 1/2
		
		6
		9
			
			12
			18
				
				24
				36
					
					Full-court
					Team practice

Bowling	3/4	1 1/2	3	6	
Canoeing	3	6	12	24	Continuous paddling

Football
  recreational
  school team
	
	2
	4 1/2
		
		4
		9
			
			8
			18
				
				16
				36
					
					Team practice

Golf	1 1/2	3	6	12	Walking; steady play
Gymnastics school team	 3	 6	 12	 24	 Team practice
Handball	4 1/2	9	18	36	Steady play
Horseback riding	1	2	4	8	
Judo or karate	2	4	8	16	No long breaks
Racquetball	4 1/2	9	18	36	Steady play
Rowing crew team	 6	 12	 24	 48	 Actual rowing time
Skating (ice or roller)	3 1/2	7	14	28	Actual skating time

Skiing
  cross-country
  downhill
	
	8
	4 1/2
		
		16
		9
			
			32
			18
				
				64
				36
					
					Actual skiing time
					Actual skiing time

Soccer
  recreational
  school team
	
	4
	5
		
		8
		10
			
			16
			20
				
				32
				40
					
					Actual playing time
					Team practice

Softball
  recreational
  school team
	
	1
	3
		
		2
		6
			
			4
			12
				
				8
				24
					
					Team practice

Tennis
  doubles
  singles
	
	2
	3 1/2
		
		4
		7
			
			8
			14
				
				16
				28	

Volleyball
  recreational
  school team
	
	1
	3
		
		2
		6
			
			4
			12
				
				8
				24
					
					Team practice

Wrestling school team	 5	 10	 20	 40	 Team practice

9 Chapter Review

Reviewing Concepts and Vocabulary

Number your paper from 1 to 4. Copy the number of each statement on a sheet of paper. Next to each number, write the word (or words) that correctly completes the sentence.

1. Sports that you can do by yourself are called _____.
2. Catching, throwing, and kicking are examples of _____.
3. The largest age group that plays team sports is _____.
4. Sports that can be done when you grow older are _____ sports.

Number your paper from 5 to 10. Next to each number, choose the letter of the best answer.

Column I	Column II
5. agility	a. use of senses and muscles together
6. balance	b. strength times speed
7. coordination	c. starting a movement quickly
8. power	d. covering a distance in a short time
9. reaction time	e. changing directions quickly
10. speed	f. maintaining an upright posture

Number your paper from 11 to 16. On your paper, write a short answer for each statement or question.

11. What are some of the ways to self-assess your skill-related physical fitness?
12. What is the difference between skill and skill-related physical fitness?
13. Which sports are best for developing each of the five health-related parts of physical fitness?
14. Why might team sports not be good as an only choice for your lifetime activity plan?
15. What are some guidelines for choosing sports?
16. Why is it important to be physically fit when participating in sports?

Thinking Critically

Write a paragraph to answer the following questions.

Do Web sites dedicated to sports describe ways to be active, or do they provide information for spectators? Do differences for different types of sports exist in the Web sites? Log on to the Web. Use a search engine such as Google (www.google.com) or Yahoo (www.yahoo.com) to locate Web sites for several sports. First, look up a popular team sport. Next, look up a popular individual sport. Third, look up a sport you consider to be a lifetime sport. Determine whether the top Web sites are for spectators or participants.

Unit Review on the Web

www.fitnessforlife.org/student/9/6

Unit III review materials are available on the Web at the address listed in the Web icon.

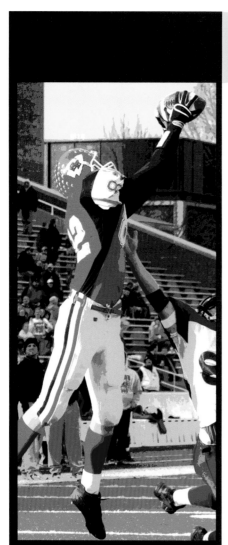

Project

Keep a record of your daily participation in active sports for one week. Record the minutes of activity in these activities each day. How might you adjust your physical activity to better maintain or improve your cardiovascular fitness level? What short-term goals might you have for minutes each day in active sports? (Do not include active aerobics and active recreation because they are included in the last chapter.) Make a written plan for the following week, incorporating changes that might help you reach your goals. Use the worksheets provided by your teacher.

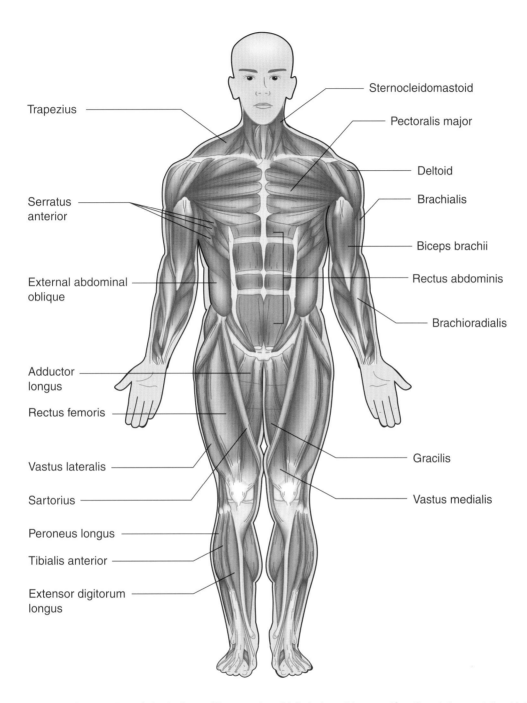

Trapezius

Serratus anterior

External abdominal oblique

Adductor longus

Rectus femoris

Vastus lateralis

Sartorius

Peroneus longus

Tibialis anterior

Extensor digitorum longus

Sternocleidomastoid

Pectoralis major

Deltoid

Brachialis

Biceps brachii

Rectus abdominis

Brachioradialis

Gracilis

Vastus medialis

Muscles of the body. The major muscles of the body are illustrated and labeled on this page (front) and the next (back). The specific muscles used in the chapters that follow will be described with each exercise. Refer to these two muscle charts for exact muscle locations.

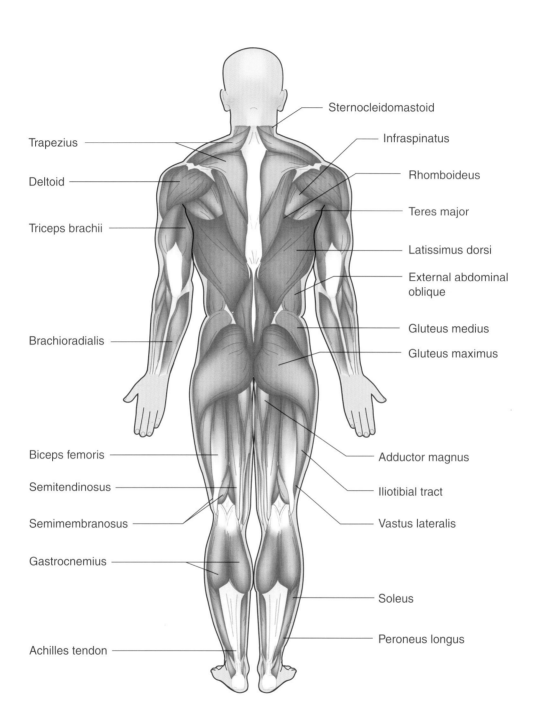

Sternocleidomastoid

Trapezius

Deltoid

Triceps brachii

Brachioradialis

Biceps femoris

Semitendinosus

Semimembranosus

Gastrocnemius

Achilles tendon

Infraspinatus

Rhomboideus

Teres major

Latissimus dorsi

External abdominal oblique

Gluteus medius

Gluteus maximus

Adductor magnus

Iliotibial tract

Vastus lateralis

Soleus

Peroneus longus

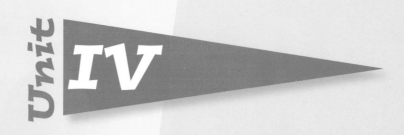

Physical Activity Pyramid:
Level 3 Activities

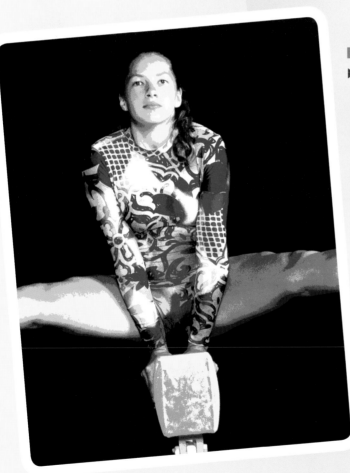

Healthy People 2010 Goals

▶ Increase the number of teens who do regular exercise for flexibility.

▶ Increase the number of teens who do regular exercise for strength and muscular endurance.

▶ Decrease steroid use among teens.

▶ Reduce risk of back problems.

▶ Reduce risk of osteoporosis.

▶ Reduce risk of pain from muscle injury.

Unit Activities

▶ Jump and Stretch Routine

▶ The Basic 10: Flexibility Exercise Circuit

▶ Partner Resistance Exercises

▶ Fundamentals of Weight and Resistance Training

▶ Homemade Weights

▶ Muscular Endurance Exercise Circuit

10

Flexibility

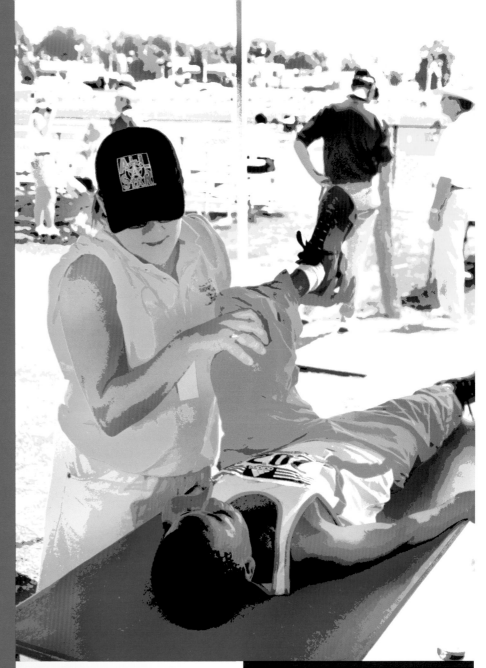

In this chapter...

Activity 1
Jump and Stretch Routine

Lesson 10.1
Flexibility Facts

Self-Assessment
Arm, Leg, and Trunk Flexibility

Lesson 10.2
Improving Flexibility

Taking Charge
Building Intrinsic Motivation

Self-Management Skill
Building Intrinsic Motivation

Activity 2
The Basic 10: Flexibility Exercise Circuit

Activity 1

JUMP AND STRETCH ROUTINE

Regular physical activity strengthens your heart and improves other parts of your cardiovascular system. Jumping rope is an activity that most people can perform to improve cardiovascular fitness. Stretching exercises improve the flexibility of your muscles and joints. This workout includes only basic jump-rope skills, but you may want to add other, more difficult skills as your ability improves. The stretching exercises require a partner.

Lesson 10.1

Flexibility Facts

Lesson Objectives

After reading this lesson, you should be able to

1. Describe the characteristics of flexibility.
2. Explain how you benefit from good flexibility.
3. Explain why it is important to balance strength and flexibility exercises.
4. Explain how the fitness principles of overload, progression, and specificity apply to flexibility.

Lesson Vocabulary

hypermobility (p. 156), joint laxity (p. 156), range of motion (ROM) (p. 155)

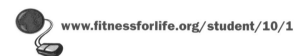

www.fitnessforlife.org/student/10/1

In this lesson, you will learn about the importance of being flexible and how to improve flexibility by applying fitness principles. You will also learn to evaluate flexibility.

What Is Flexibility?

Flexibility is the ability to move your joints through a full range of motion (ROM). A joint is a place in the body where bones come together. The best known joints include the ankles, knees, and hips in the legs; the knuckles, wrist, elbows, and shoulders in the arms; and the joints between the vertebrae in the spine. Some joints, such as the knees and elbows, work like a hinge,

permitting movement in only two directions. Other joints, such as the hip and shoulder, work like a ball and socket, allowing movement in all directions. **Range of motion (ROM)** is the amount of movement you can make in a joint.

Benefits of Good Flexibility

Flexibility is sometimes referred to as the forgotten part of health-related fitness. This is because most people tend to focus on the other parts of health-related fitness to the exclusion of flexibility. We know, however, that having good flexibility has many health benefits, both when you are young and when you grow older. Some of these benefits are described here.

Improved Function

Everyone needs a minimum amount of flexibility to maintain health and mobility, and some people need additional flexibility. For example, dancers and gymnasts must be very flexible to perform their routines; plumbers, painters, and dentists often need to bend and stretch; and some musicians need very flexible fingers and wrists.

Flexibility is important to many athletes because it allows a longer backswing in throwing and striking movements. A long backswing enables a faster forward swing. In the case of weightlifting, shot put, and some other sports, the greater backward movement is believed to allow a faster forward movement, producing more power.

Improved Health and Wellness

Stretching exercises can help prevent injury and muscle soreness and have a beneficial effect on a number of conditions. For example, flexible musicians are less likely to have pain in the joints. Stretching exercises can often alleviate menstrual cramps in women. They can prevent or provide relief from leg cramps and shin-splints (pains in the front of the shins caused by overuse). Stretching short muscles helps improve posture, which helps prevent or relieve back pain and reduces fatigue. Stretching a muscle can help it relax. In chapter 17 you will learn how stretching exercises can help relieve stress.

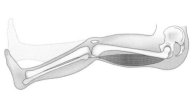
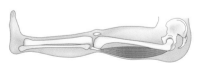

a   *b*   *c*

(a) *Poor joint range of motion—knee does not fully extend because of short hamstring muscles;* (b) *good range of motion—knee fully extends because of long hamstrings;* (c) *too much range of motion—knee bends backward.*

Characteristics of Flexibility

Just as heredity and other factors influence your success in sports and recreational activities, similar factors influence your flexibility. Some of these are discussed here.

Body Build and Flexibility

Some people will not be able to score as well on flexibility tests as others no matter how much they stretch. Anatomical differences in our bodies help determine what we can and cannot do. Rather than comparing your scores on flexibility tests with those of others, compare your scores with your own previous scores and seek to improve.

Can short people touch their toes more easily than tall people? In most cases this is not true because a shorter person does tend to have relatively short legs and trunk but also tends to have short arms (although there are exceptions). In contrast, a tall person tends to have longer legs and trunk, as well as longer arms. There are some people who have exceptionally long arms or legs whose body build may make it easier for them to score well or not so well on flexibility tests, but this is the exception rather than the rule.

Generally, females tend to be more flexible than males. Also, younger people tend to be more flexible than older people. As people grow older their muscles typically grow shorter because they are used less, and

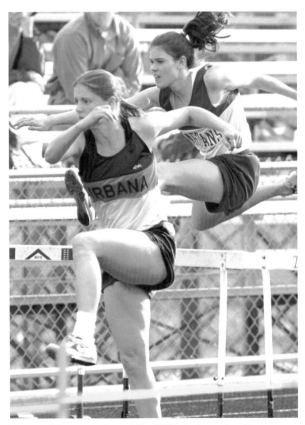

These athletes need good flexibility to jump hurdles.

their joints allow less movement because of conditions such as arthritis. One important reason for doing regular stretching exercises when you are young is to reduce the risk of joint problems when you are older. Good flexibility enhances performance in a variety of tasks for people of all ages.

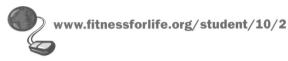

www.fitnessforlife.org/student/10/2

Hypermobility

Some people have an unusually large range of motion in certain joints, and people often refer to them as being double jointed. This condition is called **hypermobility,** the ability to extend the knee, elbow, thumb, or wrist joint past a straight line, as if the joint could bend backward. Hypermobility is usually an inherited trait and tends to be more common in some groups than others. Some people who have hypermobile joints are prone to joint injuries and may be more likely to develop arthritis, a disease in which the joints become inflamed. For the most part, however, those with hypermobile joints do not have problems, other than a slight disadvantage in some sports. For example, when doing the push-up exercise, the elbows of a hypermobile person might easily lock when the arms straighten, making it difficult to unlock the elbows to begin the downward movement.

Joint Laxity

When the supporting tissue around a joint allows the bones to move in ways other than intended, it is described as **joint laxity,** or looseness. Laxity occurs when the ligaments around the joint are overstretched, most likely from injury or incorrect exercise. If laxity occurs in a knee joint, it may lead to knee sprains and torn cartilage or a dislocated kneecap. Ligaments cannot be strengthened by doing exercises. However, strengthening the muscles around the joint can help reduce looseness. In addition to the reasons described in the previous section, joint laxity is another cause of hypermobility.

Balancing Strength and Flexibility

You should do strength and flexibility exercises together. Everyone needs strong muscles, but exclusive use of

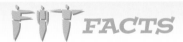

About twice as many females as males are hypermobile, and more females meet minimum fitness standards for flexibility than males.

strength exercises can lead to a loss of normal range of motion and a condition sometimes called being muscle-bound. On the other hand, if you only do flexibility exercises, then your joints may become susceptible to injury because you need strong muscles to reinforce the ligaments that hold the bones together.

A balanced exercise program includes both strength and flexibility exercises for all your muscles so that they can apply equal force on all sides of a joint. People commonly use the flexors (muscles on the front of the body) a great deal because many daily activities emphasize the use of those muscles. For example, the majority of people have strong biceps muscles (on the front of the arm), pectoral muscles (on the front of the chest), and quadriceps muscles (on the front of the thigh). The pull of these strong muscles results in the body hunching forward. To avoid becoming permanently hunched over, you need to make certain that these strong, short muscles on the front of the body get stretched. At the same time, you must strengthen the weak, long, relatively unused muscles on the back of the body. Table 10.1 shows the muscles most in need of flexibility exercises in most people.

Are there any muscles that do not need stretching? For most people, the answer is yes. For example, most people eventually begin to develop a hunched-over posture often called humpback at some point in life. Because the upper back muscles become overstretched in people with this postural problem, they should avoid further stretching of those muscles. Another example

FITNESS Technology

When you perform flexibility self-assessments, you will use low-tech devices such as a yardstick or a ruler. In some cases you may use a flexibility box that includes a built-in measuring stick. When experts do research on flexibility, they use more sophisticated instruments such as goniometers, which measure joint angles. Some goniometers are electronic and computerized. Your school may have an inexpensive goniometer, such as the one in the picture, that you can use when assessing joint range of motion.

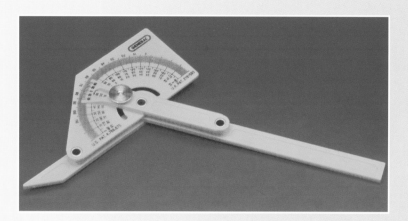

might be the abdominal muscles. It is important to keep your abdominal muscles strong but most people do not need to stretch them, In fact, if the abdominals are stretched they begin to sag and the abdomen protrudes, leading to poor posture.

Each person must evaluate his or her own needs to avoid stretching already overstretched muscles and avoid strengthening muscles that are already so strong that they are out of balance with their opposing muscles. Keeping muscles on opposites sides of a joint in balance helps them pull with equal force in all directions. Such a balance helps align your body parts properly, ensuring good posture.

Table 10.1

Muscles That Need the Most Stretching

Muscle(s)	Reason for stretching
Chest muscles	To prevent poor posture
Front of shoulders	To prevent poor posture
Front of hip joint	To prevent swayback posture, backache, or a pulled muscle
Back of thigh (hamstrings)	To prevent swayback posture, backache, or a pulled muscle
Inside of thigh	To prevent back, leg, and foot strain
Calf muscles	To avoid soreness and Achilles tendon injuries, which may occur from running and jumping
Lower back	To prevent soreness, pain, and back injuries

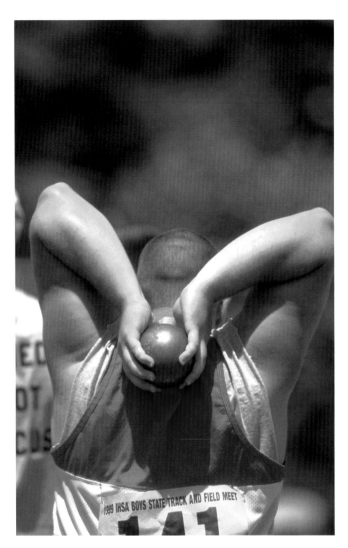

The boy in the picture is stretching the specific muscles needed to put the shot. To develop overall flexibility, you must stretch all the muscles that need stretching.

Fitness Principles and Flexibility

The principles of overload, progression, and specificity apply to flexibility, just as they apply to the other components of health-related fitness.

Principle of Overload

You need to stretch your muscles longer than normal to increase your flexibility. To stretch a muscle, you need to lengthen it more than you do in your daily activities. To achieve this kind of stretch, you usually need a force greater than your own opposing muscles. For example, if you want to stretch your chest muscles, you cannot get an overload just by pulling your arms back and holding them in that position. You need additional force, such as your own body weight, when you put

your arms on either side of a doorframe and lean forward. You can use another body part, a partner, or a weight to assist in the stretch. Be sure to give feedback when a partner helps you stretch so that he or she can apply the proper amount of force.

Principle of Progression

You need to gradually increase your exercise intensity. You can increase intensity by stretching farther as you gain flexibility. Up to a point, you may also progress by gradually increasing the amount of time you hold the stretch or the number of repetitions you perform. Eventually you will achieve your flexibility goals. Then you need to maintain the flexibility you have achieved.

Principle of Specificity

Flexibility exercises improve only the specific muscles at the specific joints that you stretch. To develop overall flexibility, you must stretch all the muscles that need stretching.

Maintaining Flexibility

Once you have reached an acceptable level of flexibility for your muscles, you must continue to move all of your joints and muscles through this new and improved range of motion on a regular basis. If you do not use the range of motion you have available in a joint, the muscles will begin to shorten again and you will lose that flexibility.

Lesson Review

1. What are the characteristics of flexibility?
2. How do you benefit from good flexibility?
3. Why is it important to balance strength and flexibility exercises?
4. How do the fitness principles of overload, progression, and specificity apply to flexibility?

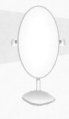

Self-Assessment

Arm, Leg, and Trunk Flexibility

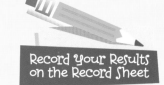
Record Your Results on the Record Sheet

This self-assessment helps you evaluate the flexibility of some of your muscles and joints. Use these general directions for the tests that follow. Then score yourself using table 10.2.

▶ Perform each exercise as described and illustrated here.

▶ Stretch and hold the position for 2 seconds while a partner checks your performance.

Use the record sheet to help you score this test. Record only the first trial.

▶ You are expected to do these tests in class only once, unless your instructor tells you otherwise. You will want to retest yourself periodically. The record sheet provides space to write the results of your future retests.

Table 10.2

Rating Chart: Flexibility

Fitness Rating	Score
Good	8-10
Marginal	5-7
Low	0-4

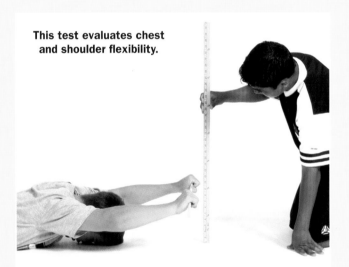

This test evaluates chest and shoulder flexibility.

Arm Lift

1. Lie facedown. Hold a ruler or stick in both hands. Keep your fists tight, palms facing down.
2. Raise your arms and the stick as high as possible. Keep your forehead on the floor and your arms and wrists straight.
3. Hold this position while your partner checks the height of the stick from the floor with a ruler.
4. Record 1 checkmark in the correct column. Pass = 10 inches or more.

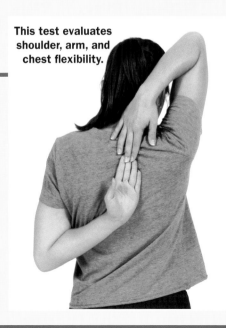

This test evaluates shoulder, arm, and chest flexibility.

Zipper

1. Reach your right arm and hand over your right shoulder and down your spine, as if you were pulling up a zipper.
2. Hold this position while you reach your left arm and hand behind your back and up your spine to try to touch or overlap the fingers of your right hand.
3. Hold the position while your partner checks it.
4. Repeat, reaching your left arm over your shoulder.
5. Record 1 checkmark for each side. Pass = touch or overlap fingers.

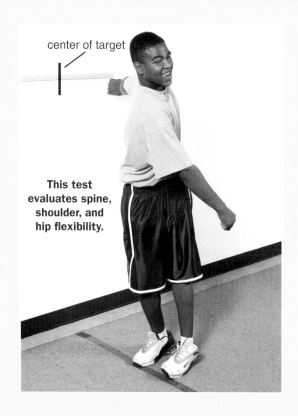
center of target

This test evaluates spine, shoulder, and hip flexibility.

Trunk Rotation

1. Stand with your toes on the designated line. Your right shoulder should be an arm's length (fist closed) from the wall and directly on a line with the target spot.
2. Drop your right arm and extend your left arm to your side at shoulder height. Make a fist, palm down.
3. Without moving your feet, rotate your trunk to the left as far as possible. Your knees may bend slightly to permit more turn, but don't move your feet. Try to touch the target spot or beyond with a palm-down fist.
4. Hold the position while your partner checks it.
5. Repeat, rotating to the right.
6. Record 1 checkmark for each side. Pass = touch center of target or beyond.

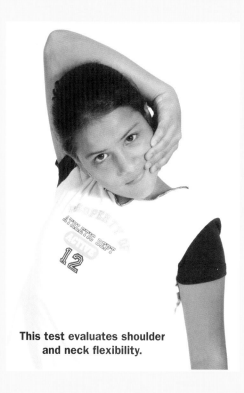
This test evaluates shoulder and neck flexibility.

Wrap Around

1. Raise your right arm and reach behind your head. Try to touch the left corner of your mouth. You may turn your head and neck to the left.
2. Hold the position while your partner checks it.
3. Repeat with your left arm.
4. Record 1 checkmark for each side. Pass = touching corner of mouth.

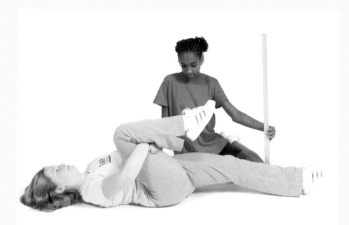

This test evaluates the flexibility of the muscles on the front of the hip, the hamstrings, and the lower back.

Knee to Chest

1. Lie on your back. Extend your left leg. Bring your right knee to your chest. Place your hands on the back of your right thigh. Pull your knee down tight to your chest.
2. Keep your left leg straight and both the leg and lower back flat on the floor.
3. Hold the position. Have your partner check that your knee is on your chest and use a ruler to measure the distance that your left calf is from the floor.
4. Repeat with your left knee.
5. Record 1 checkmark for each side. Pass = calf 1 inch or less from floor.

This test evaluates the flexibility of the calf muscles and range of ankle movement.

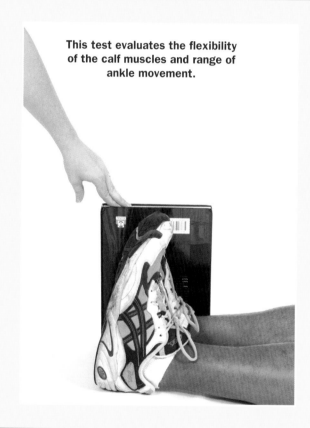

Ankle Flex

1. Sit erect on the floor with your legs straight and together. You may lean backward slightly on your hands if necessary.
2. Flex your ankles by pulling your toes toward your shins as far as possible.
3. Hold this position while your partner checks the angle that the soles of your feet make with the floor. The partner will align a T square or a book with the floor, and see whether the soles are at least perpendicular to the floor.
4. Record 1 checkmark in the correct column. Pass = soles angled 75 degrees or more.

Safety Tip: Warm up before taking a flexibility test. Warm muscles are less likely to be injured and will stretch farther.

Improving Flexibility

Lesson Objectives

After reading this lesson, you should be able to

1. Explain the differences among static stretching, PNF stretching, and ballistic stretching.
2. Describe the fitness target zones for static and ballistic exercise.
3. List the guidelines for doing flexibility exercises safely.

Lesson Vocabulary

ballistic stretching (p. 163), CRAC (p. 163), PNF stretching (p. 163), range of motion (ROM) exercise (p. 162), static stretching (p. 162)

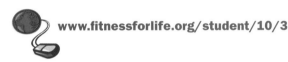

www.fitnessforlife.org/student/10/3

In this lesson, you will learn about the types of exercise used for flexibility. In addition, you will see how to apply the FIT formula to maintain or build flexibility. Finally, you will learn safety guidelines and try some stretching exercises for various muscle groups.

The Physical Activity Pyramid

As you learned in lesson 10.1, flexibility in the joints of the body is essential for good health as well as for efficient, effective functioning. For best results you must perform exercises especially designed to improve flexibility, because other activities may do little to improve it. Selecting activities and including exercises for flexibility from the Physical Activity Pyramid is the most effective way to improve your flexibility.

Types of Flexibility Exercises

Properly selected exercises can improve your flexibility and provide many other benefits such as helping to relieve muscle cramps. Range of motion exercise and stretching exercise are two main types of flexibility exercises.

Range of Motion (ROM) Exercise

The term **range of motion (ROM) exercise,** usually called ROM exercise, refers to flexibility exercises that

Rest or inactivity

Exercise for flexibility

Exercise for strength and muscular endurance

Level 3

Active aerobics

Active sports and recreation

Lifestyle physical activity

are used to maintain the range of motion already present in your joints. ROM exercises are probably the safest type of flexibility exercise to use in a warm-up routine. Some experts think that when you stretch your muscles too much in the warm-up, the muscles are more likely to be injured in the workout or sport that follows. So ROM exercise, or moderate stretching exercises, are recommended for the warm-up. More intense stretching is necessary to improve flexibility, but as noted in chapter 1 this type of stretching should be done in flexibility workouts when the body is warm rather than in the warm-up.

If you are as flexible as you need to be, then you should move your body to maintain that flexibility. Without attempting to stretch muscles any farther, it is wise to move all of the joints through their complete range of motion at least three times a week. Every day is even better. For example, if your self-assessment scores are in the good zone where you wish to be, then you should regularly exercise to maintain that level of flexibility.

Stretching Exercise

Whereas a ROM exercise maintains your current level of flexibility, a stretching exercise is designed to increase your range of motion by stretching farther than your current range of motion. The three types of stretching exercises are static, PNF, and ballistic.

Static stretching is stretching slowly as far as you can without pain, until you feel a sense of pulling or tension, then holding the stretch for several seconds (15 or more for best results). Done correctly, static stretching increases your flexibility and can help you relax. Static stretching exercises are safer than ballistic stretching exercises because you are less likely to stretch too far and injure yourself. Static stretching can be especially beneficial for people who have bad backs, previous muscle or joint injuries, or arthritis. Even athletes should perform static stretches at the beginning and end of their exercise programs to warm up and cool down. By themselves, static stretches might not build enough flexibility for an athlete, so athletes may need to add PNF and ballistic stretches.

PNF stretching (PNF stands for proprioceptive neuromuscular facilitation) is a stretching technique used by physical and occupational therapists. It has recently become popular among athletes. PNF stretching is a variation of static stretching that is more effective for improving flexibility. A PNF stretch involves contracting the muscle before you stretch it so that you can stretch it farther. Some variations of PNF require a partner to assist you, but one form is easy for you to use with or without a partner. It is called **CRAC** (contract-relax-antagonist-contract). After you contract a muscle that you want to stretch, the muscle automatically relaxes. Contracting the opposing muscles (antagonist) during the stretch also makes the muscle you are stretching relax. CRAC does both of these. Some samples of CRAC are included in the activity at the end of this chapter.

Ballistic stretching is a series of quick but gentle bouncing or bobbing motions that are not held for a long time. If you are active in sports, part of your exercise program should include movements used in your sports. If you move or stretch muscles quickly in a sport (for example, fast throwing or sprinting), then some of your flexibility exercises should resemble the sport's movement. Those who use ballistic stretching should start with static stretching before doing the ballistic stretches. Take care to stretch gently; stretching too quickly or overstretching can cause injury.

Some teachers and coaches have been opposed to all ballistic stretching because of the possibility of overstretching if it is not done carefully. However, studies show that ballistic stretching does not cause as much muscular soreness as static stretching. If you are an athlete and wish to achieve a high performance level of flexibility, you may wish to apply the principle of specificity by using a ballistic stretching exercise that closely mimics the backswing so common to sports. You can see an example of this type of stretch at baseball games when the batter takes a few easy swings with a weighted bat or does trunk twists with a bounce in each direction before getting in the batter's box. Another example is the track athlete who stretches the Achilles tendon with a few gentle bounces on the heels.

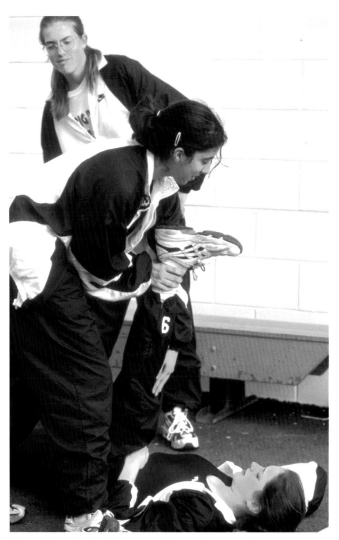

The athletes in the photo are using static stretching as they warm up before working out.

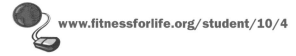

www.fitnessforlife.org/student/10/4

The FIT Formula for Flexibility

To improve flexibility as a result of increasing the length of your muscles, you must exercise in the fitness target zone for flexibility. Flexibility has two different target zones, one for static exercise (including PNF) and one for ballistic exercise. The FIT formula for static stretching and PNF is located in the second column of table 10.3, and the FIT formula for ballistic stretching is located in the third column of table 10.3.

Guidelines for Flexibility Exercises

To get the most benefit and the most enjoyment from your exercise program, it is important to perform the exercises correctly and observe certain cautions to avoid injury. Before you begin stretching, follow these guidelines and cautions to help you safely achieve and maintain flexibility.

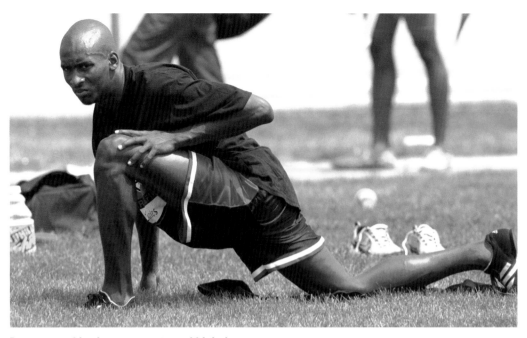
Proper stretching is necessary to avoid injuries.

▶ **Start with a general body warm-up.** Stretching is most effective in building flexibility when the muscles are warm. If stretching is used in a warm-up, it is wise to warm up your muscles with mild cardiovascular exercise such as walking or slow jogging before you begin stretching. If you are planning a more intense flexibility workout, it is best to do it after you have done other exercise that gets the muscles warm.

▶ **Use static stretching or PNF when beginning or for general health.** If you do not exercise regularly or if you do not need a high performance level of flexibility, do static or PNF rather than ballistic stretching. Ballistic stretching is only needed by those interested in high level performance.

▶ **Do not overstretch or ballistically stretch an injured muscle.** If you have a recent injury to a muscle or joint, such as a back problem, do not stretch ballistically; do only static or PNF stretches.

▶ **If you do ballistic stretching, do not bounce too far.** Stretch gently to avoid injury.

▶ **Do not stretch joints that are hypermobile, unstable, swollen, or infected.**

▶ **Do not stretch until you feel pain.** The old saying "no pain, no gain" is wrong. Stretch only until the muscle feels tight and a little uncomfortable.

▶ **Avoid dangerous exercises.** As you learned in chapter 2, you should avoid some popular exercises because they can cause injury. Avoid rolling your head and neck in a full circle, tipping your head backward to stretch your neck, backbends (unless you are a trained gymnast), arm circles with your palms down, and standing toe touches or windmills.

▶ **Avoid stretching muscles that are already overstretched from poor posture.**

Table 10.3

Fitness Target Zones for Flexibility

	Static or PNF	Ballistic
Frequency	• Stretch each muscle group daily, if possible, but at least 3 days a week—ROM stretch before and after workouts.	• Stretch each muscle group daily, if possible, but at least three days a week. *Caution: Before doing ballistic stretching, read about ballistic stretching on page 163 and the guidelines on pages 164 to 165.*
Intensity	• You must stretch the muscle beyond its normal length. • You must have a partner or equipment, or you can use your own body weight to provide an overload.	• You must stretch the muscle beyond its normal length. • Use slow, gentle bounces or bobs, using the motion of your body part to stretch the specific muscle. *Caution: No stretch should cause pain, especially sharp pain. Be especially careful when doing ballistic stretching.*
Time	• Hold each stretch for 15 to 30 sec. Rest for 10 sec. • Stretch each muscle group. Start with 1 set of 1 rep and progress to 3 or 4 sets, 1 rep each.	• Bounce against the muscle slowly and gently 10 to 15 times. Rest for 10 sec between sets. • Stretch each muscle group. Start with 1 set and progress to 3 sets.

Taking Charge: Building Intrinsic Motivation

Some people need to be rewarded by others to stay physically active. When they are no longer rewarded, they use it as an excuse to stop being active. They have extrinsic motivation—motivation given by others. People who have intrinsic motivation are self-motivated—they are active because they want to be. The more intrinsic rewards you get from physical activity, the more likely you are to remain active.

James pulled on his track shirt and stuffed his jeans and T-shirt into his locker. "I can't wait for track season to be over," he told Leon. "If the coach makes us do sprints again today, I'm going to pretend I sprained my ankle or something."

"I like sprints," Leon said as he tied the laces on his running shoes. "You get to see what you can do when you go all out."

"I'm already all out—all out of here as soon as possible! If I weren't going to get a letter jacket at the end of track this year, I'd quit now."

"What about next year? Are you going out for track again?" Leon asked.

"Nah. I can barely beat you and Angelo now in the 400. If I can't run faster than you two, how am I going to place in meets with other schools? I'm slowing down. It's time to quit while I'm ahead."

"Why don't you try out for something different next year? I'm thinking about soccer," Leon said. "I figure all this running would help me there. And it would motivate me to jog all summer to keep in shape."

"Yeah, maybe I'll try out for the soccer team, too. If I jogged with you this summer, maybe I'd stay motivated."

For Discussion

How does James show that he's extrinsically motivated? How does Leon show that he is intrinsically motivated? What could James do to become more intrinsically motivated? Fill in the questionnaire provided by your teacher to evaluate your own motivation to be physically active. Consider the guidelines on page 166.

▶ **Be sure to overload when stretching.** To benefit from static or PNF stretching, you need gravity, force, or a partner to provide sufficient overload. If you use a partner, he or she should be extremely careful not to cause overstretch. You must tell your partner when the tension is tight enough.

▶ **Consider contracting then relaxing the muscle before your stretch.** Your stretch can be more effective if you contract the muscles before you stretch them.

▶ **Consider contracting the antagonist (opposite) muscle while you stretch.** Your stretch can be more effective if you contract the muscles opposite of the muscles you are trying to stretch so that the stretched muscle can relax more and stretch farther as in PNF stretching.

▶ **Start slowly.** Regardless of the type of flexibility exercise you choose for your program, start slowly. Like muscular endurance exercises, even though some flexibility exercises seem easy, it does not take much to make your muscles sore. Begin slowly, and gradually increase the time and the number of repetitions and sets.

Lesson Review
1. What are the differences among static stretching, PNF stretching, and ballistic stretching?
2. What are the fitness target zones for static and ballistic exercise?
3. What are the guidelines for doing flexibility exercises safely?

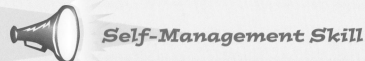

Self-Management Skill

Building Intrinsic Motivation

Intrinsic motivation refers to doing something because you enjoy it rather than doing it for a reward such as a grade or an award. People with good intrinsic motivation to be physically active are interested in it because they enjoy it. They feel confident in their abilities and typically do not feel tense or nervous when doing activities. Extrinsic motivation refers to doing an activity for some external reward or to avoid punishment. Exercise is unfortunately often used as punishment. Extrinsic motivation techniques, including punishment, can lead to lower intrinsic motivation and less enjoyment. Follow these guidelines to help you build intrinsic motivation for physical activity:

▶ **Do a self-assessment to determine your current intrinsic motivation level.** A worksheet that includes a self-assessment is available from your teacher.

▶ **Use the self-assessment to plan strategies for improvement.** If you are low in intrinsic motivation, the remainder of these guidelines will be especially useful.

▶ **Choose goals that will allow success.** If you are successful, you are more likely to enjoy an activity. Choose activities that encourage success. Set small, attainable goals that you can accomplish. Optimal challenge, having a goal that is not too hard nor too easy, is important.

▶ **Avoid negative self-talk.** Do not tell yourself that you are incompetent or ineffective. Instead, use positive self-talk. Tell yourself that you will improve with practice.

▶ **Focus on physical activity goals rather than fitness goals.** Fitness goals take time to achieve. Keep records and focus on doing activities that you schedule. Giving effort is the important thing.

▶ **Select activities that match your abilities.**

▶ **Find friends of similar abilities and interests.**

▶ **Consider non-competitive activities.** If competition is not fun for you, select activities that are noncompetitive such as lifestyle activities, active aerobics, or active recreation activities.

▶ **Avoid situations that make you tense or in which leaders use exercise as punishment.**

▶ **Avoid situations that focus on external rewards such as money or trophies.**

▶ **Consider outdoor activities that are refreshing and relaxing.**

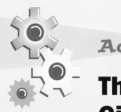

Activity 2

The Basic 10: Flexibility Exercise Circuit

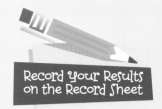
Record Your Results on the Record Sheet

The American College of Sports Medicine (ACSM) recommends that you perform 8 to 10 basic exercises to stretch all of the major muscle groups of the body. The exercises included in this activity will allow you to stretch each of the major muscle groups.

This flexibility program will help improve your range of motion. If you did not get a good fitness rating on your evaluation, or if you have been inactive or have joint injuries, choose the static and PNF exercises. If you got a good rating and exercise regularly, then you may add some ballistic exercises to your program. If you add ballistic exercises, be sure to begin with the static and PNF exercises before progressing to the ballistic ones. Review the guidelines on pages 164 to 165, and then follow these directions. Write your results on your record sheet.

▶ Refer to table 10.3 on page 164 for the appropriate number of repetitions (reps), sets, and time.

▶ Perform each of the exercises below and record the date and number of sets or reps on your record sheet. Your instructor will probably specify the number of sets and reps.

▶ For a PNF exercise, hold a maximum isometric contraction for 3 seconds, relax, then stretch for 15 seconds or more.

▶ You may do a PNF exercise as a static exercise by omitting the contraction phase and doing only the stretch phase for 15 seconds or more.

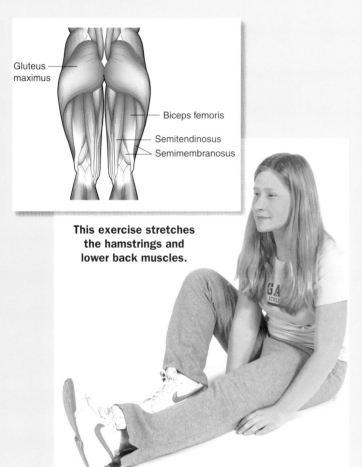

Gluteus maximus
Biceps femoris
Semitendinosus
Semimembranosus

This exercise stretches the hamstrings and lower back muscles.

Back-Saver Sit and Reach (PNF or Static)

1. Assume the back-saver sit and reach position, with the right knee bent and left leg straight.
2. Bend your left knee slightly and push your heel into the floor as you contract the hamstrings hard for 3 seconds. Relax.
3. Immediately grasp your ankle with both hands and gently pull your chest toward your knee. Hold the position for 15 seconds.
4. Repeat the exercise on the other leg.

Note: For static stretch, omit step 2.

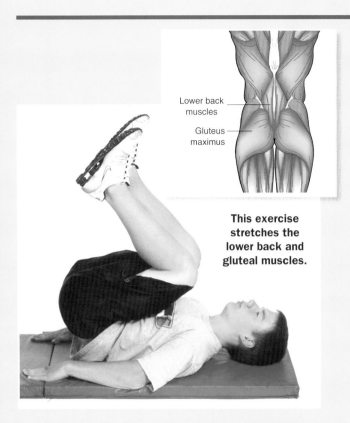

Lower back muscles

Gluteus maximus

This exercise stretches the lower back and gluteal muscles.

Knee to Chest (PNF or Static)

1. Lie on your back with your knees bent and your arms at your sides.

2. Lift your hips until there is no bend at the hip joint. Squeeze the buttocks muscles hard for 3 seconds. Relax by lowering your hips to the floor.

3. Immediately place your hands under your knees and gently pull your knees to your chest. Hold the position for 15 seconds or more.

Note: For a static stretch, omit step 2.

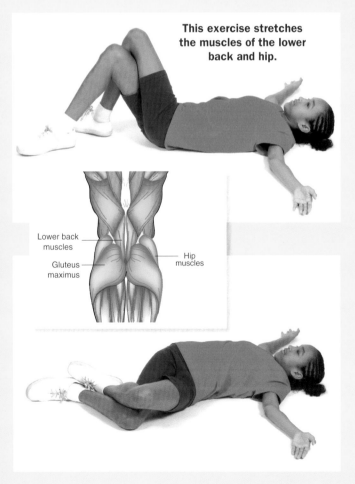

This exercise stretches the muscles of the lower back and hip.

Lower back muscles

Gluteus maximus

Hip muscles

Spine Twist (Static)

1. Lie on your back with your knees bent (hook-lying position), arms extended at shoulder level.

2. Cross your left leg over your right.

3. Keep your shoulders and arms on the floor as you rotate your lower body to the left, touching your right knee to the floor. Stretch and hold the position for 15 seconds or more.

4. At the end of the stretch, reverse the position of your legs (cross your right over your left), then rotate to the right and hold the position.

168

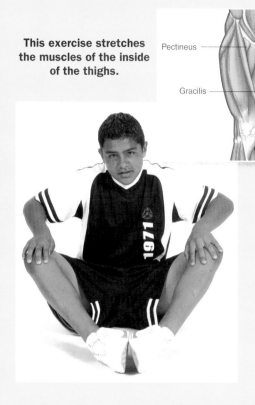

This exercise stretches the muscles of the inside of the thighs.

Pectineus — Adductor longus — Adductor magnus — Gracilis

Sitting Stretch (PNF or Static)

1. Sit with the soles of your feet together, your elbows or hands resting on your knees.

2. Contract the muscles on the inside of your thighs, pulling up as you resist with your arms pushing down. Hold the position for 3 seconds. Relax your legs.

3. Immediately lean your trunk forward and push down on your knees with your arms to stretch the thighs. Hold the position for 15 seconds or more.

Note: For a static stretch, omit step 2.

Zipper (PNF or Static)

1. Stand or sit. Lift your right arm over your right shoulder and reach down the spine.

2. With your left hand, press down on your right elbow. Resist the pressure by trying to raise that elbow, contracting the opposing muscles. Hold the position for 3 seconds. Relax.

3. Immediately stretch by reaching down your spine with your right arm, as your left arm assists by pressing on your elbow. Hold the position for 15 seconds or more.

4. Repeat the exercise with your other arm.

Note: For a static stretch, omit step 2.

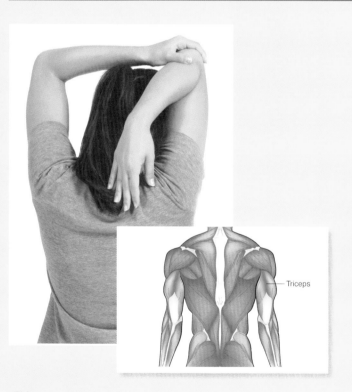

Triceps

This exercise stretches the triceps and latissimus muscles.

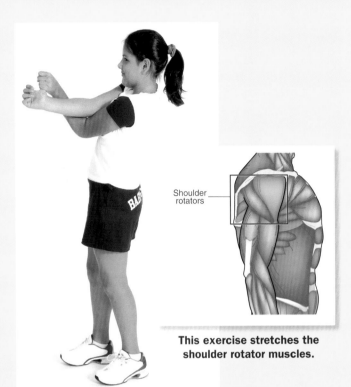

Arm Pretzel (Static or Ballistic)

1. Stand or sit. Cross your right arm over your left. Turn your right palm toward the back of your left hand and point your thumb down.

2. Grasp your right thumb with your left hand and pull down gently. Stretch and hold the position for 15 seconds or more.

3. Reverse arm positions and stretch your left shoulder.

Shoulder rotators

This exercise stretches the shoulder rotator muscles.

Hip Stretch (Static or Ballistic)

1. Take a long step forward on your right foot and kneel on your left knee. The right knee should be directly over your ankle and bent at a right angle.

2. You should feel a stretch across the front of the left hip joint and in the front of the thigh muscles.

3. Place your hands on your right knee for balance. Stretch by shifting the weight forward as you tilt your pelvis and trunk backward slightly. Keep your back knee in the same spot to stretch the hip and thigh muscles. Hold the position for 15 seconds or more.

4. Repeat the exercise with your other leg.

Note: For a ballistic stretch, do a gentle bouncing motion forward as you tilt the pelvis back.

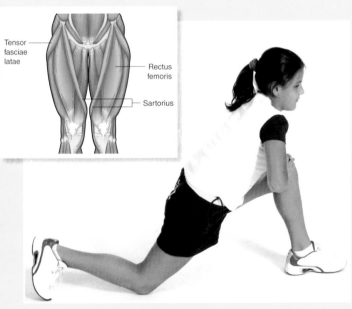

Tensor fasciae latae

Rectus femoris

Sartorius

This exercise stretches the muscles on the front of the thigh (quadriceps) and the muscles on the front of the hip.

Arm Stretch (Static)

1. Sit or stand and cross your right arm over your left with the palms facing. Lace your fingers together.
2. Raise your arms overhead to your ears. Straighten your elbows, stretching up and back. Hold the position 15 seconds or more.

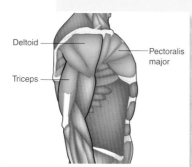

Deltoid

Pectoralis major

Triceps

This exercise stretches the muscles of the shoulders, arms, and chest.

Chest Stretch (PNF, Static, or Ballistic)

1. Stand in a forward stride position in a doorway. Raise your arms slightly above shoulder level. Place your hands on either side of the doorway.
2. Lean your body into the doorway. Resist by contracting your arm and chest muscles. Hold the position for 3 seconds. Relax.
3. Immediately lean further forward, letting your body weight stretch the muscles. Hold the position for 15 seconds or more.
4. For a ballistic stretch, gently bounce your body forward.

Note: For a static stretch, omit steps 2 and 4.

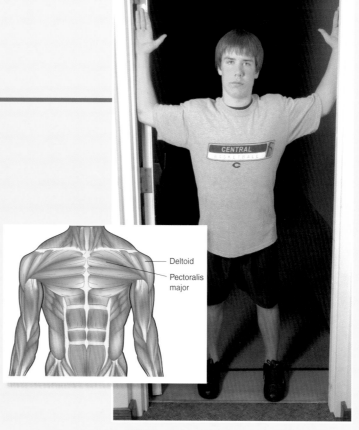

Deltoid

Pectoralis major

This exercise stretches the chest and shoulder muscles.

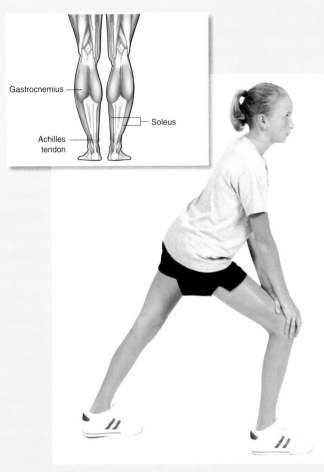

Gastrocnemius

Soleus

Achilles tendon

This exercise stretches the calf muscles and the Achilles tendon.

Calf Stretch (Static or Ballistic)

1. Step forward with your right leg in a lunge position. Keep both feet pointed straight ahead and your front knee directly over the front foot. Place your hands on your right leg for balance.

2. Keep the left leg straight and the heel on the floor. Adjust the length of your lunge until you feel a good stretch in the left calf and Achilles tendon. Hold the position for 15 seconds or more.

3. Repeat the exercise with your other leg.

Note: For a ballistic stretch, gently bounce heel toward floor.

10 Chapter Review

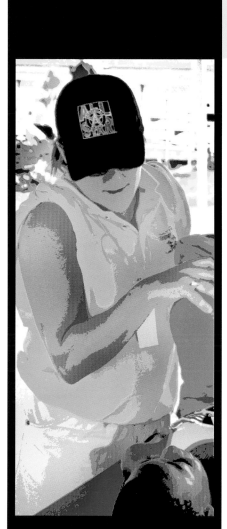

Project

Keep a record of your daily participation in flexibility exercises for one week. Record the minutes of these exercises each day. How might you adjust your physical activity to better maintain or improve your flexibility level? What short-term goals might you have for performing specific flexibility exercises each day? Make a written plan for the following week, incorporating changes that might help you reach your goals. Use the worksheets provided by your teacher.

Reviewing Concepts and Vocabulary

Number your paper from 1 to 7. Next to each number, write the word (or words) that correctly completes the sentence.

1. _____ in the body's joints is essential for good health, wellness, and efficient, effective functioning.
2. The amount of movement you can make at a joint is called your _____.
3. Exercises that involve moving beyond your range of motion are _____.
4. Doing _____ will help you maintain movement ability in your joints.
5. A _____ involves contracting, then relaxing the muscle before you stretch it.
6. _____ is stretching slowly as far as you can without pain, then holding the stretch for several seconds.
7. Gentle bouncing motions are part of _____.

Number your paper from 8 to 12. Next to each number, choose the letter of the best answer.

Column I	Column II
8. hypermobility	**a.** pain in the front of the shins
9. arthritis	**b.** place where bones come together
10. joint	**c.** looseness of the joints
11. laxity	**d.** the ability to extend the knee, elbow, thumb, or wrist joint past a straight line
12. shinsplints	**e.** disease in which joints are inflamed

Number your paper from 13 to 15. On your paper, write a short answer for each statement or question.

13. Why do you have to be especially careful when a partner helps you stretch?
14. Why should you do some mild cardiovascular exercise before stretching?
15. What are the two main kinds of exercise that increase flexibility?

Thinking Critically

Write a paragraph to answer the following question.

During the first two weeks of volleyball practice, three players suffered shoulder muscle tears and two players experienced extreme back pain. The coach thinks the injuries may be because of a lack of flexibility. Why do you think flexibility may be a factor, and what advice would you give the coach?

11

Muscle Fitness: Basic Principles and Strength

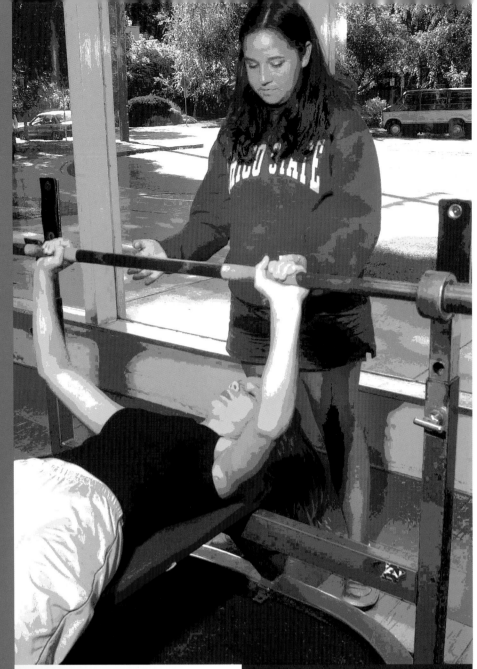

In this chapter...

Activity 1
Partner Resistance Exercises

Lesson 11.1
Muscle Fitness Basics

Self-Assessment
Determining Your Modified 1RM and Grip Strength

Lesson 11.2
Building Strength

Taking Charge
Preventing Relapse

Self-Management Skill
Preventing Relapse

Activity 2
Fundamentals of Weight and Resistance Training

Activity 1

PARTNER RESISTANCE EXERCISES

To build strength and muscular endurance, you have to work your muscles against a resistance. Resistance can be provided by free weights, machines, or your own body weight. But in these exercises, you are going to use a partner's body weight as resistance. Choose a partner who is about your height and weight, then try these exercises. A word of caution: To avoid injuring each other, be gentle when you provide resistance or try to move your partner's body parts.

Muscle Fitness Basics

to a force that acts against your muscles. It is usually measured in terms of pounds. You can lift your own body weight, use free weights, or use a weight machine. Some machines use other forces, such as hydraulic pressure, air pressure, or friction to provide resistance. Various activities in levels 1 and 2 of the Physical Activity Pyramid can be helpful in promoting muscle fitness development, but for best results you should use muscle

Lesson Objectives

After reading this lesson you should be able to

1. Explain the difference between strength and muscular endurance.
2. Describe some of the health benefits of muscle fitness.
3. Describe the various types of muscles and muscle fibers.
4. Describe some of the methods of progressive resistance exercise used to improve muscle fitness.

Lesson Vocabulary

absolute strength (p. 180), calisthenics (p. 180), fast-twitch muscle fibers (p. 177), hypertrophy (p. 176), intermediate muscle fibers (p. 177), isokinetic exercise (p. 180), isometric contraction (p. 177), isotonic contraction (p. 177), one repetition maximum (1RM) (p. 180), progressive resistance exercise (PRE) (p. 175), relative strength (p. 180), reps (p. 176), set (p. 177), slow-twitch muscle fibers (p. 177)

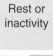

Rest or inactivity

Exercise for flexibility

Exercise for strength and muscular endurance

Level 3

Active aerobics

Active sports and recreation

Lifestyle physical activity

 www.fitnessforlife.org/student/11/1

Muscle fitness is comprised of two health-related parts of physical fitness: strength and muscular endurance. Muscular endurance is the ability to contract muscles many times without tiring or to hold a muscle contraction for a long time. The person in the picture needs good muscular endurance to carry the backpack for a long time. Strength indicates the amount of force a muscle can exert. The amount of weight a muscle group can lift one time measures strength. The number of times a muscle group can repeat an exercise or how long a muscle group can hold a contraction without tiring measures muscular endurance.

Both muscular endurance and strength are developed by a **progressive resistance exercise (PRE).** The exercises are called progressive because you gradually or progressively increase the amount of overload you apply to the muscles. This is consistent with the basic principles of overload and progression. Resistance refers

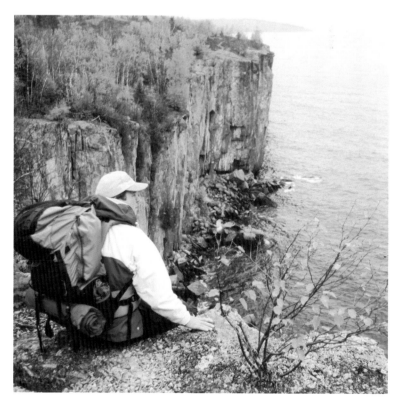

Hiking with a backpack requires good muscular endurance.

fitness exercises using PRE from level 3 of the Physical Activity Pyramid.

Strength and endurance use resistance in different ways. Strength is developed by doing an exercise for only a few times, but with a lot of resistance. The girl lifting the boxes needs strength. Muscular endurance is developed by doing an exercise many times, but with less resistance, such as the light backpack the girl is wearing in the picture.

Strength training tends to increase the size of muscles as they become stronger. This increase in muscle size is called **hypertrophy.** Because muscular endurance training uses less weight, endurance training does not cause as much hypertrophy.

The Muscular Endurance–Strength Continuum

Exercises used to develop muscular endurance and strength differ only in the number of repetitions and the amount of resistance. The relationship between endurance and strength can be illustrated by a continuum. The continuum shown here represents pounds of resistance one one edge and number of repetitions on the other edge.

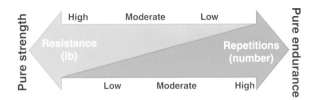

Muscular endurance–strength continuum.

The continuum shows the resistance and repetitions that a person might use to build muscle fitness. You can see that you would use high resistance with few repetitions to develop strength, and a low resistance with a high number of repetitions for endurance. Using the resistance and the number of repetitions from the middle of the continuum would develop both strength and endurance. This continuum also shows that usually when you train for strength you will develop some endurance, and when you train for endurance you will develop some strength.

Muscle Fitness Terminology

You probably will hear the terms *reps* and *sets* in relation to muscular endurance exercises. The diagram on the next page can help you understand these terms. Repetitions, or **reps,** are the number of consecutive times you

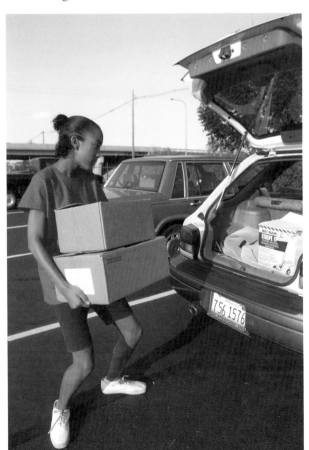

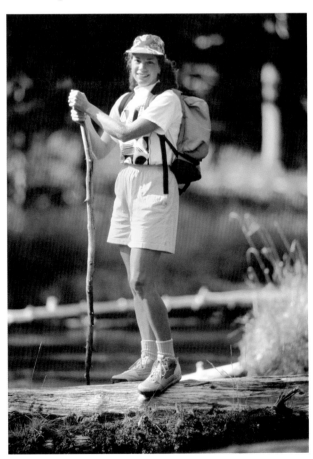

The girl lifting boxes (left) uses strength while the girl wearing the light backpack (right) uses muscular endurance.

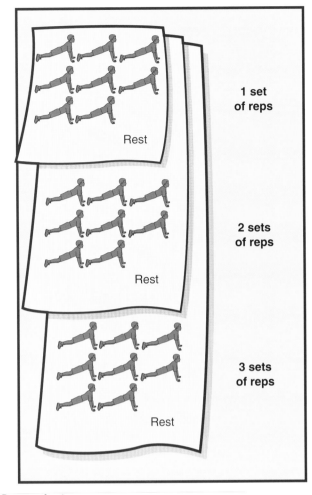

1 set
of reps

Rest

2 sets
of reps

Rest

3 sets
of reps

Rest

Reps and sets.

do an exercise. A **set** is one group of repetitions. For example, suppose you do an exercise 8 times, then rest; repeat it 8 times, then rest; and repeat another 8 times. Then you will have completed a total of 3 sets of 8 repetitions each.

The Structure of Muscles

The muscles of the body create the movement that allows you to do the activities described in this book. In this section you will learn more about how the muscles work.

Muscle Types

Your body has three types of muscles: smooth, cardiac, and skeletal. Smooth muscles make up the walls of internal organs such as the stomach and blood vessels. Your heart is made of cardiac muscle. Both smooth and cardiac muscles are classified as involuntary muscles because you cannot consciously control their movements.

Skeletal muscles are attached to bones and make movement possible. You use these muscles to do physical activity. They are called voluntary muscles because you control them. Muscles work together to allow a

body part to function. For example, when you contract the biceps muscle (see the figure on the bottom of page 178), your arm bends at the elbow, bringing your hand close to your shoulder. At the same time the triceps relaxes to allow the biceps to do its work.

As the diagram shows, muscles are attached to bones on either side of a joint. The bones act as levers to which the muscles apply force. An **isotonic contraction** is a muscle contraction that pulls on the bones and produces movement of body parts. Isotonic exercises involve isotonic contractions in which body parts move. The two types of isotonic muscle contractions are concentric and eccentric. The first picture shows the biceps muscle doing a concentric, or shortening, contraction. In the second picture, as the arm is slowly straightened the biceps is doing an eccentric, or lengthening, contraction. An **isometric contraction** occurs when muscles contract and pull with equal force in opposite directions, so no movement can occur. Isometric exercises involve isometric contractions and body parts do not move. An example of an isometric contraction would be pushing your hands and arms together in front of your body. You push hard with both hands against the resistance of each other, but no movement exists. (See chapter 15 for examples of isometric exercises.)

Muscle Fibers

Muscle fibers are long, thin, cylindrical muscle cells. Skeletal muscles such as those in the arms and the legs are made of many muscle fibers. The strength and endurance of skeletal muscles depends on whether the muscles are made of slow, fast, or intermediate fibers and how much exercise they get.

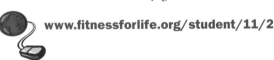 **www.fitnessforlife.org/student/11/2**

Slow-twitch muscle fibers contract at a slow rate and are usually red in color. These fibers generate less force than fast-twitch muscle fibers but they are able to resist fatigue. For this reason, a muscle with many slow-twitch fibers has good endurance. Slow-twitch fibers are also involved in cardiovascular activities such as running for distance. **Fast-twitch muscle fibers** contract quickly and are white in color. They generate more force when they contract, and for this reason muscles with many fast-twitch fibers are important for strength activities. **Intermediate muscle fibers** have characteristics of both slow- and fast-twitch fibers. They contract quickly and have good endurance. You use them for activities involving both strength and cardiovascular fitness. The types of fibers in your muscles are determined by your genes; however, you can increase the strength and endurance of your muscles with proper training.

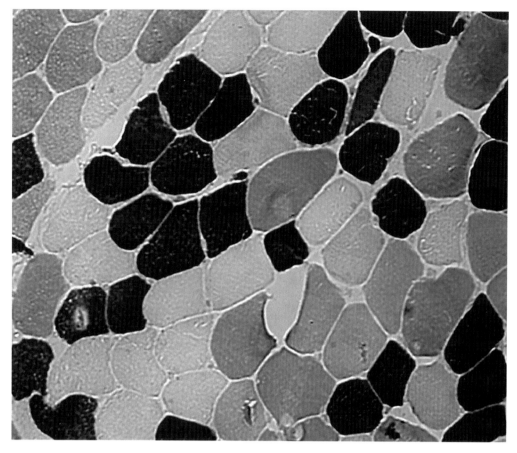

A photomicrograph that shows slow-twitch (black) and fast-twitch (gray and white) muscle fibers.
Reprinted with permission from J.H. Wilmore and D.L. Costill, 2004, **Physiology of sport and exercise, 3rd ed, (Champaign, IL: Human Kinetics), p. 45.**

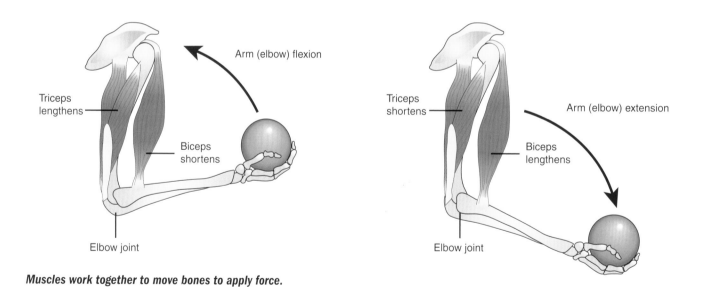

Muscles work together to move bones to apply force.

FIT FACTS

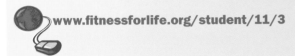

Birds, like humans, have both fast-twitch and slow-twitch muscle fibers. The flying muscles (breast muscles) of a duck or a goose are dark in color because they contain many slow-twitch fibers (typically red in color). The breast of a chicken is made up of mostly fast-twitch fibers (typically white in color) because the chicken needs power to fly up a few feet onto a perch; chickens typically do not fly long distances. For this reason, the breast of a chicken is mostly white meat while the wing muscles have more dark meat.

www.fitnessforlife.org/student/11/3

Resistance Exercise: Training Method or Sport?

Training is another term often used for exercise, especially for exercises used to build muscle fitness. For example, the term *weight training* is used to describe using weights to perform PRE. A difference exists between training done to improve muscle fitness and activities such as weightlifting.

Weight Training

This form of exercise is done to improve muscular strength and endurance. It can be used by anyone to improve health and fitness. It can also be used for those interested in improving performance for sports or for meeting job requirements. Weight training is not a competitive event.

Resistance Training

This type of training is the same as weight training except that a machine that provides resistance is used rather than weights.

Circuit Training

Circuit training has been described previously. It can be done to improve many different kinds of fitness such as flexibility and cardiovascular fitness. The circuit training exercises at the end of this chapter include PRE exercises designed to build muscle fitness. Other exercise circuits that build muscle fitness are included in chapters 12, 13, and 15.

Weightlifting

This is an Olympic sport involving the use of free weights; the athletes try to lift a maximum load. There are only two exercises in weightlifting: the snatch, and the clean and jerk.

Powerlifting

This is another competitive sport using free weights. There are only three exercises in powerlifting: the bench press, the squat, and the deadlift. The athletes try to make one maximal lift for each type of lift.

Bodybuilding

This sport can also be done competitively. The athletes are primarily concerned about the appearance of their bodies. They are judged based on how large and well defined their muscles are rather than how much they can lift. They train with more repetitions than weightlifters and powerlifters.

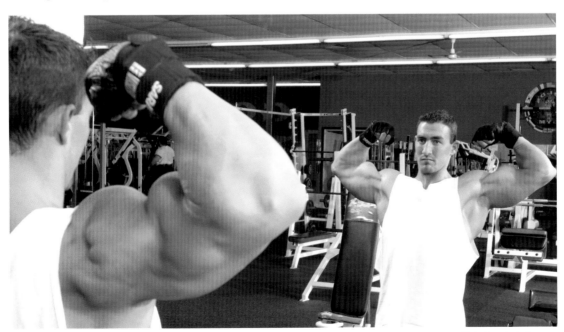

The sport of bodybuilding can be done competitively. The athletes are judged based on how large and well defined their muscles are rather than how much they can lift.

Muscle Fitness Assessment

You can assess muscle fitness in many ways. A **one repetition maximum (1RM)** test is considered to be the best test for strength. A true 1RM test requires a person to determine the amount of weight that can be lifted or resistance that can be overcome in one repetition. For example, if a person could lift 100 pounds once, but not twice, 100 pounds would be the 1RM for the muscle group being tested. The 1RM test results can be used in several ways. First, the results give you a good idea of your strength. Second, the assessment can be performed for each of the major muscle groups of the body. Finally, 1RM results can be used to determine how much weight or resistance you should use when performing the exercises shown later in this chapter.

The true 1RM test is commonly used by athletes and adults, but most experts recommend that a modified self-assessment be used by teens. The modified 1RM self-assessment provides a good estimate of true 1RM and does not require the lifting of maximal weight or the use of maximal resistance. Teens are advised to use only a percentage of 1RM both in testing strength and performing strength exercises. In the self-assessment in this chapter you will perform the modified 1RM test that uses multiple repetitions or lower than maximal weight (resistance) to estimate 1RM. This self-assessment is safe for teens when performed properly. You can do a 1RM test for many muscle groups, but two assessments, one for the upper body (arm press) and one for the lower body (leg press), are most often used. A dynamometer is often used to test isometric strength. You will learn more about these tests in the self-assessment for this chapter.

For muscular endurance, various exercises—often called **calisthenics**—are typically used for self-assessment. In these assessments the number of repetitions is counted. Examples include the push-up and curl-up. You will get the opportunity to try several self-assessments of muscular endurance in the next chapter.

Absolute Versus Relative Strength

Absolute strength is measured by how much weight or resistance you can overcome regardless of your body

FITNESS Technology

In recent years, tremendous technological advances have been made in resistance exercise machines. Innovations have included adjustable benches and chairs so that machines fit people of all sizes. Systems for changing resistance have made machines easier to use. Another innovation is isokinetic resistance machines. **Isokinetic exercise** is a type of isotonic exercise in which the velocity of movement is kept constant through the full range of motion. New isokinetic machines are now available. They use special hydraulics or electronics to regulate movement velocity and to allow full exertion at all angles of joint movement during an exercise. With traditional free weights or resistance machines, the resistance is often greater at the first part of a movement than at the end of the movement. Also, the speed of the movement may be greater at one point than another. Other advantages include extra safety and the advantage of building power, a part of fitness important to athletic performance. Isokinetic machines are often used by researchers and in rehabilitating injuries. Disadvantages are the expense of the machines and that many isokinetic machines do not allow eccentric contractions, which are often used in sports performances.

www.fitnessforlife.org/student/11/4

size. Big people typically have more absolute strength than smaller people. On average males are larger than females, so the average absolute strength for males is higher than for females. Your 1RM score is an example of absolute strength. **Relative strength** is strength adjusted for your body size. The most common method for determining relative strength is to divide your weight into your absolute strength score to get a "strength per pound of body weight" score. Relative strength scores are considered to be fairer assessments of strength for those who do not have large bodies. The ratings in the self-assessment in this chapter are for relative strength.

www.fitnessforlife.org/student/11/5

Lesson Review

1. What is the difference between strength and muscular endurance?
2. What are some of the health benefits of muscle fitness?
3. What are the various types of muscles and muscle fibers?
4. What are some of the methods of progressive resistance exercise used to improve muscle fitness?

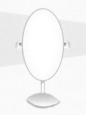

Self-Assessment

Determining Your Modified 1RM and Grip Strength

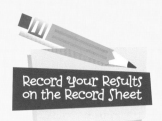

Record Your Results on the Record Sheet

PART 1: Estimating Your 1RM

As you know, 1RM means one repetition maximum. It represents the maximum weight a group of muscles can lift one time (or resistance they can overcome). Because beginners should begin gradually (without heavy lifting), a modified method has been developed that allows you to determine your 1RM without overexerting your muscles. The results you get will allow you to see how strong you are.

The modified 1RM can be done with free weights or machines, but the instructions that follow will be for machine use. Resistance machines are recommended for these self-assessments, especially for beginners, because they are safer. Two tests are used most often, and the ones performed in this self-assessment activity are for the upper body (arm press) and the lower body (leg press). If a person performing the arm press on a resistance machine can lift 50 pounds one time, but not more than one time, this number would represent the 1RM for the arm press. Similarly, if the person could move a resistance of 150 pounds one time with the leg press, but not more than one time, 150 would the 1RM for the leg press. As mentioned earlier in this chapter, 1RM scores for the arm press and leg press will be *estimated* to avoid maximal lifting, something that is discouraged for teens.

Follow these directions for each of the two self-assessments:

▶ Choose a weight (resistance) that you think you can lift 5 to 10 times but is too heavy for you to lift more than 10 times. Do not use a weight that you can lift fewer than 5 times.

▶ Using correct technique, lift the weight as many times as you possibly can. Count the number of lifts and write the number on your record sheet. If you were able to do more than 10 lifts, wait until another day before you try a heavier weight for that exercise. Go to the next muscle group exercise.

▶ If you can tell that you will not be able to lift the weight at least 5 times, stop and choose a lighter weight.

▶ If you were able to do 5 to 10 lifts and no more, then refer to table 11.1. Find the weight you lifted in the left-hand column. Now find the number of reps you did in the top row. Your 1RM score is the number in the box where the horizontal weight row and the vertical rep column intersect.

▶ Divide each of the two 1RM scores by your body weight to get a strength per pound of body weight score. The strength per pound of body weight score adjusts for body size (relative strength). For example, a person weighing 150 pounds and has a 1RM of 100 pounds on the arm press has a score of .67 pounds per pound of body weight. Use tables 11.2 and 11.3 to determine your fitness rating. Fitness ratings are only determined for the arm and leg press.

▶ If time allows, perform this procedure to determine your 1RM for other exercises included in the activity at the end of this chapter. Do the 1RM self-assessment for as many exercises as time allows. You do not need to determine a strength per pound of body weight score for these exercises. Use the 1RM scores to help you determine how much resistance to use for your PRE program.

Safety Tips: Proper form is essential for safety. Before you do the 1RM test, read the descriptions of the exercises and the directions that follow. Before performing the assessment, practice each of the two exercises and have a teacher check your form. During the assessment, have a partner spot you and follow the resistance training guidelines on page 189.

Table 11.1

Predicted 1RM Based on Reps to Fatigue

Weight	Repetitions						Weight	Repetitions					
	5	6	7	8	9	10		5	6	7	8	9	10
30	34	35	36	37	38	39	140	157	163	168	174	180	187
35	40	41	42	43	44	45	145	163	168	174	180	186	193
40	46	47	49	50	51	53	150	169	174	180	186	193	200
45	51	53	55	56	58	60	155	174	180	186	192	199	207
50	56	58	60	62	64	67	160	180	186	192	199	206	213
55	62	64	66	68	71	73	165	186	192	198	205	212	220
60	67	70	72	74	77	80	170	191	197	204	211	219	227
65	73	75	78	81	84	87	175	197	203	210	217	225	233
70	79	81	84	87	90	93	180	202	209	216	223	231	240
75	84	87	90	93	96	100	185	208	215	222	230	238	247
80	90	93	96	99	103	107	190	214	221	228	236	244	253
85	96	99	102	106	109	113	195	219	226	234	242	251	260
90	101	105	108	112	116	120	200	225	232	240	248	257	267
95	107	110	114	118	122	127	205	231	238	246	254	264	273
100	112	116	120	124	129	133	210	236	244	252	261	270	280
105	118	122	126	130	135	140	215	242	250	258	267	276	287
110	124	128	132	137	141	147	220	247	255	264	273	283	293
115	129	134	138	143	148	153	225	253	261	270	279	289	300
120	135	139	144	149	154	160	230	259	267	276	286	296	307
125	141	145	150	155	161	167	235	264	273	282	292	302	313
130	146	151	158	161	167	173	240	270	279	288	298	309	320
135	152	157	162	168	174	180	245	276	285	294	304	315	327

"Predicted 1RM Based on Reps to Fatigue". This chart is used as modified from the *Journal of Physical Education, Recreation, and Dance,* January 1993, page 89. JOPERD is a publication of the American Alliance for Health, Physical Education, Recreation and Dance, 1900 Association Drive, Reston, VA 22091.

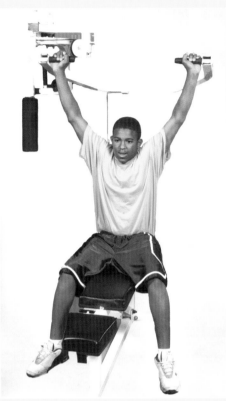

This test evaluates the strength of triceps and pectoral muscles.

Seated Arm Press

1. Sit on the stool of a seated press machine, the handles even with your shoulders. Grasp the handles with your palms facing away from you. Tighten your abdominal muscles.
2. Push upward on the handles, extending your arms until the elbows are straight.

 Caution: Do not arch your back. Do not lock your elbows.

3. Lower to the starting position.
4. If a seated press machine is not available, you can substitute the bench press. This exercise is described in the activity at the end of the chapter.

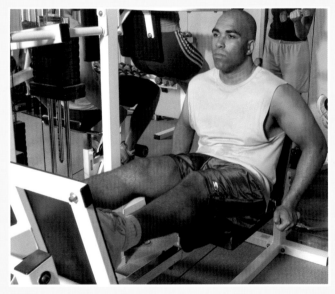

This test evaluates the strength of the quadriceps, the gluteals, and calf muscles.

Leg Press

1. Adjust the seat distance on a leg press machine for leg length comfort. The closer the seat, the greater the range for working and the greater the intensity. Sit with your feet resting on the pedal.
2. Push the pedal until your legs are straight.

 Caution: Do not lock your knees.

3. Slowly return to your starting position.

Table 11.2

Rating Chart: Arm Press (1RM)

	15 YEARS AND YOUNGER		15-17 YEARS OLD		18 YEARS AND OLDER	
	Males	Females	Males	Females	Males	Females
Good fitness	.80+	.60+	1.00+	.70+	1.10+	.85+
Marginal fitness	.67-79	.50-59	.75-.99	.60-69	.80-1.09	.67-.84
Low fitness	<.66	<.49	<.74	<.59	<.79	<.66

Table 11.3

Rating Chart: Leg Press (1RM)

	15 YEARS AND YOUNGER		15-17 YEARS OLD		18 YEARS AND OLDER	
	Males	Females	Males	Females	Males	Females
Good fitness	1.50+	1.10+	1.75+	1.30+	1.90+	1.40+
Marginal fitness	1.35-1.49	.95-1.09	1.50-1.74	1.10-1.29	1.65-1.89	1.30-1.39
Low fitness	<1.34	<.94	<1.49	<1.09	<1.64	<1.29

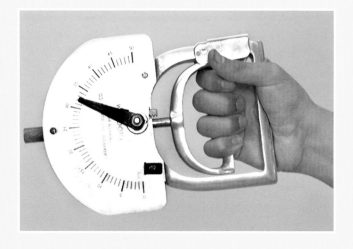

PART 2: Grip Strength

1. A dynamometer is a device used to measure isometric strength. There are many different types of dynamometers that vary in appearance. Learn to adjust the dynamometer used in this assessment to fit your hand size, if it is adjustable. Many dynamometers allow you to make the grip bigger or smaller by turning the grip handle.

2. Squeeze as hard as possible. You may not touch your body with your arm or hand, but you may bend or extend the elbow.

3. Record the best of two scores for each hand.

Write your scores on the record sheet and add them together. Look up your rating on table 11.4 and then record it.

Table 11.4

Rating Chart: Grip Strength

	15 YEARS AND YOUNGER		15-17 YEARS OLD		18 YEARS AND OLDER	
	Males	Females	Males	Females	Males	Females
Good fitness	191+	121+	226+	136+	253+	156+
Marginal fitness	158-190	99-120	191-225	114-135	209-252	116-155
Low fitness	<157	<98	<190	<113	<208	<115

Lesson 11.2

Building Strength

Lesson Objectives

After reading this lesson, you should be able to

1. Describe health and wellness benefits of strength.
2. Describe some myths about strength and tell why they are wrong.
3. Explain the FIT formula for developing strength.
4. Describe some basic guidelines for safe PRE.

Lesson Vocabulary

double progressive system (p. 187), muscle-bound (p. 187)

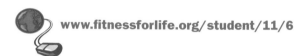

www.fitnessforlife.org/student/11/6

In this lesson you will learn about the benefits of strength, some common misconceptions about strength training, and how to apply the FIT formula for building strength using both isotonic and isometric exercises. Isotonic exercises using weights or resistance machines are considered to be best for building strength, but isotonic calisthenics and isometric exercises can also be effective when performed with enough intensity.

Health and Wellness Benefits

Strength is the amount of force a muscle can exert. If your muscles regularly work against heavy loads, they will stay strong. If you do not use your muscles, they become weak. Strong muscles help you jump, lift, push, and do activities of daily life. Strength enables you to work and play with less fatigue. Muscular strength can help prevent some health problems. For example, strong abdominal muscles can reduce the risk of backache. Exercises for muscle strength also strengthen bones and reduce the risk of osteoporosis (described in chapter 3). Osteoporosis occurs when bones become porous and weak. Resistance exercises that build strength are especially good for strengthening bone.

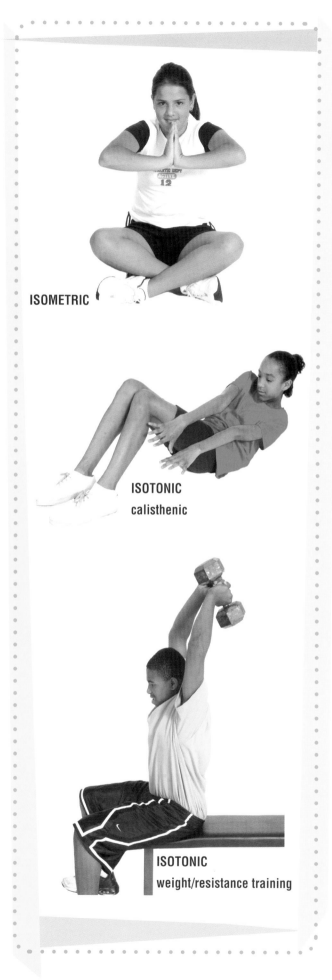

ISOMETRIC

ISOTONIC
calisthenic

ISOTONIC
weight/resistance training

Another benefit of strength is that it can help prevent muscle injuries and muscle soreness. Strong muscles can help you look your best and give your body a firm appearance. Muscles also burn more calories than fat does, so having strong and fit muscles can help in fat control. Strong muscles also help you maintain good posture.

Strength for Preteens and Teens

Until recently, experts felt that muscle fitness exercises such as those done in weight training were inappropriate for preteens and teens. Recent evidence suggests that, when done properly, PRE can have health benefits for teens similar to those for adults. Still, concerns exist about doing too much PRE too soon, especially for some people.

We know that for preteens and young teens, the body does not produce enough hormones to allow the body to build big muscles (hypertrophy), even with PRE. For these people, PRE can result in strength improvement but these improvements may not result in noticeable increases in muscle size. The strength gains are mostly because the body learns to use more muscle fibers when lifting rather than because of increases in muscle size. Placing emphasis on PRE may be discouraging for many teens because even if they give a lot of effort they may not see many benefits. This is especially true if the goal is to build big muscles. Even older teens who are late developers may have difficulty building large muscle until they get older.

The American College of Sports Medicine (ACSM) and other groups (see address by the Web icon in the FitFact) recommend a program involving moderate resistance that builds both strength and muscular endurance if the goal is to improve health. This program is effective for teens of both sexes. A program recommended for most teens, especially those just beginning PRE, is described later in this chapter. Those who intend to perform sports that require strength and power and who have experience in PRE can choose a program of greater intensity when done under the supervision of a qualified teacher or coach. Programs for teenagers should be designed especially for their age group. Teens are encouraged to avoid seeking advice from people who are unknown to them including people who have a good physique, or figure. Just because a person has a body that looks strong does not mean that he or she uses healthy exercise practices. In fact, many violate sound exercise guidelines and more than a few use unhealthy supplements.

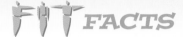

In addition to the ACSM, several other groups of experts have now prepared statements indicating that resistance training can be safe for teens when performed properly. Some of the groups include the American Academy of Pediatrics (medical doctors who specialize in youth) and the American Orthopaedic Society of Sports Medicine (medical doctors who specialize in bone problems associated with sports and activity). Self-assessments and muscle fitness exercises as described in this book follow guidelines outlined by these organizations.

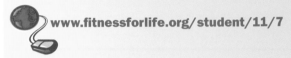

www.fitnessforlife.org/student/11/7

Myths and Misconceptions

The amount of strength you need to stay healthy and to do what you want depends on your own personal needs and interests. For example, people who have jobs requiring a lot of lifting need more strength than people who work at a desk. Despite the fact that muscle fitness exercise has many benefits, many people still hold misconceptions about them.

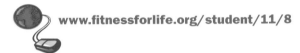

www.fitnessforlife.org/student/11/8

No Pain, No Gain

Some people still cling to the myth that exercise must hurt if it is going to result in improvement. Some of the worst offenders are people who are hooked on strength-building exercises. In fact, you should listen to your body. If you feel pain, it is your body's way of telling you that it is hurting. When doing PRE, it is true that you will become quite fatigued and feel a sensation sometimes called the exercise burn. It is important to learn the difference between this feeling and pain. If in doubt, it is best to back off to avoid injury.

Body Dysmorphia

Body dysmorphia is a term used to identify a condition that occurs when people become obsessed with building muscle. This psychological disorder, sometimes referred to as reverse anorexia, often begins with reasonable amounts of exercise to build muscle fitness. At some point those with this problem get carried away wanting to build more and more muscle. The disorder is an obsessive-compulsive disorder and often requires treatment by a professional. In more than a few cases, people with this disorder do unhealthy behaviors such as taking drugs or doing unhealthy exercises. Injury rates are high among people with this condition. Doing reasonable PRE can enhance health. Becoming obsessed with fitness can lead to unhealthy conditions.

Muscle Fitness for Females

Some people think that only males need to be concerned about their strength. This notion is false. Both males and females need strength to be healthy, to avoid injury, to look good, and to save themselves or others in an emergency.

Some girls and women fear that strength training will cause their bodies to look masculine. However, the hormones in female bodies prevent them from developing large, bulky muscles even when their exercise amounts are similar to those described in this book. Women and girls who perform strength exercises do develop strong muscles. Both men and women look more attractive with strong muscles because they are more likely to have good posture and firm bodies. Building good strength can help build your self-confidence as well.

Muscle-Bound

Some people think that strength training will cause them to be **muscle-bound**—that is, to have tight, bulky muscles that prevent them from moving freely. It is not resistance training, but rather incorrect training, that causes inflexibility. Training muscles only on one side of a joint or failing to stretch muscles are two examples of incorrect exercise that can cause a muscle-bound condition. Another example of incorrect training is failure to move your joints through their full range of motion when you lift weights or do other resistance exercises. For example, your elbow joint can bend to allow your hand to reach your shoulder and to let your arm straighten completely. When you do a biceps curl with weights, bring the weight all the way to the shoulder, then straighten the elbow each time you lower the weight. *Caution: Do not bend your elbow or any other joint backward beyond a full range of motion. You can damage the joint if you move it in a way that it was not designed to move.*

Fitness Principles and Strength

The three basic fitness principles can be applied to strength exercises. You have read about these principles—overload, progression, and specificity—in previous chapters.

Principle of Overload

A muscle must contract harder than normal to become stronger. In other words, the muscles must work against a greater load than they normally have in regular daily activity. Experts say a muscle must be contracted to at least 60 percent of 1RM if it is going increase strength. Less than 60 percent will build muscle fitness but will build a combination of strength and muscular endurance.

Principle of Progression

Overload gradually—increase the load over a period of time—to get the best improvement in muscle strength. You can injure yourself if you try to lift too much weight too soon. Also, lifting too much weight will not result in as much strength gain as would occur if you progressed gradually. To progress, you must continue increasing the resistance until you are as strong as you want to be. The concept of progressive resistance exercise is based on the principles of overload and progression.

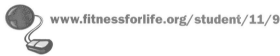

www.fitnessforlife.org/student/11/9

The **double progressive system** is the most often used method of applying the principle of progression for improving muscle fitness. In this system, you begin by performing a low number of repetitions (reps) in each set. As you improve, you gradually increase the number of reps you perform in a set. This part is the first progression. When exercising to build strength, you stop increasing reps when you reach 10. You drop back to doing a lower number of reps and increase weight or resistance. The gradual increase in weight or resistance is the second progression (double progression). You can use this system when performing your personal PRE program.

When you add resistance after lowering repetitions, it is recommended that you increase 5 to 10 percent. For teens this increase will typically be 2 to 5 pounds. You can use this information when you apply the FIT formula later in this chapter.

Principle of Specificity

You must exercise the specific muscles you wish to develop. If you wish to strengthen the muscles on the back of the thigh, you must specifically overload the particular group of muscles, called the hamstrings, by doing an exercise such as one involving knee flexion. The ACSM suggests that you perform 8 to 10 exercises to build each of the specific muscle groups in the body.

In the activity at the end of this chapter, basic exercises are presented for building 10 basic exercises (called the Basic 10).

The principle of specificity also means that you should do some strength exercises resembling the movement that you want to eventually use. For example, to strengthen the arm, a baseball pitcher might make a pitching motion against an elastic band.

Principle of Rest and Recovery

Although not discussed in earlier chapters, an additional principle is important for strength. The principle of rest and recovery indicates that you need to allow muscles time to rest and recover after a workout. For this reason, you should allow at least a day between strength workouts. This is why strength exercises are typically performed two to three days a week. Because you need to perform 8 to 10 exercises to build all of the important muscles of the body, some people choose to workout every day but do different exercises on different days. Many choose to do four or five upper body exercises one day and four or five lower body exercises the next.

The FIT Formula and Strength

For pure strength development, low repetitions and high weight or resistance produces best results. To improve strength, adults may use a resistance of 60 to 90 percent of their 1RM and perform as few as 3 reps per set. For teens, except in exceptional cases, experts recommend lower resistance and more reps (see table 11.5). The program for teens outlined in this chapter, including the program for younger teens, builds both parts of muscle fitness, strength and endurance, and is consistent with the ACSM guidelines for developing the health benefits associated with PRE.

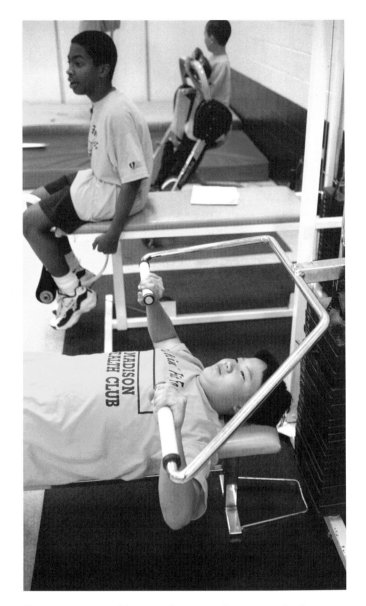

Experts recommend lower resistance and more reps for teens.

Table 11.5

Fitness Target Zones for Strength

	Isotonic Exercise	Isometric Exercise
Frequency	**Teens 13-14 and older teen beginners:** 2 days/wk on non-consecutive days **Older teens and adults:** 2-3 days/wk on non-consecutive days	Non-consecutive days; 2+ days/wk
Intensity	**Teens 13-14 and older teen beginners:** 40-60% 1RM or resistance allowing 10+ reps **Older teens:** 40-80% 1RM or resistance allowing 8+ reps* **Adults:** 60-90% 1RM or resistance allowing 3+ reps	Contract the muscle as tightly as possible for the required length of time.
Time	**Teens 13-14 and older teen beginners:** 1 set of 10-15 reps **Older teens:** 1 or 2 sets of 8-12 reps **Adults and adult athletes:** 1-3 sets of 3 to 8 reps For all groups rest between sets 1 to 2 min.	Hold the contraction for 7-10 sec. Rest for 1+ min. This is 1 set. Do 2+ sets.

* Older teens and experienced athletes may train using lower repetitions after consulting with a qualified teacher or coach.

It is easy to tell what percentage of your 1RM you are using when doing isotonic weight and resistance training, but it is more difficult to determine how much you are doing when you perform isometrics or calisthenics. For isometrics you simply contract the muscles as hard as you can for each exercise. Some calisthenics cannot provide enough overload to build strength, especially for strong people. Calisthenics are most effective for building muscular endurance and will be discussed in more detail in the next chapter.

Resistance Training Guidelines

When performed correctly resistance training is safe and will lead to improvement in your muscle fitness and physique. Follow these safety guidelines created especially for teens:

▶ **Use the three S method.** Use slow, smooth, and steady movements. Constantly remind yourself to take several seconds to make each movement. Stop at both ends of the movement. Avoid quick, sudden movements.

▶ **Exercise through a full range of motion.** For example, when doing the biceps curl, lift the weight all the way up and lower it all the way down.

▶ **Always use spotters when working with free weights.** You might be tempted to work on your own, but having a partner is much safer.

▶ **Start with a moderate program.** As you improve, increase the difficulty and keep working your way up.

▶ **Do not hold your breath when you lift.** Holding your breath can cause you to black out. Some resistance

trainers recommend exhaling on the lift and inhaling on the return movement.

▶ **Avoid overhead lifts with free weights.** If possible, use machines for these lifts. If you must use free weights, have a partner with you.

▶ **Avoid positions that cause the lower back to arch or the wrists to bend backward.** These positions can cause injuries and are not optimal for building strength.

▶ **Never use weights carelessly.** Concentrate on your technique and on what you are doing.

▶ **Never compete when you do resistance training.** For example, do not have a contest to see who can lift the most weight. Genetic differences have a lot to do with how strong a person can be. You need only be concerned with trying to improve your strength gradually and enjoying the exercise, not lifting more than someone else.

Resistance Machines Versus Free Weights

Throughout this book a wide variety of exercises are presented. Some involve free weights, some require machines, and some require no equipment at all. You are encouraged to consider resistance exercises such as calisthenics, elastic bands, or isometrics because they can be done at home without expensive equipment. You may also want to consider the advantages and disadvantages of resistance machines and free weights before making a choice of which to use. Table 11.6 provides a summary of the characteristics of both exercise methods.

Table 11.6

Resistance Machines Versus Free Weights

	Resistance Machines	Free Weights
Safety	· They are safer because weights cannot fall on the lifter. · A spotter is often not needed.	· You have a greater chance of injury from falling weights. · You can easily lose control of the weights, so you need a spotter.
Cost	· They are very expensive to own. · If you do not own the machines, you must join a club to use them.	· They are relatively inexpensive.
Versatility	· They can easily isolate specific muscle groups.	· Using them requires more balance, muscle coordination, and concentration. · You use more muscles, and the movements are more like moving heavy loads in daily life.
Convenience	· They require a lot of floor space. · You must go to where they are.	· They take up little space. · Some weights are small enough to be carried around. · They can easily scatter and get lost or stolen.

Taking Charge: Preventing Relapse

Anyone can begin a program to increase physical fitness. However, just beginning a program is not enough. Some people are active for a while and then drop out for a while. This behavior is called a relapse. Those who stay active all of their lives learn how to avoid relapses that can lead to becoming a couch potato.

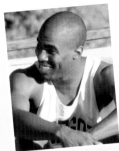

Luis missed his old school, especially his old friends. Now he usually came straight home after school instead of heading for the neighborhood court to play a little three-on-three basketball with his buddies. For the first month after he moved, Luis ate dinner, did his homework, and then clicked on the television to fill the time.

Early one evening, his mom said, "Luis, why are you lying around? You like to be active. So get up and get moving!"

Luis yawned. "Where am I going to go? Who am I going to go with? I don't have any friends here."

"What about that boy who lives down the hall? I saw him leave with a gym bag the other day. He must have been going somewhere you'd like to go."

"Well, maybe," Luis said. "But maybe he was going to play handball or something like that—something I don't know how to do."

"And maybe he was going to play basketball, huh? And maybe it wouldn't kill you to learn how to play handball or another new sport, right?"

Luis smiled up at his mom. "Maybe. What's his apartment number?"

"3B—and while you're there, ask his mom whether she knows about any exercise classes around here for old people like me, okay?"

For Discussion

What caused Luis to have a relapse into inactivity? What could he do if it turns out that the boy down the hall likes to swim and hates basketball? What are some other things that cause relapses? What can be done to avoid them? Fill out the questionnaire supplied by your teacher to find out how you might respond if something begins to interfere with your level of physical activity. Consider the guidelines on page 191.

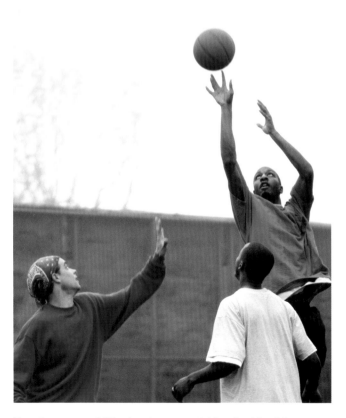

Even in a new neighborhood you can get involved in pick-up games by finding out who else plays and asking them where a game can be found.

Lesson Review

1. What are some of the health and wellness benefits of having good strength?
2. What are some myths about strength? Why they are wrong?
3. What types of exercises can you do to improve your strength? Should teens do something different than adults?
4. What is the FIT formula for strength?
5. What are six guidelines that teens should follow for resistance training?

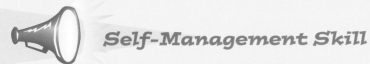

Self-Management Skill

Preventing Relapse

Relapse means that you stop doing something that you want to keep doing or think you should keep doing. For example, you might start a PRE program but stop doing it because you feel you can't take the time or for other reasons. Follow these guidelines to help you stick with something once you have started it:

▶ **Do a self-assessment.** It may help you see whether you are likely to stick with something and may give you ideas for how to stick with it if you have had problems in the past.

▶ **Use the information from the self-assessment to determine areas that can be improved.**

▶ **Write down your goals for doing the behavior.** Put them on the refrigerator or some place where you will see them every day. You have had good reasons to accomplish these goals or you would not have started to make a change in the first place. Keep focused on your goals.

▶ **Monitor your behavior by keeping a log or chart.** Use the log or chart to reinforce or reward yourself. Tell yourself that you have stuck with it so far and you can keep it up.

▶ **Tell other people what you are trying to accomplish.** Ask them to encourage you regularly.

▶ **Select a regular exercise time.** If you are trying to stick with exercise or another similar behavior, select a time of day and try to do the behavior at the same time every day.

▶ **Do not let one setback be a reason for a long-term relapse.** If you miss a day, tell yourself, "it is all right to take a day of once in a while." Repeat this saying to yourself periodically.

▶ **Consider a variety of activities.** For a behavior such as being physically active, consider trying different activities from time to time for variety.

Resolving Conflict: Developing and Enforcing Rules

Joining a health club or taking advantage of a school's weight room is a great way to build muscular fitness. However, encountering conflict during a workout is discouraging and may be a reason to avoid using weights and exercise machines. Problems have occurred in some exercise facilities, including failure to clean equipment after use, failure to put away weights, and extended use of equipment (staying on too long). Some people say they feel out of place in certain areas of the exercise room (such as the free weight area used by bodybuilders or athletes).

The best way to prevent relapse for those just beginning a muscular fitness program is to have clear rules that help all users feel comfortable and welcome. If your school or health club does not have clearly posted rules, you can ask the supervisor if you can help develop some rules. The following are some important steps in developing rules:

▶ Develop a committee with members that represent all users.

▶ Survey users to determine what conflicts currently exist.

▶ Develop preliminary rules (guidelines). Avoid having unnecessary rules. Focus on those that help avoid or resolve conflict, such as methods of keeping equipment clean (cleaning after use), time limits on machines, and putting away equipment after use. Some gyms have dress codes.

▶ Ask users for comments before finalizing preliminary rules.

▶ Post rules or disseminate them in other ways.

▶ Recommend ways to enforce the rules. If the exercise room or club has rules but they are not enforced, the committee may want to develop guidelines for enforcement.

The negotiating and discussion techniques described on page 147 may be useful for a committee that is developing or revising rules or guidelines for resolving conflict in an exercise room or health club.

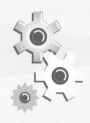

Fundamentals of Weight and Resistance Training

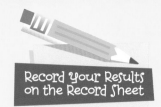

Record Your Results on the Record Sheet

This activity will introduce you to safe training with free weights. As you learned earlier in the chapter, free weights can be less safe than using resistance machines. But you can injure yourself using either free weights or resistance machines if you do not exercise properly. In this activity you will learn correct lifting and spotting techniques. Spotting is providing assistance to a partner by being prepared to catch the weight if the partner loses control of the weight or gets off balance.

Because the potential for injury is great, it is essential that you work through each of the mastery levels listed next. To keep track of your progress, an observer will check off your mastery of correct spotting and lifting techniques as well as your maturity and cooperation in assisting and giving coaching (feedback). Record your results on your record sheet. Warm up and stretch before beginning this activity.

▶ **Level 1 mastery: lifting technique, no weight.** Perform each exercise without any weights by using a wand or stick instead of a barbell. Concentrate on correct form (placement of body parts) when you are working. Give useful coaching when you are watching your partners.

▶ **Level 2 mastery: spotting technique, no weight.** While your partner performs the lift with the wand, you and another partner practice correct spotting technique. Pay particular attention to your leg and hand positions.

▶ **Level 3 mastery: lifting and spotting, light weights.** Perform each exercise using light weights, 5 lifts each. Practice your lifting and spotting techniques, and continue to give each other coaching on both lifting and spotting techniques.

▶ **Level 4 mastery: your normal workout using free weights.** Select the appropriate percentage of 1RM and the appropriate number of sets and repetitions (see table 11.5 on page 188). Perform each of the Basic 10 exercises. *Note: The same abdominal and back exercises as used with resistance machines are used for free weights.*

 www.fitnessforlife.org/student/11/10

Safety Tips:
▶ Make all moves slowly.
▶ Exhale on the lift; inhale on the return to starting position. Do not hold your breath.
▶ Handle all weights with care and awareness of the potential for serious injury.

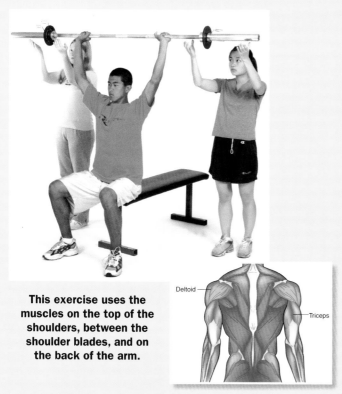

This exercise uses the muscles on the top of the shoulders, between the shoulder blades, and on the back of the arm.

Deltoid

Triceps

Seated Overhead Press

Weights: barbell, dumbbells

This exercise requires two spotters. Spotters stand by the lifter's shoulders on either side of bench. Keep your hands with the palms up under the bar. Be ready to take the bar if the lifter loses control, especially at the top of the lift if the barbell begins to move backward or if the lifter begins to tremble.

1. Sit on end of a bench in front stride (split-foot) position.
2. Hold the barbell at chest height in preparation for pushing the bar vertically. Grasp the barbell with your hands facing away from your body, hands slightly wider than your shoulders.
3. Tighten your abdominal, back, and arm muscles. Tip your head back slightly.
4. Push the bar straight up, directly overhead, keeping your arms perpendicular.
5. Lower the barbell to the starting position. Use the seated arm press exercise on the resistance machine (page 183) to determine your 1RM for this exercise.

 Caution: Do not let the bar go forward or backward. Do not lock your elbows. Do not arch your back.

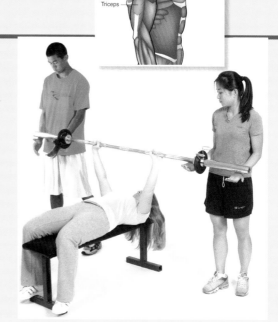

Pectoralis major

Triceps

This exercise uses the muscles on the front of the chest (pectoral) and the backs of the arms (triceps).

Bench Press

Weights: barbell, dumbbells

This exercise requires two spotters. Spotters stand by the lifter's shoulders on either side of bench. Place the bar in the hands of the lifter. Keep your hands with the palms up under bar. Be prepared to take it if the lifter loses control.

1. Lie on your back on a bench with your feet on floor, lower back flat. Extend your arms perpendicularly to the floor, into the up position.
2. Grasp the bar with a palms-up grip, hands slightly wider than shoulder-width, elbows straight, bar approximately over your collarbones.

 Caution: Do not lock your elbows.

3. Lower the bar until it touches your chest, even with a line just below your armpits. When the bar touches your chest, your forearms should be perpendicular to the floor and your elbows should point neither at your feet nor out to the sides but halfway in between (45 degrees).
4. Push the bar up to the starting position, arms perpendicular to the floor. The bar follows a slightly curved path.

 Caution: Do not bounce the bar off your chest. Do not arch your back or lift your hips. Keep your arms perpendicular to the floor. If the weight gets in front of or behind your arms, you will lose control and get pinned. Use the bench press on the resistance machine (page 236) to determine your 1RM for this exercise.

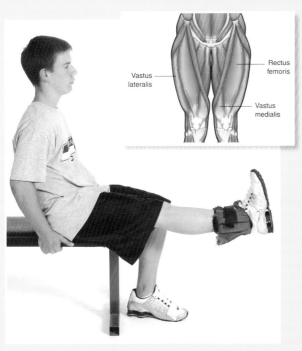

Knee Extension

Weights: weighted boot or ankle weight

One person can assist the lifter to put on the boot or ankle weight.

1. Put the weight on one foot or ankle. Sit on a bench, with your lower leg hanging over the edge. Grasp the bench with your hands.

2. Lift the weighted boot by extending your knee until your leg is straight.

 Caution: Do not lock knees when you extend and do not kick the leg upward–lift slowly.

3. Repeat the exercise on the other leg. Use the knee extension on the resistance machine (page 23) to determine your 1RM for this exercise.

This exercise uses the muscles on the top of the thigh (quadriceps).

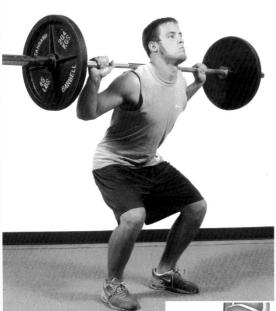

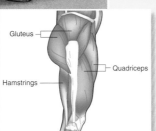

Half Squat

Weights: barbell, dumbbells

Note: This exercise can only be done if a squat rack is available.

1. Stand in a side-stride position with your feet shoulder-width apart or slightly wider, toes straight ahead or slightly turned out. Keep your head up and your back straight.

2. Hold the barbell across the back of your shoulders at the base of your neck, hands slightly wider than your shoulders, palms facing away from your body. Point your elbows toward the floor, and your forearms perpendicular to the floor.

3. Squat until your knees are at a right angle, then rise. Keep heels flat on floor. Do not let knees come ahead of the toes. Focus on a spot on the wall slightly higher than standing height. Remain looking at this spot for the duration of the lift, when lowering and straightening.

 Caution: Do not round the back. Do not lean too far forward at the hips or let knees get in front of toes. Do not squat too deeply. Use the leg press exercise on the resistance machine (page 183) to determine your 1RM for this exercise.

This exercise uses the muscles on the front of the thighs (quadriceps) and the buttocks muscles (gluteals).

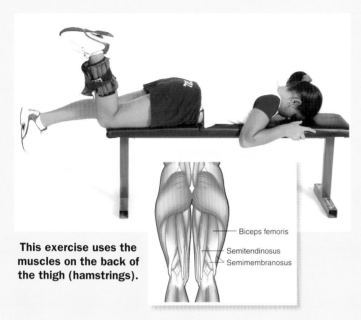

This exercise uses the muscles on the back of the thigh (hamstrings).

Biceps femoris
Semitendinosus
Semimembranosus

Hamstring Curl

Weights: weighted boot or ankle weight
    One person can assist the lifter to put on the boot or ankle weight.

1. Put the weight on one foot or ankle. Lie face-down on a bench, with your kneecaps hanging over the edge. Grasp the bench with your hands.
2. Lift the weighted boot by flexing your knee to a right angle.

 Caution: Do not lock knees when you extend.

3. Repeat the exercise on the other leg. Use the hamstring curl on the resistance machine (page 237) to determine your 1RM for this exercise.

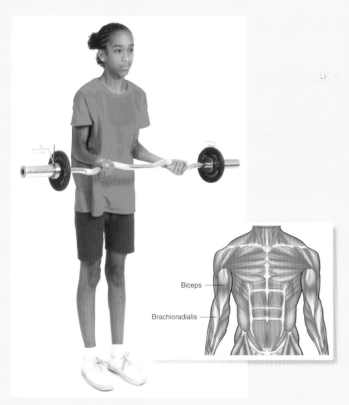

Biceps
Brachioradialis

This exercise uses the muscles on the front of the arm (biceps) and other elbow flexor muscles.

Biceps Curl

Weights: barbell, dumbbells
    Spotters are not required, but they can place the barbell in the lifter's palms-up hands.

1. Stand erect, feet in side-stride position. Tighten your abdominal and back muscles.
2. Grasp the bar with your palms up, hands slightly wider than your shoulders.
3. Keep your elbows close to your sides and lift the weight by bending your elbows only. Raise the weight to near your chin, then return.

 Caution: Do not move other joints, especially in the back.

4. You can repeat this exercise with your palms down to work the weaker elbow muscles. Use the biceps curl on the resistance machine (page 237) to determine your 1RM for this exercise.

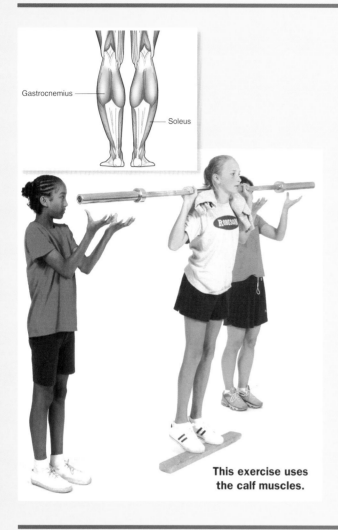

This exercise uses the calf muscles.

Heel Raise

Weights: barbell, dumbbells

This exercise requires two spotters. Spotters stand by the lifter's shoulders, one on each side.

1. Stand with the balls of your feet on a 2-inch board, toes turned in slightly.
2. Rise onto your toes, then lower to the starting position.

 Caution: Keep your spine straight.

3. Advanced lifters may also try toes out and toes straight ahead. Use the heel raise on the resistance machine (page 238) to determine your 1RM for this exercise.

Seated French Curl

Weights: dumbbell

This exercise requires one spotter.

1. Sit on the end of a bench with your arms extended overhead, palms facing up.
2. Hold one end of a dumbbell in both hands above and behind the head. Tighten your abdominal and back muscles. Slowly lower the weight toward the back of your neck until the arms are fully flexed at the elbows. Keep the elbows high.
3. Slowly return to the starting position, moving only the elbow joints. Use the triceps press (page 239) to determine your 1RM for this exercise.

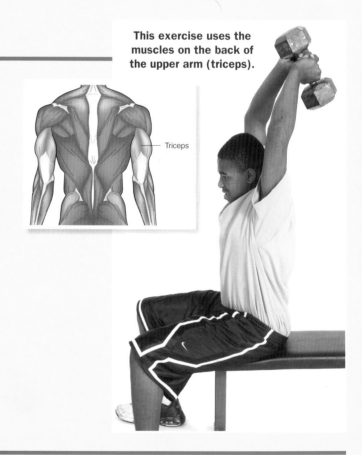

This exercise uses the muscles on the back of the upper arm (triceps).

196

Bent Over Dumbbell Row

Weights: Dumbbell
  This exercise requires no spotters.

1. Hold the dumbbell in one hand and rest the free hand on a bench to support the weight of your trunk and protect your back.
2. Pull the dumbbell upward until it touches the side of your chest near the armpit and the upper arm is horizontal with the floor.
3. Slowly lower the weight.
4. Repeat the exercise with other arm. Use the seated row (page 239) to determine 1RM for this exercise.

This exercise uses the biceps, the shoulder muscles, and the muscles between the shoulder blades.

Trapezius
Posterior deltoid
Biceps
Brachioradialis

Back Extension Exercise (Trunk Lift)

1. Lie facedown on a table (or bench). Slide forward until your upper body extends over the edge at the waist. With a partner holding your legs, allow the upper body to lower.
2. From the low position, lift your upper body until it is even with the edge of the table.

⚠️ **Caution:** Do not lift any higher.

3. Lower to the beginning position. Repeat the exercise up to 10 times.

Safety Tip: As you do these exercises, move only as far as the directions specify.

Erector spinae

This exercise uses the back muscles.

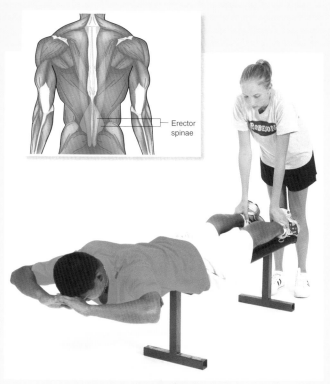

197

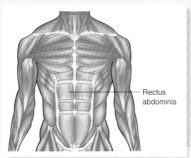

Rectus abdominis

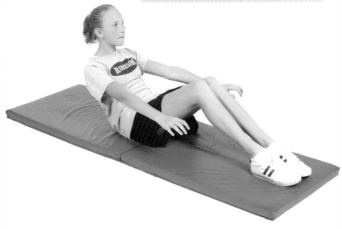

This exercise uses the abdominal muscles.

Abdominal Exercise (Curl-Up)

The curl-up, sometimes referred to as the crunch, is a good substitute for the straight-leg sit-up, bent-knee sit-up, and hands-behind-the-head sit-up.

1. Lie on your back with your knees bent and your feet close to your buttocks.
2. Hold your hands and arms straight in front of you and curl your head, shoulders, and upper back off the floor.
3. Slowly roll back to the starting position.

⚠️ **Caution:** Do not hold your feet while doing a trunk curl.

As you improve, you might hold your arms across your chest. When you become very good, you might place your hands on your face (cheeks).

11 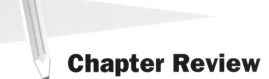 Chapter Review

Reviewing Concepts and Vocabulary

Number your paper from 1 to 4. Next to each number, write the word (or words) that correctly completes the sentence.

1. _____ is the amount of force a muscle can exert.
2. _____ refers to an increase in muscle fiber size.
3. A person can become _____ if he or she does strength training improperly by developing some muscles while ignoring others.
4. When you do calisthenics to develop strength, you use your body weight as the _____.

Number your paper from 5 to 10. Next to each number, choose the letter of the best answer.

Column I	Column II
5. isometric exercise	**a.** muscle fitness exercise that regulates velocity
6. weightlifting	**b.** the maximum amount of weight a group of muscles can lift one time
7. progressive resistance	**c.** exercises in which the muscles do not move
8. isokinetic exercise	**d.** muscle fitness exercises that involve movement
9. 1RM	**e.** the gradual increase of weight used in strength training
10. isotonic exercise	**f.** a sport, not a method of training

Number your paper from 11 to 15. On your paper, write a short answer for each statement or question.

11. How do strong muscles help you look better and prevent health problems?
12. Why can't preteens build as much muscle size as older teens?
13. Why should you assess your strength before you start a strength-training program?
14. Why should you gradually increase the amount of weight you use?
15. How often should you do your strength training program?

Thinking Critically

Click on the Web icon that provides additional information concerning muscle fitness myths (page 186). This Web site provides information about muscle fitness training for preteens and teens. It also leads you to the Web sites of the ACSM and the President's Council on Physical Fitness and Sports. Read some of the articles at these sites (on resistance training for preteens and teens) and write a short paper on the topic. Report your results to your class.

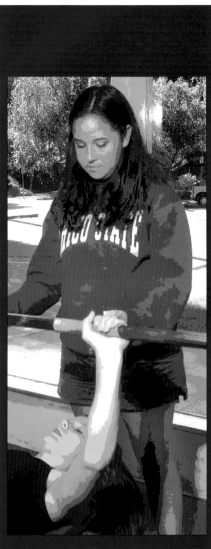

Project

Keep a record of your daily participation in resistance exercises for strength development for one week. Record the minutes of these exercises you do each day. How might you adjust your physical activity to better maintain or improve your strength? What short-term goals might you have for performing specific strength exercises each day? Make a written plan for the following week, incorporating changes that might help you reach your goals. Use the worksheets provided by your teacher.

12

Muscle Fitness: Muscular Endurance and General Muscle Fitness Information

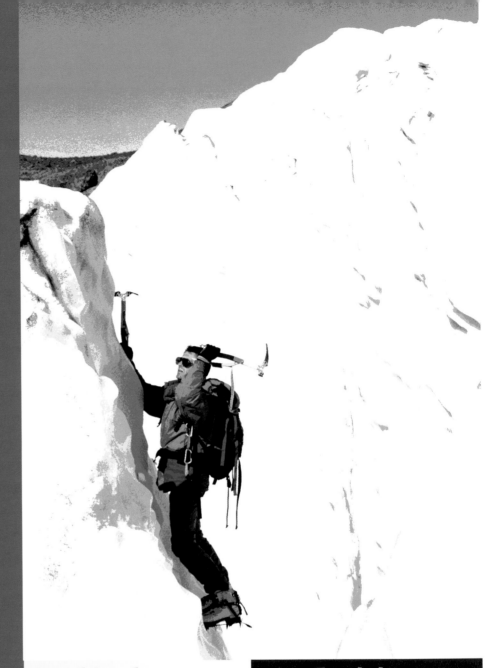

In this chapter...

Activity 1
Homemade Weights

Lesson 12.1
Improving Muscular Endurance

Self-Assessment
Muscular Endurance

Lesson 12.2
Muscle Fitness

Taking Charge
Managing Time

Self-Management Skill
Managing Time

Activity 2
Muscular Endurance Exercise Circuit

Activity 1

HOMEMADE WEIGHTS

In chapter 11 you learned how to properly perform free-weight exercises to build muscular endurance and strength. If your school has weights and keeps the weight room open for recreational use, you can perform weight training at school. Of course, you can buy weights or join a health club so that you have the equipment to do free-weight training, but either can be expensive. An alternative is to use homemade weights made of bottles filled with water and a broomstick or piece of plastic pipe. If done properly, this alternative can be a safe and inexpensive way to do free-weight training.

Improving Muscular Endurance

Lesson Objectives

After reading this lesson you should be able to

1. Describe the differences among muscular endurance, cardiovascular fitness, and muscular strength.
2. Describe benefits of good muscular endurance.
3. Explain the FIT formula for building muscular endurance.
4. Describe several guidelines for building muscular endurance.

Lesson Vocabulary

electromyogram (EMG) (p. 202)

 www.fitnessforlife.org/student/12/1

In this lesson, you will learn about muscular endurance and how it improves your health and affects your life. You will also learn about the FIT formula for building muscular endurance.

In the last chapter you learned that muscular endurance, one part of muscle fitness, is different from strength, the other part of muscle fitness. It is also important to know the difference between cardiovascular fitness and muscular endurance.

Muscular Endurance Versus Cardiovascular Fitness

Cardiovascular fitness is the ability of the heart, lungs, and blood vessels to function efficiently during vigorous activity. The cyclist in the first picture needs good cardiovascular fitness to ride for a long time. Cardiovascular fitness is dependent on the heart and blood vessels to deliver blood. It is very general in nature rather than specific to one area of the body as is the case for muscle fitness. Good cardiovascular fitness allows the entire body to function.

Muscular endurance is the ability to contract muscles many times without tiring or to hold one contraction for a long time. Muscular endurance is dependent on the ability of your muscle fibers to keep working with-

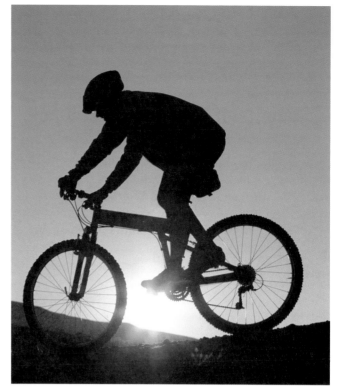

Cardiovascular fitness.

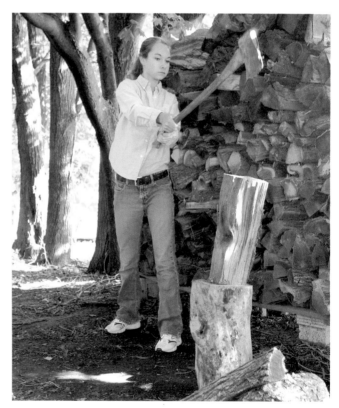

Muscular endurance.

out getting tired. You can have good muscular endurance in one part of the body, such as the legs, without having good muscular endurance in another part of the body, such as the arms. The person in the second picture needs good muscular endurance to be able to chop wood. If she has not developed good muscular endurance in the arms, she will not be able to continue chopping for a very long time even if she has good cardiovascular endurance.

Benefits of Muscular Endurance

Muscular endurance exercise improves appearance, fitness, and physical and mental health. Good muscular endurance enables people to work longer without getting tired. Those with good muscular endurance find it easier to maintain good posture. In addition, they are less likely to have backaches, muscle soreness, and muscle injuries.

Muscular endurance training also increases your lean body mass and decreases fat. This improvement in body composition can help you look and feel better. Muscular endurance developed through physical activity decreases heart rate, helping reduce the risks of cardiovascular disease. Resistance training, whether done for endurance or strength, also strengthens your bones.

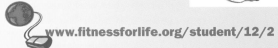

Many teens wear backpacks. To carry a backpack effectively, you need adequate strength and muscular endurance. In a typical year the U.S. Consumer Product Safety Commission reports more than 6,000 backpack related injuries, mostly to youth. In addition to improving your muscle fitness, you can do several things to reduce your risk of injury from wearing a backpack (see photo).

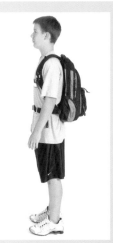

www.fitnessforlife.org/student/12/2

FIT Formula for Muscular Endurance

The frequency, intensity, and time recommended for muscular endurance are shown in table 12.1. You may either do calisthenics, in which you lift the weight of your body parts, or work against the resistance of weights or machines. These kinds of exercises involve isotonic muscle contractions.

It is also possible to build muscular endurance using isometric contractions. In life you have to contract posture muscles for long periods during the day. When holding things, such as a serving tray, you need extended isometric contractions. In general, however, performing isometric exercises should help you perform most isotonic exercise that you will encounter in daily life. Also it is hard to get motivated to hold isometric contractions for extended periods of time. For these reasons only isotonic exercise is included in the table. Isometric contractions can be used successfully to test your muscular endurance because it is not hard to get motivated to do one repetition and you can easily see how well you have performed. The trunk lift you performed in the self-assessment for chapter 5 is an example.

Muscular endurance exercises can be done more frequently than strength exercises. Strength exercises are typically done only 2 to 3 times a week. Muscular endurance exercises can be done on most days of the week because they do not require maximal contractions. Like cardiovascular fitness exercise, it is probably best to take at least one day a week off from exercise. Because the resistance is lower than for strength, multiple sets of muscular endurance exercises are often performed.

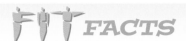

The **electromyogram (EMG)** is a machine researchers use to determine how hard a muscle contracts. Small contractions such as those for muscular endurance show a low muscle action wave, and harder contractions such as those for strength show a larger muscle action wave.

Table 12.1

Muscular Endurance Target Zones (Isotonic)

	Threshold	Target zone
Frequency	3 days/wk	3-6 days/wk
Intensity	20% 1RM	20-55% of 1RM
Time	1 set of 11-25 reps for each exercise	1-3 sets of 11-25 reps for each exercise

Rest 2 minutes between sets.

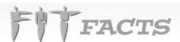

Rather than doing more than 25 repetitions of an exercise in one set, several sets of 25 repetitions or less is recommended. When people perform calisthenics with more than 25 repetitions in a set, they often perform the exercises incorrectly.

Circuit Training Programs for Muscular Endurance

Muscular endurance programs include calisthenics and resistance training. Sports, active aerobics, and active recreation are also good for developing muscular endurance. You learned about circuit training earlier. It is included again here because it is one of the most popular forms of muscular endurance training. You can easily do a muscular endurance circuit with little or no equipment or with expensive machines. As explained in chapter 8, circuit training involves moving from one exercise station to another with short breaks for changing stations. At each station, you perform a different exercise using the FIT formula described earlier. Many different exercise circuits are provided in this book, including one emphasizing muscular endurance at the end of this chapter. Later you will get the opportunity to develop your own circuit training program.

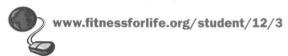

www.fitnessforlife.org/student/12/3

Guidelines for Muscular Endurance Exercise

To avoid injury and increase your enjoyment of the activities, follow these guidelines when exercising for muscular endurance:

▶ **Always warm up and stretch gently before exercising.**

▶ **Breathe normally while exercising.** Holding your breath may cause an abdominal hernia or cause you to black out.

▶ **Start with low-intensity exercises and progress slowly.** Too many reps and sets too soon will cause muscular soreness and slow your progress.

▶ **Use good body mechanics and correct technique.** To work a specific set of muscles, the movement must be done exactly right or you may actually be working the wrong set of muscles or straining other body parts.

▶ **Take your time and work rhythmically.**

▶ **Always move through a full range of motion.** This will prevent loss of flexibility. (See chapter 10 for more on flexibility and range of motion.)

▶ **Avoid working the same muscles in two consecutive exercises.**

▶ **Exercise each specific muscle group.** If you do not know how to isolate a specific muscle, ask your instructor about it. Most people tend to exercise their chest (pectoral), biceps, and other muscles on the front of the body, while neglecting the muscles on the back. Include exercises for the triceps on the backs of your arms, the hamstrings on the backs of your legs, and the muscles between your shoulder blades.

▶ **Vary your exercise routine to avoid boredom.** Many ways exist to exercise the same muscles effectively.

▶ **Consider multiple sets.** Good muscular endurance is best achieved by doing multiple sets rather than doing one set of repetitions to exhaustion.

Lesson Review
1. What are the differences among muscular endurance, cardiovascular fitness, and muscular strength?
2. What are the benefits of good muscular endurance?
3. What is the FIT formula for muscular endurance?
4. What are some of the guidelines for performing muscular endurance exercises?

FITNESS Technology

In recent years high-tech physical fitness tests that were formerly only available in laboratories have become available in schools and fitness centers. One assessment system (called TriFit) can be used to test multiple parts of fitness including blood pressure, flexibility, body composition, cardiovascular fitness, and muscle fitness. If your school has a high-tech system such as TriFit, you can use it to test various aspects of fitness to compare against your self-assessments done in this book. It is important to learn self-assessments that you can do at home in addition to high-tech tests because you can do self-assessments at home even when high-tech equipment is not available.

Muscular Endurance

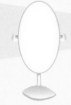

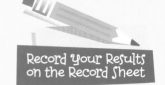
Record Your Results on the Record Sheet

Many tests can help you evaluate your muscular endurance, but the best ones assess your body's large muscles. In this self-assessment you will perform some isotonic and some isometric tests. To evaluate your muscular endurance, follow these directions:

▶ Warm up before doing these assessment activities.

▶ Write on your record sheet the number of times you complete each test. Check "yes" if you could do the test as long or as many times as indicated. Check "no" if you could not. If you cannot pass all the tests, you need to work on muscular endurance.

▶ Look up your rating on table 12.2 and write your rating on your record sheet.

Table 12.2

Rating Chart: Muscular Endurance

Fitness rating	Number of tests passed
Good	5
Marginal	3 or 4
Low	<3

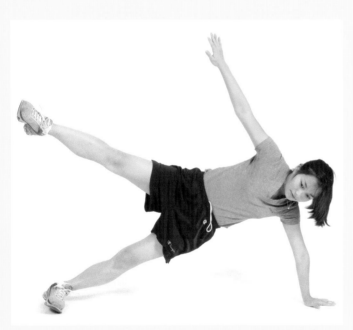

This test evaluates the isometric muscular endurance of some of the leg and arm muscles as well as trunk stabilizing muscles.

Side Stand (Isometric)

1. Lie on your side.
2. Use both hands to get your body in position so that it is supported by your left hand and the side of your left foot. Keep your body stiff.
3. Raise your right arm and leg in the air. Hold this position.
4. Return to the starting position and repeat the test on the right side. Pass (males) = hold the position for 30 seconds on each side. Pass (females) = hold the position for 20 seconds on each side.

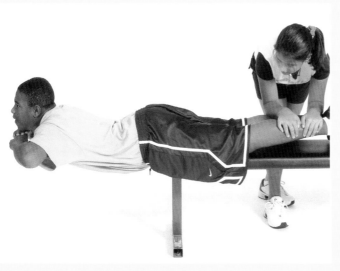

This test evaluates the isotonic muscular endurance of the upper back muscles.

Trunk Extension (Isotonic)

1. Lie facedown on a stable weight bench or the end of a bleacher that is 15 to 20 inches high. The top of your hips should be even with the end of the bench, and the upper body should hang off the end of the bench. If the surface is hard, cover it with a mat or a towel.

2. Have a partner hold your calves using one hand on each leg 12 inches above the ankles. Overlap your hands and place them (palms away) in front of your chin.

3. Start with your upper body bent at the hip so that the chin is near the floor with the palm of your lower hand against the floor. Place a small mat on the floor below the hands and chin.

4. Keeping your head and neck in line with your upper body, slowly lift your head and upper body off the floor until the upper body is in line with your lower body.

 Caution: Do not to lift the upper trunk higher than horizontal (in line with lower body).

5. Lower to the starting position so that the palm of the lower hand touches the floor.

6. Perform one lift every 3 seconds. You may want to have a partner say "up-down" to help you. Pass (males) = 20 repetitions. Pass (females) = 15 repetitions.

Sitting Tuck (Isotonic)

1. Sit on the floor with your knees bent and arms outstretched.

2. Lean back and balance on your hips. Keep your knees bent near your chest (feet off the floor).

3. Straighten your knees so the body forms a V. You may move your arms sideways for balance.

4. Bend your knees to your chest again. Repeat the exercise as many times as you can. Count each time you push your legs out. Pass (males) = 25 repetitions. Pass (females) = 20 repetitions.

Safety Tip: Avoid arching your lower back repetitively to avoid straining or pulling the muscles in that area.

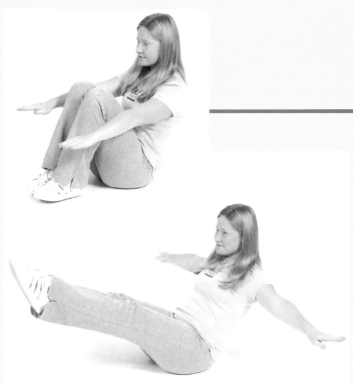

This test evaluates the isotonic muscular endurance of the abdominal muscles and some of the hip and leg muscles.

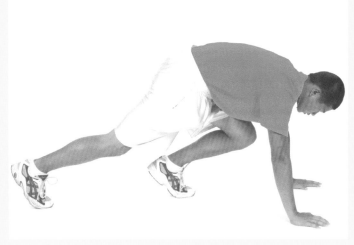

Leg Change (Isotonic)

1. Assume a push-up position with weight on your hands and feet.
2. Pull your right knee under your chest, and keep the left leg straight.
3. Change legs by pulling your left leg forward and pushing your right leg back.

 Caution: Do not let your lower back sag.

4. Continue changing legs.
5. Repeat this exercise for 1 minute and count the number of leg changes. Pass = 25 changes.

This test evaluates the isotonic muscular endurance of the hip and leg muscles.

Bent Arm Hang (Isometric)

1. Hang from a chinning bar with your palms facing away from your body.
2. You may stand on a chair or with the help of a partner, lift your chin above the bar.
3. On a signal, the partner will let go or remove the chair. Count how long you can hang. The time begins when the chair is removed and ends when the chin touches or goes below the bar, or the head tilts backward. Pass (males) = hold for 16 seconds. Pass (females) = hold for 12 seconds.

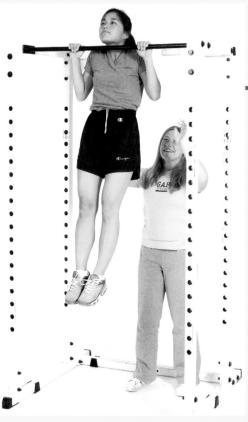

This test evaluates the isometric muscular endurance of the arm, shoulder, and chest muscles.

Lesson 12.2

Muscle Fitness

Lesson Objectives

After reading this lesson, you should be able to

1. Describe some methods of doing inexpensive PRE for health, fitness, and wellness.
2. Describe some of the methods of training for improving performance.
3. List several ergogenic aids and describe their effects and safety.

Lesson Vocabulary

anabolic steroids (p. 209), androstenedione (p. 210), committed time (p. 212), core exercises (p. 207), creatine (p. 210), ergogenic aid (p. 209), free time (p. 212), periodization (p. 208), plyometrics (p. 208)

 www.fitnessforlife.org/student/12/4

In this book the focus is on building muscle fitness to improve your health, fitness, and wellness. This includes building enough strength and muscular endurance to help you feel good and look your best. Many of the exercises you have learned so far require equipment that can be quite expensive. In this chapter you will learn ways to develop muscle fitness using inexpensive equipment. Some people may want to develop muscle fitness for enhanced performance. Some methods used to increase sports performance will be discussed. In addition, you will learn about supplements that are sometimes used and abused by those interested in building muscle fitness.

Building Muscle Fitness Using Inexpensive Equipment

You have already learned how to use calisthenics to build muscle fitness. Calisthenics done in an exercise circuit often require little or no equipment and can be done almost anywhere. Other types of inexpensive muscle fitness exercises include rubber band exercises, homemade weights, ball exercises, and partner resistance exercises.

Rubber (Elastic) Band Exercises

These exercises use rubber bands to provide the resistance for exercise. The rubber bands are inexpensive to buy and can be used to perform many different exercises. The bands can be easily transported so that you can do the exercises almost anywhere. Rubber band exercises are often used by physical therapists to help people rehabilitate after an injury. You had the opportunity to try rubber band exercises in chapter 5.

Homemade Weights

You do not have to buy expensive weights to overload the muscles. As you learned earlier in this chapter, you can use food cans, milk bottles filled with water, and other products found in the home to perform your exercises.

Exercise Balls

Large, air-inflated balls are often used to perform exercises to build muscle fitness. They are sometimes called stability balls because they are used by physical therapists to help people build muscles that stabilize the body to build good posture. The balls are typically 2 to 3 feet in diameter, as is the one in the picture.

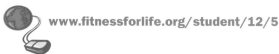 www.fitnessforlife.org/student/12/5

Partner Resistance Exercises

These exercises are basically calisthenics done with a partner. They require little or no equipment and can be fun to perform. A disadvantage is that you cannot perform them by yourself. You had a chance to try some of these exercises as an activity in chapter 11.

Core Exercises

Exercises that build the muscle of the trunk are sometimes called **core exercises.** Many of these exercises

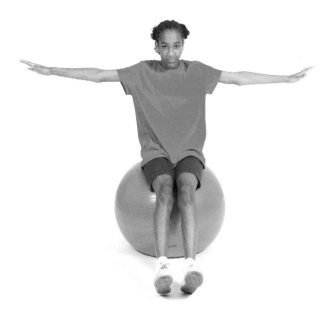

Exercise balls are often used to build muscle fitness.

have been described earlier in the book. For example, the exercises for the care of the back and for good posture in chapter 3 are core exercises. Ball exercises as just described can also be effective in building the back, abdominal, and trunk muscles.

Methods of Building Muscle Fitness for Enhanced Performance

Isotonic, isometric, and isokinetic exercises using resistance machines, free weights, calisthenics, and inexpensive equipment are the types of muscle fitness activities that are used by most people interested in health, fitness, and wellness. Some people will want to build extra muscle fitness to help them improve performance in sports and for jobs such as police work, fire safety, or military training. Some special techniques used to enhance performance are discussed here.

Plyometrics

Plyometrics is a type of exercise designed to improve power. You learned earlier that power is a type of skill-related physical fitness that is a combination of strength and power. People with power can use their strength quickly. Power is important for track and field, football, volleyball, and many other sports.

Plyometrics was pioneered by Olympic track and field coaches from the former Soviet Union. This kind of training involves such activities as hopping drills and jumping off of or onto boxes. The idea is to stretch the muscle or have it do an eccentric (lengthening) contraction immediately followed by a concentric contraction of the muscle. For example, when you jump off of a box and land on the ground, the muscle lengthens, or does an eccentric contraction. When you jump back on the box, the muscle shortens, or does a concentric contraction. This type of training builds power that improves jumping abilities. Experts agree that you should first

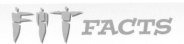

Pilates is one form of core training that has gained popularity. It was named for Joseph Pilates, who developed exercises and exercise machines. Recently the courts ruled that the Pilates exercise is a generic name like yoga and karate. For this reason anyone can call himself or herself a Pilates expert. Though many Pilates instructors may be quite knowledgeable about exercises, many may not. You can do Pilates training, and other forms of core training, without expensive exercise machines.

build high performance levels of flexibility and strength through stretching and isotonic exercises before trying plyometrics. This type of exercise causes soreness and the risk of injury is high. Most experts feel that plyometrics is not a good method of training for preteens and young teens or beginning exercisers of any age. This type of activity should be done only after extensive conditioning using other methods described in this book, and it is most appropriate for older, well-trained athletes. Consult with a qualified coach before performing this type of activity.

 www.fitnessforlife.org/student/12/6

Periodization

Periodization is not a type of training like isometrics or plyometrics. It is way of scheduling your muscle fitness exercise program. In periodization you schedule several different periods of exercise. During each period, you change the way you do your exercise. For example, over 15 weeks of training a person might do three periods of five weeks each. In one period you might focus on muscular endurance exercises with relatively high repetitions and relatively low resistance. In another period you might focus more on strength using higher resistance and a lower number of repetitions. The third period might focus on a combination of strength and muscular endurance training. Many different schedules exist for periodization of training, so the three periods might occur in different orders for different people. Typically the goal is to use a variety of training periods to keep training interesting and, if often used by athletes, to gradually increase performance so that they peak, or reach their best performance level, at the right time. For example, an Olympic athlete would want to have peak performance at the Olympic games and a high school athlete might want peak performance for an important event. Periodization by a nonathlete would be done more to provide variety and continued interest rather than peaking for a specific sporting event.

 www.fitnessforlife.org/student/12/7

Interval Training

Interval training is another type of training often used to increase anaerobic performances such as sprinting and fast swimming, and for short bursts of vigorous activity such as in soccer, hockey, football, and basketball. It involves short sprints and high-intensity exercise followed by rest periods. For more information on interval training, consult the address in the Web icon or check with your physical education teacher or coach.

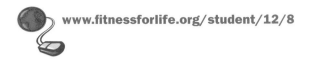

Ergogenic Aids

In the previous section you learned some methods of training that are especially appropriate for building high levels of muscle fitness for enhancing athletic performance. For centuries people, especially those interested in high level performance, have tried to find methods of enhancing performance, including methods other than exercise training.

Ergo is a Latin word meaning work. *Genic* is a word that is derived from the word generate. An **ergogenic aid** is anything that is done to help you generate work or to increase your ability to do work including performing vigorous exercise. Some ergogenic aids, or products thought to be ergogenic aids, are classified as drugs, while others are classified as food supplements. A drug is tested by the Food and Drug Administration (FDA) before it can be sold as a prescription or over the counter medicine. As you will see, many ergogenic aids can be dangerous. Some of the ergogenic aids that get the most publicity are described in the following section.

Anabolic Steroids

Anabolic steroids are synthetic drugs that resemble the male hormone testosterone. For certain diseases, doctors legally prescribe these drugs in small doses. However, some people illegally buy and use anabolic steroids to increase muscle size and strength. Not only are anabolic steroids illegal to use without a doctor's prescription, they are also extremely dangerous. The drawing illustrates some of the harmful effects of steroids. The use of anabolic steroids is prohibited by the United States Olympic Committee and by most other athletic associations.

Teenagers are at high risk for harm from steroids because their bodies are still growing. Anabolic steroids can damage the growth centers of bones, causing the long bones of the body to stop growing. This condition can prevent a person from growing to his or her full height. Many side-effects, such as hair loss, acne, deepening voice, and dark facial hair growth in women, do not go away when the drug is stopped. For athletes a major problem is the increased risk of injury to the tendons and ligaments.

THC is a steroid that was developed to fool drug tests by sport officials. Like other steroids, it is dangerous and illegal.

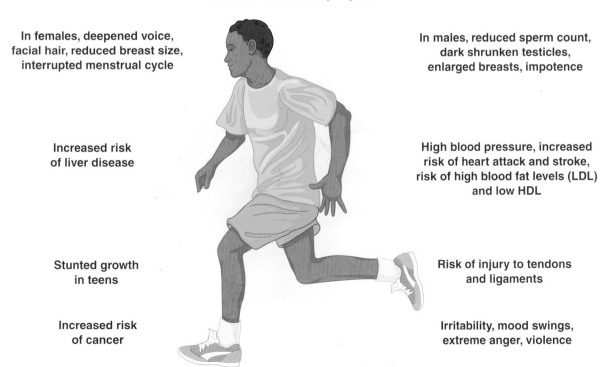

Dangers of using anabolic steroids.

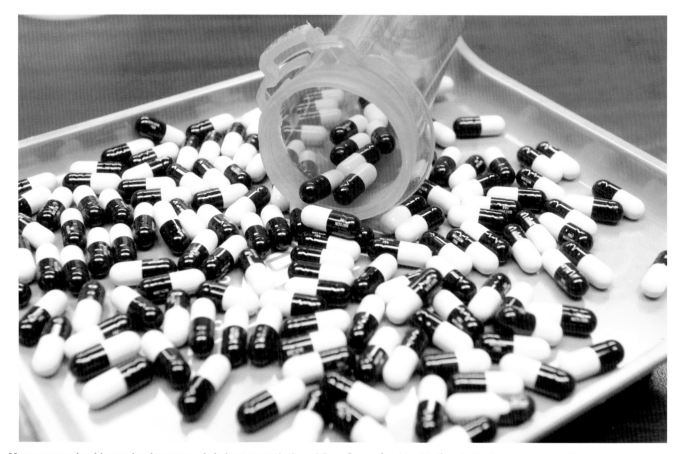

Many ergogenic aids can be dangerous. It is best to seek the advice of a professional before taking any supplement.

Androstenedione

Androstenedione is a food supplement that is sold legally in some countries including the United States, but is illegal in some other countries. Some sports organizations ban its use. Androstenedione, sometimes called andro, is converted by the body to a product similar to anabolic steroids. It gained popularity when several famous athletes indicated that they used it. A study in a leading medical journal indicated that androstenedione had little or no effect on building muscle fitness among those doing progressive resistance training. Other studies have shown that andro has many of the harmful effects of anabolic steroids.

Creatine

Creatine is a substance manufactured in the bodies of meat-eating animals including humans. It is needed for the body to perform anaerobic exercise including many types of progressive resistance exercise. Creatine can also be taken as a food supplement. Taking extra creatine as a supplement does allow your body to store more of it. Some studies have indicated that people who take appropriate amounts of creatine can train harder with shorter rest periods than those who do not take it. Though some studies suggest that this extra ability to do intense training may enhance some types of athletic performance, a recent medical journal review of all the

studies of creatine use concluded that the evidence does not support the notion that creatine enhances muscle development or improves sports performance.

Because creatine has only become popular in recent years, little or no information exists about the long-term dangers of its use. Short-term use reveals no serious health effects, although there has been some concern about possible increased risk of dehydration among athletes who use creatine.

 www.fitnessforlife.org/student/12/9

Other Supplements

Many other food supplements are used by athletes and bodybuilders in hopes of enhancing appearance or sports performance. Many are very expensive or dangerous. Human growth hormone (HGH) is an illegal drug that is exceptionally dangerous, especially for teens. It causes premature closure of bones. Its effects can be deforming and even life threatening.

Another supplement, ephedra—recently banned by the FDA—was used in weight loss products and products purported to enhance athletic performance. The product has been shown to cause several problems including irregular heart rate and other potentially dangerous effects on the nervous system and the heart.

Taking Charge: Managing Time

Why can some people always find time for an added activity while others barely have time to do their regularly scheduled activities? For a lot of people the answer is time management. Good time managers know how to make the best use of their time. They efficiently control their daily schedule in order to complete their activities without wasting time. These people are more likely to find time for regular physical activity.

Jennifer lives near some good cross-country ski trails. Her friends spend a few hours skiing every Monday and Wednesday after school in the winter. They often go skiing on weekends as well. Although they always ask her to join their fun, Jennifer usually refuses. Her common excuse is, "I just don't have the time. I really love skiing, but with three honors classes, homework, and my job at the mall, I barely have time to eat, let alone ski. I wish I could go with you, but I can't. It's impossible! I'll ski next year when my schedule is easier. Then I'll have more spare time."

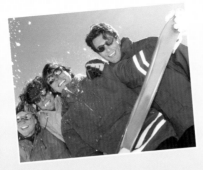

Jennifer's friends are used to her excuses. In fact, she used many of the same excuses last year. Her friends have the same classes and work hours that Jennifer works, but they complete their homework assignments and handle their jobs with time to spare. They do not understand why Jennifer cannot manage to find the time to go skiing with them.

For Discussion

What is different about how Jennifer and her friends manage their time? Consider the time management strategies presented on page 212. What strategies might Jennifer follow to better manage her time? How will these strategies help her free some time for physical activities? Complete the questionnaire provided by your teacher to find out how well you manage your time so that you have enough left for regular physical activity.

Protein supplements are very common among athletes because they are legal and easy to obtain. Your body needs protein because it is necessary for growth and development of most body tissues. Because protein is a major part of the muscles of the body, many people believe that taking extra protein will build extra muscle. Most people eat more protein in their regular diet than they really need. The United States government suggests that a healthy diet should contain about 12 to 15 percent of calories as protein. A more liberal recommendation of 10 to 35 percent of the diet as protein was recently presented by the National Institute of Medicine to allow for differences in diets for individuals.

Athletes and very active people do need to consume more calories of protein than inactive people, but because they take in many more total calories, experts agree that 12 to 15 percent of their diet is adequate to meet the body's needs. Taking more than 15 percent of the diet as protein does not result in greater gains in muscle. If not taken in excess, extra protein in the diet is relatively safe, but too much protein can cause kidney problems. Protein supplements in the form of pills, powders, and protein bars are very expensive, costing as much as 50 cents each gram. Protein in food such as meat, poultry, fish, beans, and eggs is much cheaper, costing only a few cents each gram. The calories in extra dietary protein (in excess of body needs) will be stored as fat just as will extra dietary fat and carbohydrate calories.

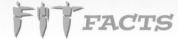

Most people think that food supplements are tested by the FDA to make sure that they are safe. This assumption is not true. Unlike medicines that must be tested before they are approved for safe use, food supplements are unregulated. The law does not require that they be tested for effectiveness or safety before they are sold. Unlike foods sold in the store that require a food label showing nutrition information, food supplements are not required to have labels and great variation exists in content of different products with the same name. For this reason, it is very important to learn the ingredients of a product and the effects of its ingredients before using it.

More information on food supplements is presented in chapter 15.

Lesson Review

1. What are some of the methods of doing inexpensive PRE for health, fitness, and wellness?
2. What are some of the methods of training for improving performance?
3. What are several ergogenic aids? Describe their effects and safety.

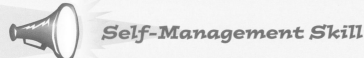

Self-Management Skill

Managing Time

How many times do you hear yourself and others say, "I don't have time"? It seems to be a common complaint. If you are one of those who seems to have too little time, how can you remedy the problem? Many experts believe that learning to manage time is one way to become more active. Because time management is so important, in this lesson you will learn how to manage your time so that you will be more active.

In the year 1900, the average person worked more than 60 hours a week. Now the average work week is approximately 40 hours. Likewise, in 1900 many young people were not enrolled in school and were already working long hours in factories and on farms. Now most teens are in school, and even those who work in addition to going to school are involved for fewer than 60 hours a week.

It would seem that free time is much more abundant now than it was years ago. But this isn't always true. Most of us make other commitments for our time when we aren't working or going to school. For example, you may have to care for brothers and sisters, or you might have made commitments to school or community activities such as clubs, band, chorus, or sports. You might have a job after school or on weekends. Time is also spent on things such as eating, sleeping, dressing, and getting to and from school or work. The time spent in all of these activities is called **committed time.**

Free time is the time left over when work or school time and committed time have been accounted for. Some people have very little free time because they have made so many commitments. The people who say they don't have time for activity often have not planned the use of their time carefully. Active people manage their time effectively so that they can commit time on a regular basis to being active. If you are in the group of people who often say, "I don't have time," the guidelines that follow can help you.

Keep Track of Your Time

The best way to start to manage your time more efficiently is to check to see what you do with it. Keeping records will help you do this. Write down what you do during the course of each day. Record when you sleep, when you eat, when you are in school, when you are at work, and when you do all of the other things you do. You might use three categories: school and work, committed time, and free time. Most people who keep records of their time are surprised with the results. For example, some people who say they don't have time to exercise spend several hours a day watching television. Others find that they spend a long time doing nothing.

Analyze Your Time Use

Once you have kept records of your time for several days, you can review your records to see how many hours you spend in each of the three categories. You can also determine exactly how you spend your committed time and your free time. This determination will help you decide whether you are using your time the way you would like to use it.

Decide What to Do With Your Time

After you determine how much time you spend in various activities, decide whether you are managing your time efficiently. Efficient time management

occurs when you get to do all the things you think are important. Here are some questions you can use to decide what is important:

- ▶ What activities did you spend more time on than you wanted to?
- ▶ How much less time could you spend on each?
- ▶ Are the activities you would like to change under your control?
- ▶ What activities do you want to spend more time on?
- ▶ How much more time would you spend on these activities?

Schedule Your Time

After you decide how you would like to spend your time, you can make a schedule to help you be sure that you have time for the things you think are important. If you feel that regular physical activity is important, you will commit time to doing it. Plan a schedule for one day, making sure you have time to do the things you think are important.

You can sometimes "kill two birds with one stone" with good scheduling. For example, you have to get to school somehow, so you might be able to spend committed time to getting to school on a bicycle or walking. You commit the time to two different purposes. Or you might commit yourself to a sports team or an activity club. This time is committed, but it is committed to a form of physical activity.

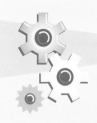

Activity 2

Muscular Endurance Exercise Circuit

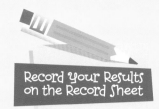
Record Your Results on the Record Sheet

This activity shows you some calisthenics that you can use to build muscular endurance. It includes only eight groups of muscles, and for most teens will be only light to moderate in intensity. When you design your own program, you can choose the intensity and exercises that are best for you. While performing these exercises, keep these points in mind:

▶ Learn how to do each exercise correctly.
▶ Do the exercises in the order and with the number of repetitions listed in table 12.3.
▶ If you cannot complete an exercise as many times as directed, just do as many as you can.
▶ Your instructor will tell you when to start and stop the exercise. If you cannot do 20 repetitions, walk or jog during the time before the next exercise.
▶ For each exercise, write on your record sheet the number of repetitions you were able to complete in the 1 minute allowed (up to 20 reps).
▶ After you have been exercising for a few weeks, repeat the circuit up to 3 times. Do the warm-up only before the first and the cool-down only after the last circuit.

Table 12.3

Sample Muscular Endurance Exercise Program

Exercise	Length of time or number of reps
Warm-up and stretch	Same as warm-up in chapter 1 (3 min)
1. Stride jump	1 every 3 sec for 1 min = 20 reps
2. Side leg raise (right leg)	1 every 3 sec for 1 min = 20 reps
3. Side leg raise (left leg)	1 every 3 sec for 1 min = 20 reps
4. Trunk (upper back) lift	1 every 3 sec for 1 min = 20 reps
5. Bridging	1 every 3 sec for 1 min = 20 reps
6. 90-degree push-up or knee push-up	1 every 4 sec for 1 min = 15 reps
7. Curl-up with twist	1 every 3 sec for 1 min = 20 reps
8. High knee jog	Right foot down every 3 sec for 1 min = 20 reps
9. Prone arm lift	1 every 3 sec for 1 min = 20 reps
Cool-down and stretch	Same as warm-up (3 min)

Safety Tips: In some exercises, such as the curl-up, your feet should not be anchored. When doing the trunk lift, you can anchor your feet as long as you limit your lift to about 12 inches.

Stride Jump

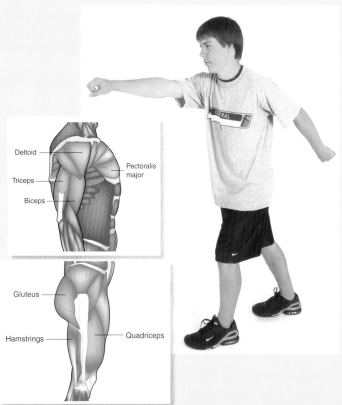

Deltoid
Triceps
Biceps
Pectoralis major
Gluteus
Hamstrings
Quadriceps

1. Stand with your left leg forward and right leg back. Hold your right arm at shoulder height straight in front of your body and your left arm straight behind you.
2. Jump, moving your right foot forward and left foot back. As your feet change places, your arms switch position. Keep your feet 18 to 24 inches apart.
3. Continue jumping, alternating feet and arms. Count 1 each time the left foot moves forward.

This exercise develops the muscles of the legs and arms. It also develops cardiovascular fitness.

Side Leg Raise

1. Lie on your right side. Use your arms for balance.
2. Lift the top (left) leg 45 degrees. Keep your kneecap pointing forward and ankle pointing toward the ceiling. If your leg is allowed to rotate so that the knee points upward, you will work the wrong muscles.
3. Lower your leg. Repeat the movement. You can use an ankle weight to increase intensity.
4. Roll over and repeat the exercise with your right leg.

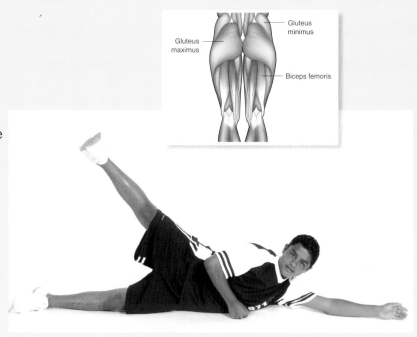

Gluteus maximus
Gluteus minimus
Biceps femoris

This exercise develops the hip and thigh muscles.

214

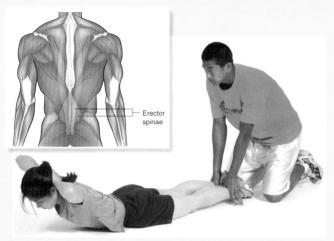

Erector spinae

This exercise develops the muscles of the upper back and helps prevent "hump back."

Trunk (Upper Back) Lift

1. Lie facedown with your hands clasped behind your neck.
2. Pull your shoulder blades together, raise your elbows off the floor, then lift your head and chest off the floor. Arch the upper back until your breastbone (sternum) clears the floor. You may need to hook your feet under a bar or have someone hold your feet down.

 Caution: Do not lift your chin more than 12 inches off the floor.

3. Lower your trunk and repeat the exercise.

Gluteus maximus

Biceps femoris
Semitendinosus
Semimembranosus

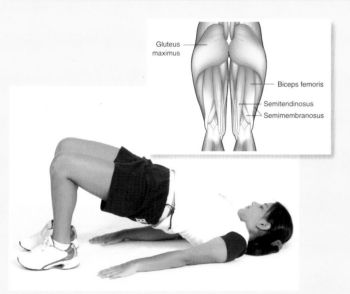

This exercise develops the muscles of the buttocks (gluteals) and the muscles on the back of the thighs (hamstrings).

Bridging

1. Lie on your back with your knees bent and your feet close to your buttocks.
2. Contract the gluteal muscles. Lift the buttocks and raise your back off the floor until the hip joint has no bend.

 Caution: Do not overarch your lower back.

3. Lower your hips to the floor and repeat the exercise.

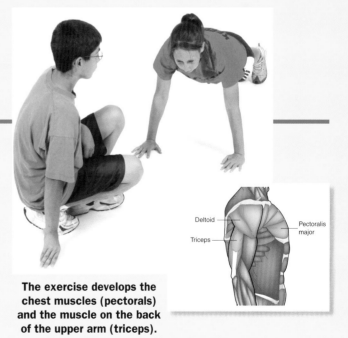

Deltoid
Triceps
Pectoralis major

The exercise develops the chest muscles (pectorals) and the muscle on the back of the upper arm (triceps).

90-Degree Push-Up

1. Lie facedown on a mat or carpet with your hands under your shoulders, your fingers spread, and your legs straight. Your legs should be slightly apart and your toes should be tucked under.
2. Push up until your arms are straight. Keep your legs and back straight. Your body should form a straight line.
3. Lower your body by bending your elbows until they are each parallel to the floor (at a 90-degree angle), then push up until the arms are fully extended. Repeat, alternating between fully extended and 90-degree arm positions.

 Caution: Do not allow your hips to sag, and do not bend at the hips more than 5 degrees.

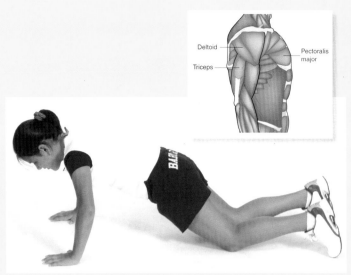

Knee Push-Up

1. If you cannot complete 20 reps of the 90-degree push-up, try this version. Lie facedown with your hands placed under your shoulders.
2. Push up, keeping your body rigid, until your arms are straight, but keep your knees on the floor.
3. Keep your body rigid, and lower it until your chest touches the floor.

 Caution: Do not allow the hips to sag and do not bend at the hips more than 5 degrees.

The exercise develops the chest muscles (pectorals) and the muscle on the back of the upper arm (triceps).

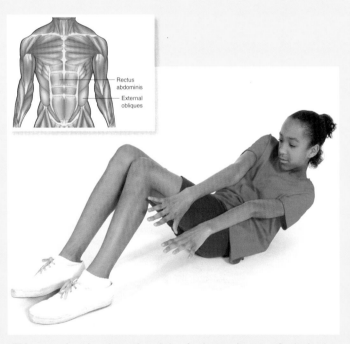

Curl-Up With Twist

1. Lie on your back with your knees bent to about a right angle (90 degrees), your feet flat on the floor. Extend your arms down along your sides.
2. Flatten your lower back to the floor. Tuck your chin and lift your head. Then raise your shoulder blades, twisting to the left and reaching with both arms outside your left leg. Curl up until both shoulder blades are off the floor.
3. Curl down to the starting position and repeat the exercise twisting to the right. Continue alternating right and left twists.

 Caution: Always flatten your lower back and tuck your chin as you curl up and curl down. Do not let anyone hold your feet.

This exercise develops the abdominal muscles, particularly the oblique abdominal muscles.

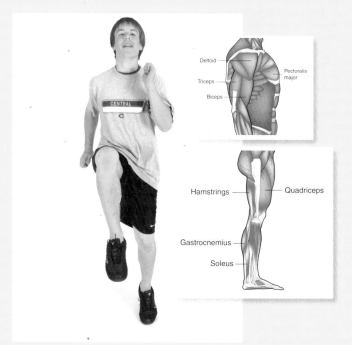

Deltoid
Triceps
Biceps
Pectoralis major

Hamstrings
Quadriceps
Gastrocnemius
Soleus

This exercise develops the muscles of the arms and the legs and is also good for cardiovascular fitness.

High Knee Jog

1. Jog in place. Try to lift each knee so that your upper leg is parallel with the floor.
2. Count 1 each time the right foot touches the floor. Try to do 1 to 2 jog steps per second.

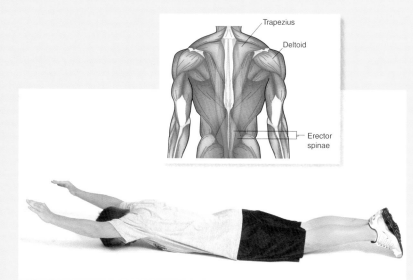

Trapezius
Deltoid
Erector spinae

This exercise develops the muscles of the back and the back of the shoulder joint, and it helps prevent poor posture.

Prone Arm Lift

1. Lie facedown on the floor with your arms extended and held against your ears.
2. Keep your forehead and chest on the floor and lift your arms so the hands are 6 inches off the floor.
3. Lower your arms and then repeat the exercise. Keep your arms touching your ears and keep your elbows straight.

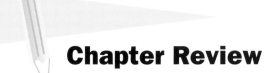

12 Chapter Review

Reviewing Concepts and Vocabulary

Number your paper from 1 to 5. Next to each number, write the word (or words) that correctly completes the sentence.

1. A part of fitness called _____ requires a fit heart and circulatory system.
2. If you have poor _____ your leg muscles might get tired when you run.
3. _____ training is a way of performing muscular endurance exercises that involves changing stations with short breaks in between.
4. _____ is the real name of the supplement sometimes called andro.
5. The real name for the product called HGH is _____.

Number your paper from 6 to 10. Next to each number, choose the letter of the best answer.

Column I	Column II
6. plyometrics	a. short, high-intensity exercise followed by breaks
7. ephedra	b. a product manufactured by meat-eating animals
8. periodization	c. varying your muscle fitness program schedule
9. creatine	d. a training technique involving jumping
10. interval training	e. a product that can alter heart rate

Number your paper from 11 to 15. On your paper, write a short answer for each statement or question.

11. What are some of the basic guidelines for building muscular endurance?
12. How many days a week should you train for muscular endurance?
13. What self-assessments can you do to determine whether you have enough muscular endurance?
14. What kinds of physical activities can you do to build muscular endurance?
15. What is an ergogenic aid?

Thinking Critically

Write a paragraph to answer the following question.

Your friend Derrick is excited about an article he read in a muscle magazine. He tells you that he is going to take some steroids to make his muscles big and strong. What would you tell your friend? What would you recommend he do to strengthen his muscles safely?

Unit Review on the Web

www.fitnessforlife.org/student/12/10

Unit IV review materials are available on the at the address listed in the Web icon.

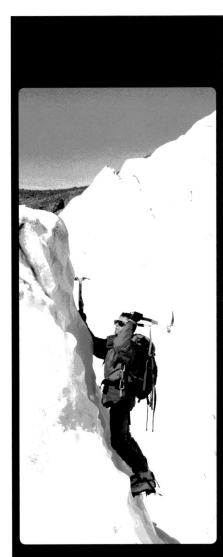

Project

Keep a record of your daily participation in resistance exercises for muscular endurance development for one week. Record the minutes of these exercises each day. How might you adjust your physical activity to better maintain or improve your muscular endurance? What short-term goals might you have for performing specific muscular endurance exercises each day? Make a written plan for the following week, incorporating changes that might help you reach your goals. Use the worksheets provided by your teacher.

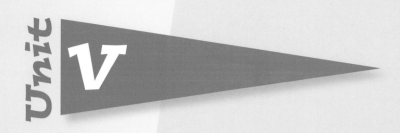

Unit V

Healthy Choices

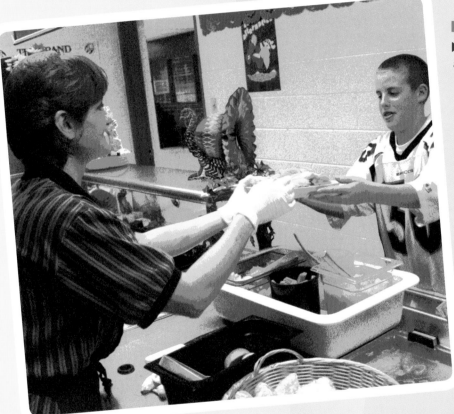

Healthy People 2010 Goals

▶ Reduce the number of teens who are overweight or obese.

▶ Increase the number of people who are at a healthy weight.

▶ Increase servings of fruit, vegetables, and whole grain products in the daily diet.

▶ Decrease amount of fat, especially saturated fat, in the daily diet.

▶ Reduce daily salt intake.

▶ Increase the number of people who get adequate calcium in the daily diet.

▶ Increase the number of teens who eat healthy meals and snacks.

▶ Increase regular physical activity levels of teens.

▶ Increase the number of people who meet national dietary guidelines.

▶ Increase the number of teens and young adults who receive health risk information.

▶ Improve health literacy and increase public health information dissemination.

Unit Activities

▶ Your Exercise Circuit

▶ Muscle Fitness Exercises With Resistance Machines

▶ Jollyball

▶ Cooperative Aerobics

▶ Continuous Rhythmical Exercise

▶ Active Learning: Isometric Exercise Circuit

13

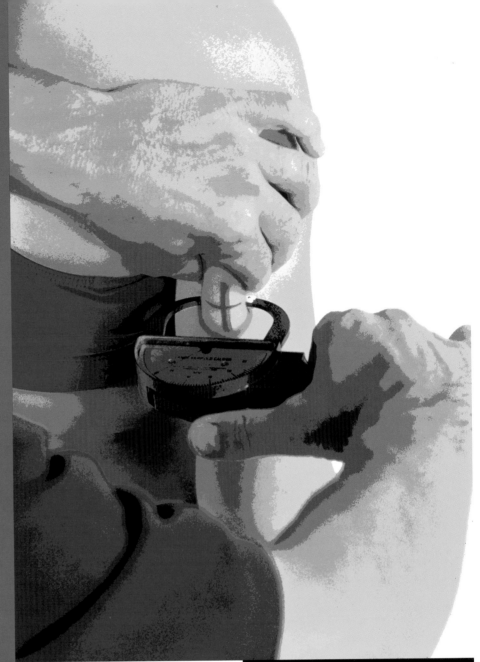

Body Composition

In this chapter...

Activity 1
Your Exercise Circuit

Lesson 13.1
The Facts About Body Composition

Self-Assessment
**Skinfold Measurements and
Height–Weight Charts**

Lesson 13.2
Controlling Body Fatness

Taking Charge
Improving Physical Self-Perceptions

Self-Management Skill
Improving Physical Self-Perceptions

Activity 2
**Muscle Fitness Exercises With
Resistance Machines**

Activity 1

YOUR EXERCISE CIRCUIT

In previous chapters you learned about various exercise circuits. These circuits were preplanned to help you learn various exercises for specific parts of health-related physical fitness. Now that you have had some experience with circuits, you can plan your own total fitness exercise circuit for building all parts of health-related physical fitness. Guidelines to consider in developing your circuit include choosing exercises for all parts of health-related fitness, not having two stations in a row that work the same muscles, and being sure that you include only safe exercises. Your teacher can provide you with a worksheet to help you in developing your own exercise circuit.

Lesson 13.1

The Facts About Body Composition

Lesson Objectives

After reading this lesson, you should be able to

1. Describe a healthy level of body fatness.
2. Explain how the level of body fatness is related to good health.
3. Explain how body fatness can be assessed.

Lesson Vocabulary

anorexia athletica (p. 224), anorexia nervosa (p. 223), basal metabolism (p. 221), body composition (p. 221), bulimia (p. 224), essential body fat (p. 223), overfat (p. 222), skinfolds (p. 224), underfat (p. 222)

www.fitnessforlife.org/student/13/1

Body fatness is a part of health-related physical fitness. Body fatness refers to the percentage of your total body that is comprised of fat tissue. For good health, it is important to have optimal amounts of body fat. In this lesson you will learn what level of body fat is best for you, how your body fatness affects your health, and how to assess your body fatness.

Body Composition

Together, all the tissues that make up your body are called your **body composition.** For a typical person, 15 to 25 percent of the body composition is fat and 75 to 85 percent is lean body tissue. Lean tissue includes muscles, bones, skin, and body organs such as the heart, liver, kidneys, and lungs.

People who do regular physical activity typically have a larger percentage of lean body weight, especially from muscle and bone, and less body fat than those who do not do such activity. Having a relatively low percentage of your total body weight as fat is desirable. However, for good health, it is important that your body composition include some body fat.

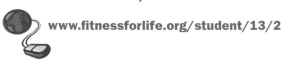

www.fitnessforlife.org/student/13/2

FIT FACTS

More than 60 percent of all adults are considered to be too fat or obese. Fewer children are considered to be too fat (13 percent) but this number is nearly three times as many as 20 years ago. About 11 percent of teens are considered to be too fat or obese. Type II diabetes, once thought to be an adult disease, is becoming more common among youth, partly because it is linked to overfatness and obesity (see chapter 3).

Factors Influencing Body Fatness

In chapter 1, you learned about some of the factors that influence physical fitness. Many factors also influence body fat levels.

Heredity

You inherit your body type from your parents. Some people are born with a tendency to be lean, muscular, or fat. Inherited tendencies make keeping body fat levels in the good fitness zone easy for some people but difficult for others. You need to consider heredity when you are determining your goals for body fatness.

Metabolism

Your **basal metabolism** is the amount of energy your body uses just to keep you living. This energy is measured in units called calories. Your basal metabolism does not include the calories you burn in work, recreation, studying, or even sitting and watching television. Some people have a higher basal metabolism than others. This means that their bodies, at complete rest, burn more calories than the bodies of those with low metabolism. People with a high metabolism can consume more calories than others can without increasing their level of body fat.

Metabolism is affected by heredity, age, and maturation. Most young people have a high metabolism because their bodies are growing and building muscle. As you grow older, your rate of metabolism becomes slower. Then most people need to reduce the number of calories in the diet to avoid gaining fat. How might the rates of metabolism of the people in the picture on page 222 be likely to differ?

Maturation

As you grow older and the hormone levels in the body begin to change, levels of body fat also change. During the teen years, female hormones cause girls to develop

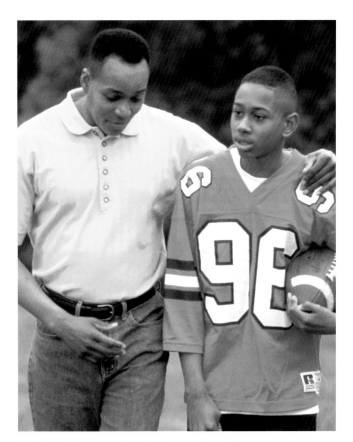

Age, heredity, and maturation affect metabolism.

Body Fat: How Much Is Good?

About one half of your body fat is located deep within your body. The remaining fat is between your skin and muscles. A fit person has the right amount of body fat—neither too much nor too little.

Weight Versus Fat

The terms *underweight* and *overweight* do not provide a great deal of information about fitness or about a person's body composition. Underweight and overweight refer to how much you weigh compared to others. Muscles weigh more than fat. Thus, you can weigh more than someone else of the same size because you are more muscular and have less body fat than the other person. For example, the runners in the picture have strong muscles. They may weigh more than other people who appear to be the same size. On the other hand, you can weigh less than someone else of the same size because you have smaller bones.

The terms **overfat** and **underfat** are very useful because they describe how much of your total body weight is made up of fat. Underfat means having too little body fat; overfat means having too much body fat. Obesity is a term used to describe people who are overfat.

higher levels of body fat than boys. Because of male hormones, teenage boys have greater muscle development than girls.

Early Fatness

Children who are too fat develop extra fat cells that make it more difficult to control fat levels later in life. Keeping body fatness within the good fitness zone during the childhood and teen years will help keep body fat levels in check throughout life.

Diet

The amount of energy in foods is measured in calories. A typical teenage male needs to consume about 2,500 to 3,000 calories a day to maintain an ideal level of body fat. A typical teenage female needs about 2,000 to 2,500 calories a day. Most males need more calories than females because they are larger and have more muscle mass.

Physical Activity

Your body burns calories for energy. The more vigorous activity you do, the more energy your body uses and the more calories you need. An inactive person uses less energy each day than an active person and therefore needs to consume fewer calories.

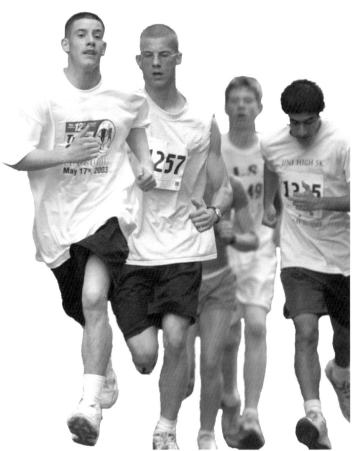

People who are muscular can weigh more than others of the same size because they have more muscle and less body fat.

Body Fat in Females and Males

From the late teens on, females generally have a higher percentage of body fat than do males. Teenage girls should not have less than 11 percent or more than 25 percent body fat. Over 35 percent fat is considered obese for females. Teenage boys should not have under 6 percent or over 20 percent body fat. Over 30 percent is considered obese for males.

Overfatness, Health, and Wellness

Having too much fat can be unhealthy. Scientists report that people who are overfat have a higher risk of heart disease, high blood pressure, diabetes, cancer, and other diseases. Being overfat also reduces a person's chances of successful surgery. Health costs for obese people are about $1,500 a year more than for people with healthy body fat levels. In addition, an overfat person tires more quickly and easily than a lean person. For this reason, an overfat person might be less efficient in work and recreation. Many experts believe that the reason why so many adults are too fat is that they try to achieve an unrealistic weight or fat level. For example, many people try to be as lean as a movie star or an athlete shown in a commercial. When they cannot attain or maintain exceptionally low body fat levels, they give up and become too fat. The experts suggest it is better to set less extreme goals that are achievable and that will result in maintaining a healthy body fat level throughout life.

Too Little Body Fat

Just as having too much body fat can be a health risk, having too little body fat is also a health risk. Eating disorders such as anorexia nervosa, anorexia athletica, and bulimia have many negative health consequences and can be fatal. Identifying the symptoms of eating disorders early is extremely important. Conditions associated with an excessive desire to lose fat and maintain very low body fat levels can be serious health problems.

Many experts believe that our nation's obsession with leanness as seen on TV, in the movies, and in magazines contributes to eating disorders. Six to 8 percent of girls in grades 9 to 12 are considered to be overweight, but more than one third (33 to 36 percent) of all girls in these grades think they are too fat. This statistic shows that many girls use an unrealistic standard in judging their body composition.

The minimum amount of body fatness is called **essential body fat** because if fat levels in the body drop below this amount, health problems result. The chart on this page shows several reasons why your body needs some body fat.

Being underfat can result in abnormal functioning of various body organs. In fact, exceptionally low body fat levels can result in serious health problems, particularly among teenagers. Females with especially low levels of body fat experience health problems related to the reproductive system and risk loss of bone density.

The Importance of Body Fat

- ▶ Fat is an insulator; it helps your body adapt to heat and cold.
- ▶ Fat acts as a shock absorber; it can help protect your body organs and bones from injury.
- ▶ Fat helps your body use vitamins effectively.
- ▶ Fat is stored energy that is available when your body needs it.
- ▶ Fat, in reasonable amounts, helps you look your best, thus increasing your feelings of well-being.

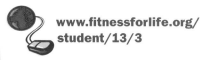

www.fitnessforlife.org/student/13/3

Anorexia Nervosa

Anorexia nervosa is a serious eating disorder. A person who has this disorder severely restricts the amount of food he or she eats in an attempt to be exceptionally underfat. In addition, many people with anorexia do extensive physical activity to further lower their levels of body fat to extremely dangerous levels.

Anorexia is most common among teenage girls, though it is becoming increasingly common among teenage boys. People with this disorder are usually very hard workers and high achievers. They have a distorted view of their bodies and see themselves as being too fat even when they are extremely thin. A fear of maturity, and the weight gain associated with adulthood, is a characteristic of persons with this disorder. People with the disorder often try to hide their condition by wearing baggy clothing, only pretending to eat, and exercising in private. Anorexia is a life-threatening condition, and those who have the condition need immediate professional help.

Anorexia Athletica

Anorexia athletica has many symptoms that are similar to those of anorexia nervosa. It is most common among athletes involved in sports such as gymnastics, wrestling, and cheerleading, in which a low body weight is desirable. This condition can lead to anorexia nervosa. The disorder is thought to be related to the pressure to maintain a low weight and an excessive preoccupation with dieting and exercising for weight loss.

Bulimia

Bulimia is an eating disorder in which a person does binge eating, or eats very large amounts of food within a short period of time. Bingeing is followed by purging. Techniques of purging include vomiting and the use of laxatives to rid the body of food and prevent its digestion. Bulimia can result in loss of teeth, gum diseases, severe digestive problems, and other significant health problems.

Body Fat Assessment

You might wonder how to assess body fatness and make determinations about how much you should weigh. Several methods exist to make such assessments.

Laboratory Measurements of Fatness

Until recently, underwater weighing was considered to be the best way to assess your body fat level. With this technique, you are immersed in a tank of water and then weighed. Lean people weigh more under water; they sink. People with more fat weigh less under water; they float. Measurements of your lung capacity are also taken because the amount of air in your lungs influences your weight. A formula is applied to your underwater weight and lung capacity to scientifically determine your body fat level.

Recently an X-ray technique called DEXA has been developed and is considered to be the new gold standard for measuring body fatness. DEXA and underwater weighing are the most accurate methods of measuring body fat, but these procedures require time, are expensive, and must be done by an expert.

Skinfold Measurements

Your body fat levels can also be determined by measuring the thickness of **skinfolds,** the fat under the skin.

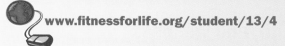

FITNESS Technology

Dual-energy X-ray absorptiometry (DEXA) is a high-tech type of X-ray machine. It takes a three-dimensional picture of the entire body that allows an attached computer to accurately determine the total amount of fat in the body. It is now considered to be the best method of determining body fatness. Studies show that skinfold measures, when done properly, can be quite accurate in predicting body fatness as determined by DEXA.

www.fitnessforlife.org/student/13/4

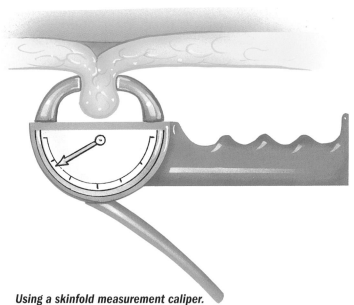

Using a skinfold measurement caliper.

Look at the picture illustrating the measurement of a skinfold. A special instrument called a caliper is used to measure skinfold thickness. You will learn to do skinfold measurements in the self-assessment in this chapter.

Body Measurements

You can also use body measurements to estimate your percentage of body fat. One procedure uses weight and waist measurements for males and height and hip measurements for females. This method is less accurate than skinfold measures.

Body Mass Index

You learned about the body mass index in chapter 5. This index is a better indicator of fat than height and weight alone, but it does not give as accurate an assessment of body fatness as DEXA, underwater weighing, or skinfold measurements. Both this procedure and the height–weight charts described in the following section can provide inaccurate measurements for people who have a lot of muscle (athletes, for example). This is because muscle weighs a lot more than fat and a very muscular person could be high in weight but not too fat. This is one reason why skinfolds or laboratory techniques are considered to be better measures for very active people.

Height–Weight Charts

A common method of assessing body weight is through the use of height–weight tables. The tables, shown in the self-assessment on page 228, list normal weight ranges for people according to age, height, and sex. Note that this procedure does not assess body fatness. As noted, measures that use weight and height only can mistakenly classify a thin, muscular person as overweight. Height–weight techniques may also mistakenly classify an overfat person who has little muscle as within a normal weight range. These tables are convenient but should not be the only source of information about body composition. You will use height–weight charts in the self-assessment in this chapter.

Waist-to-Hip Ratio

Evidence indicates that people with a very large waist compared to hip size tend to have more fat inside the body and may be at risk for health problems. This is because excessive body fat in the abdominal area is associated with high blood fat levels. You can measure the circumference of your hips and waist and calculate a ratio. It is a useful health risk indicator that can be used throughout life. You will learn more about waist-to-hip ratio in chapter 14.

Other Measurements

Computers and other machines have been developed to test body fat levels. Many are expensive and require trained people to do the assessment. Others are unreliable. Many fitness and health clubs, as well as some schools, use some of these techniques. One technique, bioelectrical impedance analysis, can be accurate when done properly. However, unless you can use the same machine from measurement to measurement, errors may occur. Advantages of skinfolds and the other methods listed are that they are relatively easy to do, they do not require expensive machines, and you can do them yourself. Research has shown that inexpensive plastic calipers such as those shown in the photos on page 226 are quite accurate if used properly by a person who is trained in using them and who practices measurement technique.

Ideal Body Weight

What is my ideal body weight? Even after learning about the different forms of body composition assess-

ment, this is the question many people ask. Experts agree that there is no such thing as an ideal body weight for all people that can be provided in a chart or a table. The self-assessments you do in this book provide you with several ways to get an idea of your body composition. The best advice is to have a long-term goal of achieving the healthy zone for body fatness (see table 13.1 on page 227).

If you are in the marginal or too much fat zone, then you should develop a plan that will gradually move you from the zone you are in to the next zone. Trying to achieve the healthy zone when you are too far from it is an unrealistic goal. If you are already in the healthy zone for body fat, a good goal is to stay there.

If you are in the healthy zone and want to be leaner to enhance your performance in a sport, you may want to achieve the high performance zone. It should be emphasized that being in the high performance zone is not necessary for good health and may not be a realistic goal for all people. Trying to be leaner than the high performance zone is not a desirable goal.

If you are in the too little fat zone, it is desirable to increase your weight by gaining body fat. Those with eating disorders often try to reduce body fat even when they already have too little for good health.

If you achieve and maintain the healthy zone for body fat, you will probably also have a desirable waist-to-hip ratio, a healthy BMI, and be in the normal weight range for your age and sex. However, as noted earlier in this chapter, it is possible to have a healthy body fat level and be above BMI and normal weight standards because people with a lot of muscle may weigh more than other people but not be overfat.

Once you have achieved a body fat level that puts you in the healthy zone, you can weigh yourself. Maintaining this weight while maintaining a fat level in the healthy zone is a desirable lifetime goal. Learning to eat well and perform regular physical activity is essential in achieving this goal.

Lesson Review

1. What is a good level of body fat?
2. How is a person's body fatness related to good health?
3. What are three methods of assessing body fat? Explain the accuracy of each method.

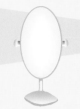

Self-Assessment

Skinfold Measurements and Height–Weight Charts

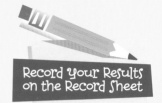

Record Your Results on the Record Sheet

One way to estimate your body fat percentage is to use skinfold measures. You can assess your body weight using height–weight charts. When you do this assessment, keep in mind these points:

▶ Your fitness scores are your personal information and should be kept confidential.

▶ Be sensitive to the feelings of others when body fat measurements are being taken. Taking the measurements privately may be appropriate.

▶ You can use your results to help build a fitness profile.

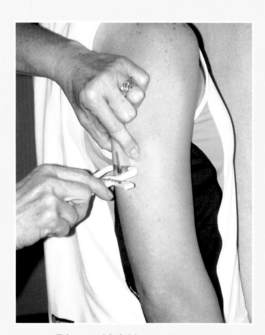

Triceps skinfold measurement.

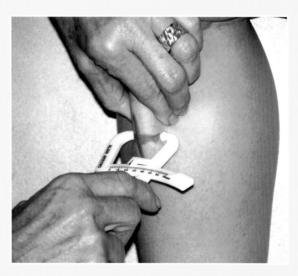

Calf skinfold measurement.

Skinfold Measurements

You can use skinfold measurements to estimate body fat percentage and target weight. For teenagers, upper arm (triceps) and calf measurements provide a good estimate of body fat percentage. Work with a partner to take each other's measurements. When you are performing the skinfold measurements on your partner use the instructions that follow. Write your results on your record sheet.

▶ **Triceps skinfold:** Pick up a skinfold on the middle of the back of the right arm, halfway between the elbow and the shoulder. The arm should hang loose and relaxed at the side.

▶ **Calf skinfold:** The person being tested stands and places the right foot on a chair. Pick up a skinfold on the inside of the right calf halfway between the shin and the back of the calf, where the calf is largest.

1. Use your left thumb and index finger to pick up the skinfold. Do not pinch or squeeze the skinfold.

2. Hold the skinfold with your left hand while you pick up and use the caliper with the right hand to get a reading.

3. Place the caliper over the skinfold about one-half inch below your finger and thumb. Hold the caliper on the skinfold for 3 seconds, and then note the measurement. Read the caliper measurement to the nearest one-half millimeter (mm), if possible.

4. Make three measurements each for the triceps and the calf skinfolds. Use the middle of the

226

Skinfold Measurements (continued)

Table 13.1

Rating Chart: Body Fatness

FATNESS RATING	% FAT	
	Males	Females
Too little fat	<6	<12
High performance	6-9.9	12-14.9
Healthy	10-19.9	15-24.9
Marginal	20-24.9	25-29.9
Too much fat	25+	30+

three measures as the score. For example, an 8, 9, and 10 give a score of 9. If your three measurements differ by more than 2 mm, take a second, or even third set of measurements.

Now you can determine your body fatness and fatness ratings.

1. Once you have had your skinfold measurements taken add the triceps and calf scores. Use the figure below to estimate your body fat percentage. Use a ruler to connect your sum

of skinfolds with the percent fat figure. For example, if you are a male and your skinfold sum is 27 mm, your body fat percentage is approximately 22 percent. Then look at the rating chart at the left to determine your rating for body fatness.

2. Once you have determined your percent body fat using skinfold measures, you can determine your target weight. Target weight is an estimate of a weight that would put you in the healthy zone for body fatness and is based on your current weight and your current sum of skinfolds. To do this you will need to use the Target Body Weight worksheet provided by your teacher. The worksheet contains tables (one for males and one for females). Using the appropriate table, find the row showing your current body weight and the column with your current sum of skinfolds. Your target weight is located in the box where the two columns intersect. If your sum of skinfolds is less than 27 mm for females and 22 mm for males, you are already at or below your target weight. People should determine their own targets based on the factors that influence body fatness discussed earlier in this chapter.

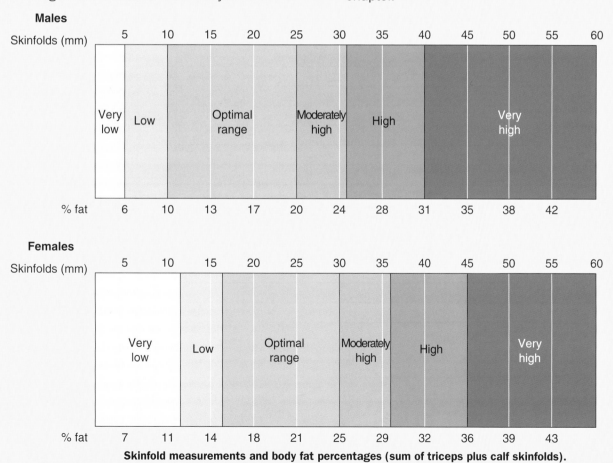

Skinfold measurements and body fat percentages (sum of triceps plus calf skinfolds).

"Triceps Plus Calf Skinfolds: Males" and "Triceps Plus Calf Skinfolds: Female" reprinted by permission of Dr. Tim G. Lohman, Department of Exercise and Sport Sciences, University of Arizona.

Height–Weight Charts

You can also use height–weight charts to estimate your appropriate weight range.

1. Remove your shoes.
2. Take your own height and weight measures or ask a partner to help you.

3. Use table 13.2 to determine the normal weight range for a person of your sex, age, and height.
4. Record your height, weight, and normal weight range on the record sheet. Compare your target weight from skinfolds and your normal weight range. Then answer the questions on your record sheet.

Table 13.2

Normal Weight Ranges

MALES					FEMALES				
HEIGHT		AGE			HEIGHT		AGE		
ft	in.	13-14	15-16	17-20	ft	in.	13-14	15-16	17-20
4	6	69-72			4	6	73-76		
4	7	73-76			4	7	76-79		
4	8	78-81			4	8	79-82		
4	9	82-85	82-85		4	9	86-89	91-94	
4	10	87-90	87-90		4	10	91-94	98-101	99-102
4	11	88-91	88-91		4	11	96-99	102-105	104-107
5	0	89-92	97-100	101-104	5	0	104-107	106-109	109-112
5	1	97-100	101-104	106-109	5	1	105-108	109-112	113-116
5	2	100-103	106-109	114-117	5	2	106-109	112-115	116-119
5	3	106-109	111-114	121-124	5	3	110-113	115-118	120-123
5	4	113-116	115-118	124-127	5	4	115-118	120-123	125-128
5	5	116-119	120-123	129-132	5	5	119-122	124-127	129-132
5	6	120-123	126-129	134-137	5	6	126-129	128-131	134-137
5	7	126-129	132-135	137-140	5	7	127-130	131-134	137-140
5	8	130-133	135-138	140-143	5	8	128-131	135-138	143-146
5	9	135-138	139-142	147-150	5	9	129-132	137-140	148-151
5	10	141-144	142-145	149-152	5	10	130-133	139-142	153-156
5	11	146-149	149-152	152-155	5	11		142-145	158-161
6	0	151-154	152-155	156-159	6	0		146-149	163-166
6	1		158-161	162-165					
6	2		160-163	167-170					
6	3			177-180					
and over									

Controlling Body Fatness

Balancing Calories

Balancing **calorie** intake and expenditure affects body fat levels. The foods you eat contain calories that your body uses for energy. Fat is stored energy (stored calories). If you take in (eat) more calories than you expend (in exercise), you will gain weight (store calories as fat). If you expend more calories than you take in, you will lose weight. If you balance the calories consumed and expended, you maintain your current weight.

Lesson Objectives
After reading this lesson, you should be able to
1. Explain how to use the FIT formula for fat control.
2. Explain how physical activity helps a person maintain a healthy body fat level.

Lesson Vocabulary
calorie (p. 229)

www.fitnessforlife.org/student/13/5

A major health goal is to help Americans achieve and maintain acceptable body fat levels throughout life. In this lesson, you will learn the FIT formula for fat control and appropriate activities for gaining weight and losing body fat.

FIT FACTS

One pound of fat contains 3,500 calories. Therefore, you can lose a pound of fat by eating 3,500 calories less than you normally eat in a given time or by burning 3,500 calories more than normal in physical activity. Eating foods that provide more calories than your body uses will cause you to gain weight. Therefore, you can gain a pound of fat by eating 3,500 calories more than you usually eat within a given time or expending 3,500 calories fewer in physical activity within a given time.

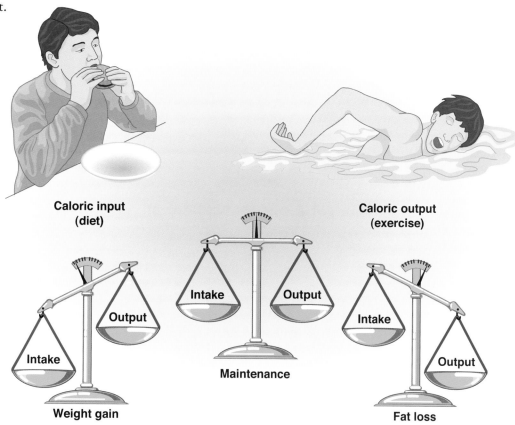

Caloric input (diet)

Caloric output (exercise)

Weight gain

Maintenance

Fat loss

Balancing caloric input and output.

The FIT Formula

As noted in the previous section, both diet and physical activity play an important role in maintaining a healthy body fat level. Because both diet and physical activity are important for fat control, each has a target zone, shown in table 13.3.

Gaining Weight

Combining proper physical activity and diet is the best weight gain method. Strength and muscular endurance exercises can help you gain weight. Resistance exercises that help build muscle are especially effective because they build muscle and muscle weighs more than fat.

Remember that physical activity burns calories. Therefore, when you are active, you need to increase your intake of calories in order to gain weight. You will learn in chapter 14 that you do not need to eat special diets or take protein supplements to gain weight; you need only eat a well-balanced diet that contains an increased number of calories.

Physical Activity and Calories

Every physical activity burns calories. You might wonder how many calories are burned by different activities. Table 13.4 shows the approximate number of calories burned each hour during vigorous recreational activities. Find the weight value nearest your own weight. Add 5 percent to the number of calories for each 10 pounds you weigh above the listed weight value. Or, subtract 5 percent from the number of calories for each 10 pounds you weigh below the listed weight value. Use this table to determine which physical activities are best for burning calories. Then see which activities appeal to you.

Physical Activity and Fat Loss

A combination of physical activity and eating fewer calories is the best way to lose fat. Research shows that a person who reduces calorie intake without increasing activity will lose both fat and muscle tissue, while a person who increases physical activity and reduces calorie consumption loses mostly body fat. Notice that physical activities from all levels of the Physical Activity Pyramid, except the top level indicating inactivity, are appropriate for helping to control body fatness.

Lifestyle Activities

Lifestyle physical activities are especially effective in long-term fat control. Studies indicate that lifestyle

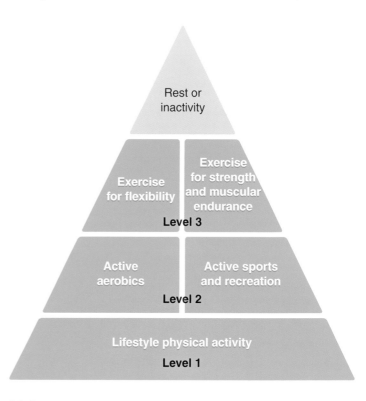

Table 13.3

Target Zones for Fat Control

	Diet	Physical activity
Frequency	• Eat 3 regular meals or 4-5 small meals daily. Regular, controlled eating is best for losing fat. Skipping meals and snacking is usually not effective.	• Participate in physical activity daily. Regular physical activity is best for losing fat. Short or irregular physical activity does little for controlling body fat.
Intensity	• To lose 1 pound of fat, you must eat 3,500 fewer calories than normal. • To gain a pound of fat, you must eat 3,500 more calories than normal. • To maintain your weight, you must keep the number of calories you eat the same.	• To lose 1 pound of fat, you must use 3,500 more calories than normal. • To gain a pound of fat, you must use 3,500 fewer calories than normal. • To maintain your weight, you must keep your level of physical activity the same.
Time	Neither diet nor physical activity results in quick fat loss. Medical experts recommend that a person lose no more than 2 pounds of weight each week without medical supervision. Both diet and physical activity can be used to safely lose 1 or 2 pounds each week.	

Table 13.4

Energy Expenditure

Activity	CALORIES USED (CAL/HR)				
	100 lb	120 lb	150 lb	180 lb	200 lb
Backpacking/Hiking	307	348	410	472	513
Badminton	255	289	340	391	425
Baseball	210	238	280	322	350
Basketball (half-court)	225	240	300	345	375
Bicycling (normal speed)	157	178	210	242	263
Bowling	155	176	208	240	261
Canoeing (4 mph)	276	344	414	504	558
Circuit training	247	280	330	380	413
Dance, ballet/modern	240	300	360	432	480
Dance, aerobic	300	360	450	540	600
Dance, social	174	222	264	318	348
Fitness calisthenics	232	263	310	357	388
Football	225	255	300	345	375
Golf (walking)	187	212	250	288	313
Gymnastics	232	263	310	357	388
Horseback riding	180	204	240	276	300
Interval training	487	552	650	748	833
Jogging (5 1/2 mph)	487	552	650	748	833
Judo/Karate	232	263	310	357	388
Racquetball/Handball	450	510	600	690	750
Rope jumping (continuous)	525	595	700	805	875
Running (10 mph)	625	765	900	1035	1125
Skating, ice/roller	262	297	350	403	438
Skiing, cross-country	525	595	700	805	875
Skiing, downhill	450	510	600	690	750
Soccer	405	459	540	575	621
Softball (fastpitch)	210	238	280	322	350
Swimming (slow laps)	240	272	320	368	400
Swimming (fast laps)	420	530	630	768	846
Tennis	315	357	420	483	525
Volleyball	262	297	350	403	483
Walking	204	258	318	372	426
Weight training	352	399	470	541	558

activities are just as effective as organized sports and games for losing fat, and more effective for permanent fat loss.

Aerobic Activities

Aerobic activities are effective for fat loss. You can do them for relatively long periods, burning many calories.

Active Sports and Active Recreation

Active sports and recreation that are equal in intensity to aerobic activities such as jogging are effective in fat loss because they can be done for long periods of time. Vigorous sports and recreational activities also burn calories but are often so intense that they cannot be performed for long periods of time.

Strength, Muscular Endurance, and Flexibility Exercises

Remember that muscle fitness exercises can help you gain weight by building muscle tissue. However, these exercises, combined with the proper diet, also can contribute to fat loss because they do burn calories. Flexibility exercises do not expend as many calories as the other four types of activities in the Physical Activity Pyramid; however, they do expend calories above resting. Any calories expended above normal can help in controlling body fatness.

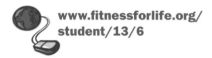

www.fitnessforlife.org/
student/13/6

Calculating Your Daily Calorie Expenditure

If you keep a record of all of the activities you perform in a day, you can determine the total calories you expended. You can use special forms (available from your teacher) to make record keeping easier. After keeping a record of the activities you do for a full day, you can use the formula at the Web site to help you calculate your daily calorie expenditure. Later you can compare your daily expenditure to your daily calorie intake (see chapter 14). To maintain weight, you must expend as much energy as you take in. To lose weight, you must expend more energy than you take in. To gain weight, you muse take in more calories than you expend.

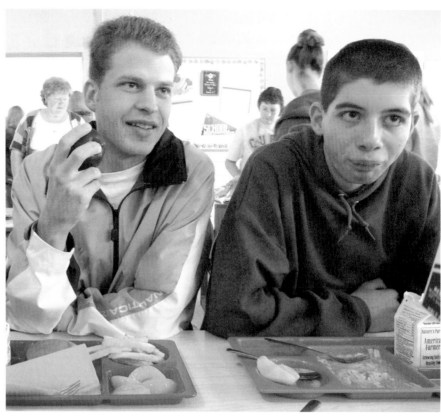

Proper nutrition and calorie intake are important to lose body fat.

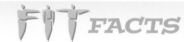

If you maintain your normal intake of calories and increase your activity by playing one half hour of tennis daily, you will lose 16 pounds in a year. If you briskly walk 15 minutes a day instead of watching TV, you will lose 5 to 6 pounds in a year.

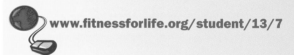

www.fitnessforlife.org/student/13/7

Table 13.5

Myths and Facts About Fat Loss

Myths	Facts
Exercise cannot be effective for fat loss because it takes many hours of exercise to lose even 1 pound of fat.	You can lose body fat over time with regular physical activity if your calorie intake remains the same. Fat lost through physical activity tends to stay off longer than fat lost through dieting alone.
Exercise does not help fat loss because it increases your appetite and encourages you to overeat.	If you are mildly active instead of inactive, your appetite should not increase. Even moderate to vigorous activity will not cause your appetite to increase so much that you overeat. People who overeat usually do so for reasons other than appetite.
Most overfat people have glandular problems.	Most overfat people eat too much, do too little physical activity, or both.
You can spot reduce by exercising a specific body part to lose fat in a particular area.	Any exercise that burns calories will cause the body's general fat deposits to decrease. One exercise does not cause one area of fat to decrease more than another.

Taking Charge:
Improving Physical Self-Perceptions

All people have a mental picture of themselves. If you think you do well in a certain activity, you will probably take part in that activity. If you feel embarrassed about your appearance or ability level while doing an activity, you probably will avoid that activity.

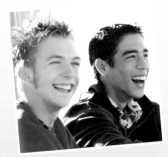

Michael was not sure that he wanted to go back to school after the summer break. It seemed as if all of his friends had grown several inches taller in the last few months, and he had stayed the same height. Michael felt embarrassed and a little jealous, even though none of his friends seemed to notice. His height certainly did not alter his ability to play tennis. In fact, friends still called him "King of the Court" because he usually won the match whenever he played.

Raul was one of the shortest in his class, but height did not stop him from being involved in activities. He realized he had never been a great basketball player, but he still liked to play with his friends from school. He discovered that height had nothing to do with his ability to go hiking, and it did not prevent him from being a good wrestler.

For Discussion

Michael's self-perception about his appearance has changed from positive to negative. What can he do to change his negative perception? How does Raul keep a positive self-perception? What else can a person do to develop a positive self-perception? Fill out the questionnaire provided by your teacher to find out about your own self-perception. Consider the guidelines on page 234.

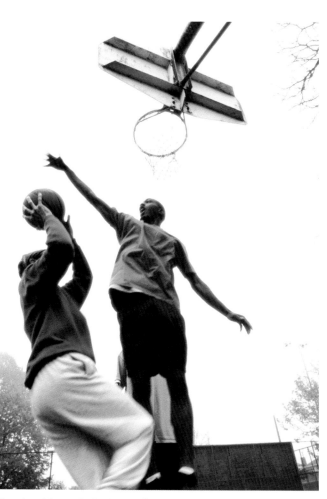

People with good physical self-perceptions are more likely to be active than those with low physical self-perceptions.

Myths About Fat Loss

Some people have incorrect ideas about physical activity and fat loss. Read table 13.5 to identify some mistaken ideas and learn some facts about losing body fat.

No matter what your body is like now, regular physical activity and proper diet will help you control body fatness. When you are fit, you look better, feel better, and have fewer health problems than people who are overfat and unfit.

FIT FACTS

Interviews with teens show that 44 percent of overweight youth were, or are, teased about their body weight. Studies show that four to five times as many teens think they are overweight than really are. Being teased or having feelings of being overweight can result in low physical self-perceptions. Teens can help other teens improve self-perceptions by being supportive rather than critical.

Lesson Review

1. How can you use the FITT formula to control your body fatness?
2. How can physical activity help you maintain a healthy body fat level?

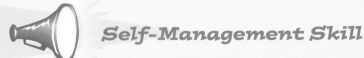

Self-Management Skill

Improving Physical Self-Perceptions

A self-perception is an awareness you have about your own thoughts, actions, or appearance. It is how you think other people view you. Some of the many kinds of self-perceptions are academic, social, and artistic. In this book the focus is on physical self-perceptions. This refers to the way you view your physical self. Four areas of physical self-perceptions are strength, fitness, skill, and body attractiveness. People with good physical self-perceptions are happy with their current strength and fitness levels, they feel that the skills that they have are adequate to meet their needs, and they like the way they look. We know that people who have positive physical self-perceptions are more likely to be active than those who do not have such good perceptions of themselves. The following list includes some guidelines that can be used to help people improve physical self-perceptions.

▶ **Assess your current physical self-perceptions.** You may use the worksheet provided by your teacher.

▶ **Consider your self-assessment results.** Use the self-assessment to determine whether you have any areas in which your physical perceptions are especially low (strength, fitness, skill, or body attractiveness).

▶ **Perform regular physical activity to improve yourself physically or practice to improve your physical skills.**

▶ **Consider a new way of thinking about yourself.** Often people set unrealistic standards such as trying to look like someone on television or in the movies. It is important to understand that in real life these people do not look the way they look on the screen. In fact, special cameras and computers are often used to change the way they look. Also you do not know whether a movie star has eating disorders or practices healthy habits. Consider your heredity and set realistic standards for yourself.

▶ **Think positively.** Almost all people have a physical characteristic that they would like to change. Studies show that the things people don't like about themselves are rarely seen as problems by other people. You are often your own worst critic, so thinking positively can help you present yourself in a positive way.

▶ **Do not let the actions of a few insensitive people cause negative feelings about yourself.** People who are insensitive to others' feelings will always exist. These people often have low perceptions of themselves and try to build themselves up by tearing other people down. Recognize that criticism from these people is their problem, not yours.

▶ **Consider how your behavior and actions influence how other people view you.** Acting happy and friendly has as much to do with how others perceive you as your physical characteristics.

▶ **Realize that all people have some imperfections.** Try to build on your strengths and improve your areas of weakness.

▶ **Find a realistic role model and be a role model for others.** Instead of trying to be like someone who is totally unlike you, try to find someone who you admire who has characteristics you can realistically achieve. Just as you look to others for models, remember that others look to you as a model. Providing a positive model for others can help you think positively about yourself.

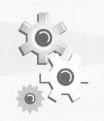

Activity 2

Muscle Fitness Exercises With Resistance Machines

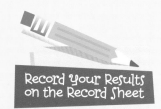
Record Your Results on the Record Sheet

Although physical activity from each of the levels of the Physical Activity Pyramid (including lifestyle activity from level 1 and active aerobics, active recreation, and active sports from level 2) is essential for improving body composition, it is also important to do exercises for muscular strength and endurance because they can significantly decrease your percentage of body fat as well as increase your lean body mass. Strength and muscular endurance exercises from level 3 of the pyramid build muscles so that you look your best.

In this activity, you will perform 10 basic exercises using resistance machines. The exercises are called the Basic 10 because they build muscle fitness in 10 of the basic, or large, muscle groups of the body. Use your 1RM values from the self-assessment in chapter 11 to determine the amount of weight or resistance you should be able to lift. If you did not have time to do the 1RM self-assessments for each exercise, complete this process before performing the exercises. Follow these instructions and guidelines to perform the exercises:

▶ Your teacher will demonstrate or have a class member demonstrate proper technique for each of the lifts. After the demonstration, travel from one machine to the next. Practice each exercise using *no resistance or weight.* Have a partner or partners evaluate your technique while you perform the exercise, and make changes if necessary. Exchange places with your partner(s). Continue this procedure at each machine. Use the guidelines on page 189 to help evaluate your partner.

▶ Next, determine 40 percent of your 1RM for each exercise. Perform 10 reps of each exercise at this resistance. Perform 1 set using proper form.

▶ If you have the opportunity to continue this program over several weeks, use the double progressive system to increase your overload (see page 187).

▶ Do exercises for the abdominal and back muscles. Some simple exercises not requiring machines are just as effective as resistance machine exercises. They are included in the Basic 10 exercises even though they do not use machines.

▶ When performing PRE, be sure to follow exercise etiquette. Carry a towel with you and wipe off the exercise bench after you do your exercise. Get off the machine between exercises so that another person can use it. Take your proper turn.

▶ You may have to wait between exercises to find an available machine. If a machine is not available, perform the curl-up or the back extension exercise on a table or bench. Once you complete these exercises, if you still have waiting time, perform a cardiovascular exercise such as bench stepping or rope jumping.

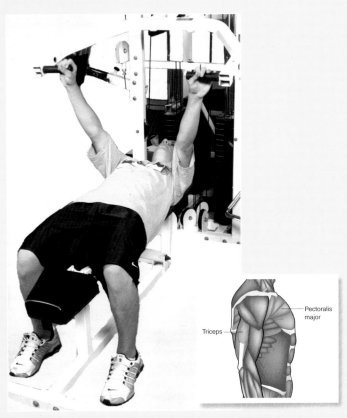

This exercise uses the pectoral and triceps muscles.

Bench Press

1. Lie on your back on the bench with your feet flat on the floor. Grasp the handles with your palms facing away from your body. Flatten your back. If possible, place your feet on the floor to help flatten your back and avoid arching it. If your feet do not reach the floor easily, you can bend your knees and place your feet on the bench to accomplish the same purpose.

   ⚠️ **Caution:** Do not place your feet on the bench if it so narrow that your feet might slip off the bench or if the bench is unstable.

2. Push upward on the handles, extending your arms completely.

   ⚠️ **Caution:** Do not lock your elbows. Do not arch your back.

3. Return to the starting position.

4. You may choose either this exercise or the seated arm press (see page 183). You may also substitute this exercise in the self-assessment if you have a bench press machine and do not have a seated press machine.

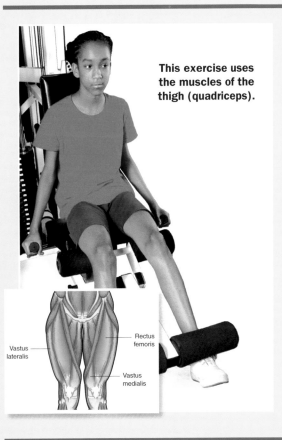

This exercise uses the muscles of the thigh (quadriceps).

Knee Extension

1. Sit on the bench. Hook one of your ankles under the pad. Grasp the handles on the bench.

2. Extend your knee. Bend the knee through its full range of motion.

3. Return to the starting position. Repeat the exercise with the other leg.

4. You may choose either this exercise or the seated leg press (see page 183).

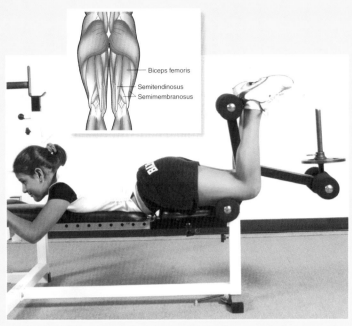

Biceps femoris
Semitendinosus
Semimembranosus

This exercise uses the hamstring muscles.

Hamstring Curl

1. Lie facedown on the bench with your kneecaps extending over the edge of the bench. Hook your heels under the cylindrical pads. Grasp the handles on the bench.
2. Bend your knees so that you lift the cylindrical pads. Bend the knees through their full range of motion. The pads will almost touch your buttocks at the top of the lift.
3. Lower to the starting position.

⚠️ **Caution:** Do not lock the knees when putting your heels under the pads. If necessary, have a partner lift the pads so that you can avoid this.

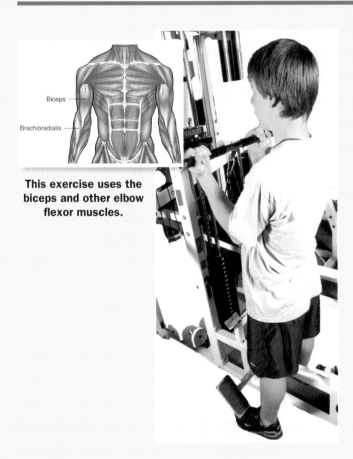

Biceps

Brachioradialis

This exercise uses the biceps and other elbow flexor muscles.

Biceps Curl

1. Stand in front of the station and grasp the handle of the low pulley, palms up. Tighten your abdominals and buttocks (gluteal muscles).
2. Pull the handle from thigh level to chest level. Bend your elbows, but keep them close to your sides.

⚠️ **Caution:** Do not move other body parts.

3. Return to the starting position.

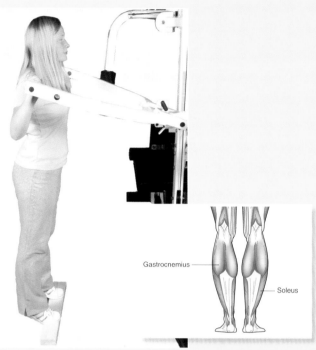

Heel Raise

1. Place a 2-inch-thick board on the floor. Stand with the balls of your feet on the board and the handles even with your shoulders.
2. Grasp the handles with your palms facing away from your body. Keep your hands and arms stationary during the lift.
3. Rise on to the balls of your feet, and then lower to the starting position.

Gastrocnemius

Soleus

This exercise uses the calf muscles.

Lat Pull-Down

1. Sit on the bench (or floor depending on the machine). Adjust the seat height so that your arms are fully extended when you grab the bar.
2. Grab the bar with your palms facing away from you. Your arms should be at least shoulder-width apart.
3. Pull the bar down to chest level.
4. Return to the starting position.

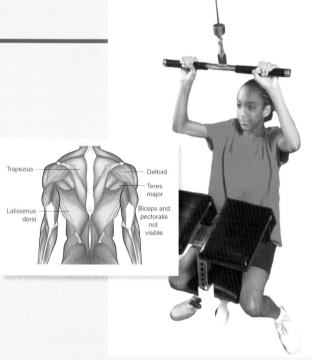

Trapezius

Deltoid

Teres major

Latissimus dorsi

Biceps and pectoralis not visible

This exercise uses the muscles of the back (latissimus dorsi), shoulder (deltoids), chest (pectoralis), and arm (biceps).

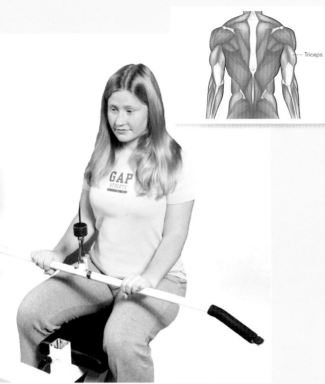

This exercise uses the muscles on the back of the
arm (triceps).

Triceps Press

1. Adjust the seat height so that your hands are on the handles just above shoulder height.
2. With your thumbs toward your body, grab the handles.
3. Keeping your back straight, push forward with your arms until they are straight.
4. Return to the starting position.

Seated Row

1. Adjust the machine so that your arms are almost fully extended and parallel to the ground.
2. Grab the handles with your thumbs up.
3. Keeping your back straight, pull straight back toward your chest.
4. Return to the starting position.

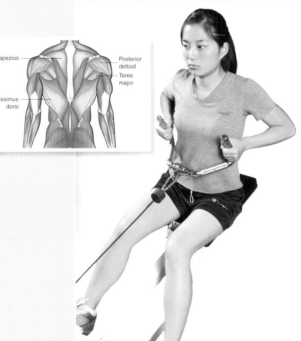

This exercise uses the muscles of the back and shoulders.

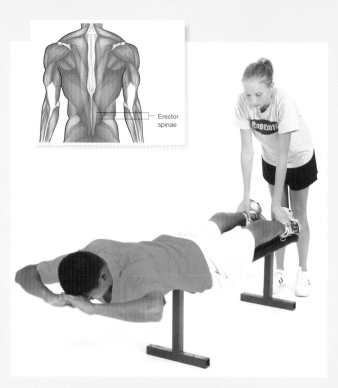

This exercise uses the back muscles.

Back Extension Exercise (Trunk Lift)

1. Lie facedown on a table (or bench). Slide forward until your upper body extends over the edge at the waist. With a partner holding your legs, allow the upper body to lower.
2. From the low position, lift your upper body until it is even with the edge of the table.

 Caution: Do not lift any higher.

3. Lower to the beginning position. Repeat the exercise up to 10 times.

Safety Tip: As you do these exercises, move only as far as the directions specify.

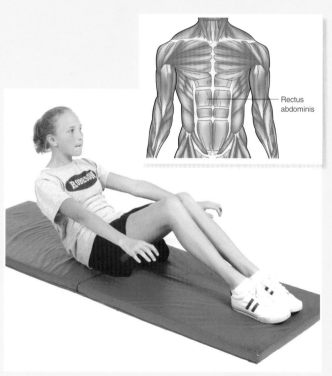

This exercises uses the abdominal muscles.

Abdominal Exercise (Curl-Up)

The curl-up, sometimes referred to as the crunch, is a good substitute for the straight-leg sit-up, bent-knee sit-up, and hands-behind-the-head sit-up.

1. Lie on your back with your knees bent and your feet close to your buttocks.
2. Hold your hands and arms straight in front of you and curl your head, shoulders, and upper back off the floor.
3. Slowly roll back to the starting position.

 Caution: Do not hold your feet while doing a trunk curl.

As you improve, you might hold your arms across your chest. When you become very good, you might place your hands on your face (cheeks).

Safety Tips:

1. Perform all movements slowly.
2. Exhale on the lift; inhale on the return to the starting position. Do not hold your breath.

240

13

Chapter Review

Reviewing Concepts and Vocabulary

Number your paper from 1 to 6. Next to each number, write the word (or words) that correctly completes the sentence.

1. An eating disorder characterized by bingeing and purging is called _____.
2. The minimum amount of body fat needed for good health is _____.
3. Your _____ is the amount of energy your body uses at complete rest.
4. A term used to describe a person who is very overfat is _____.
5. People with _____ see themselves as too fat even when they are extremely thin.
6. A technique for assessing body fat levels that involves being weighed under water is called _____.

Number your paper from 7 to 12. Next to each number, choose the letter of the best answer.

Column I	Column II
7. overfat	a. fat under the skin
8. skinfolds	b. too much body fat
9. anorexia athletica	c. all the tissues that make up your body
10. underfat	d. eating disorder most common among athletes
11. caliper	e. used for skinfold measurements
12. body composition	f. too little body fat

Number your paper from 13 to 15. On your paper, write a short answer for each statement or question.

13. Explain why maintaining essential body fat levels is important for good health.
14. Describe one myth about fat loss and explain how it is incorrect or misleading.
15. Why is a combination of diet and physical activity best for maintaining ideal levels of body fat?

Thinking Critically

Write a paragraph to answer the following question.

Each year people spend billions of dollars on weight loss or muscle building products that do not work. Look in the newspaper or a popular magazine. Find an advertisement for a weight loss product. Read the ad and make a list of its claims. Place a checkmark by those that are consistent with the information in this chapter. Place an X by those that appear to be false. Write a paragraph evaluating the advertisement.

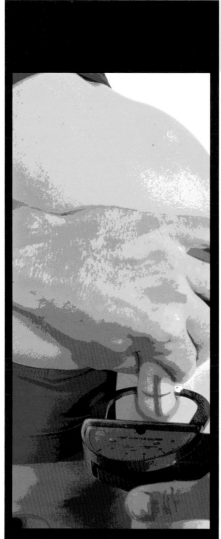

Project

Keep a record of your calorie intake and your physical activity for one week. How might you adjust your calorie intake and your amount of physical activity to better maintain or improve your levels of body fat? What short-term goals might you have for calories eaten each day and calories expended each day for the one-week period? Make a written plan for the following week incorporating changes that might help you reach or maintain ideal levels of body fat. Use the worksheets provided by your teacher.

14

Choosing Nutritious Food

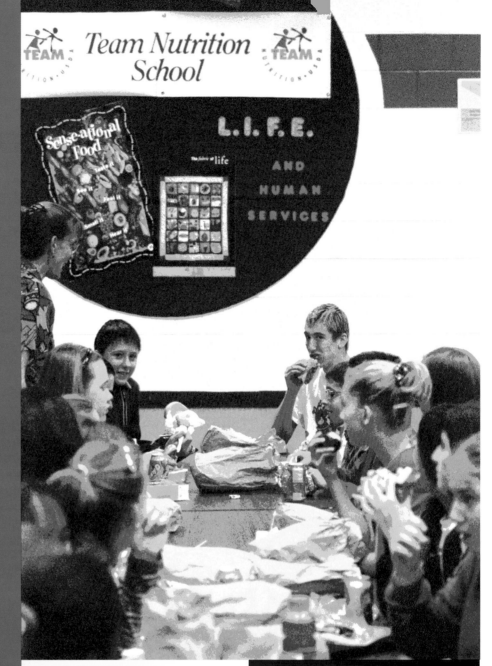

In this chapter...

Activity 1
Jollyball

Lesson 14.1
A Healthy Diet

Self-Assessment
Body Measurements

Lesson 14.2
Making Food Choices

Taking Charge
Saying "No"

Self-Management Skill
Saying "No"

Activity 2
Cooperative Aerobics

Activity 1

JOLLYBALL

In planning your lifetime physical activity program, you might want to include some sports but feel that you lack the necessary skills. Many people avoid participation in sports for the same reason. However, some sports can be modified to make them more fun for everyone regardless of skill level. For example, jollyball is the name given to several modifications of volleyball that may make the sport more fun for everyone.

Lesson 14.1

A Healthy Diet

Lesson Objectives

After reading this lesson, you should be able to

1. Describe the three types of nutrients that provide energy and the amounts of each necessary for good health.
2. Explain why vitamins and minerals are necessary to good health.
3. Describe MyPyramid and explain how it can help you plan for healthy eating.

Lesson Vocabulary

AI (p. 244), amino acids (p. 244), complete proteins (p. 244), DRI (p. 244), incomplete proteins (p. 244), micro-nutrients (p. 244), RDA (p. 244), saturated fats (p. 244), transfatty acids (p. 244), UL (p. 244), unsaturated fats (p. 244)

www.fitnessforlife.org/student/14/1

What kinds of foods are important for your health? How much food do you need to eat? In this lesson, you will learn about healthful foods. You also will learn how to select foods for a balanced diet.

Nutrients Your Body Needs

Scientists have identified 45 to 50 different nutrients—food substances required for the growth and maintenance of your cells. These nutrients have been divided into six groups—carbohydrates, proteins, fats, vitamins, minerals, and water. Each of these six types of nutrients will be discussed in this chapter.

www.fitnessforlife.org/student/14/2

Nutrients That Provide Energy

Three types of nutrients supply the energy the body needs to perform its daily tasks: carbohydrates, proteins, and fats. The United State Department of Agriculture (USDA) recommends that most of the calories in your diet come from carbohydrates. Fewer of the calories in your diet typically come from fat and protein. The rec-

FIT FACTS

Fats contain more calories per unit of weight than proteins or carbohydrates. One gram of fat contains 9 calories. One gram of carbohydrate or protein contains 4 calories.

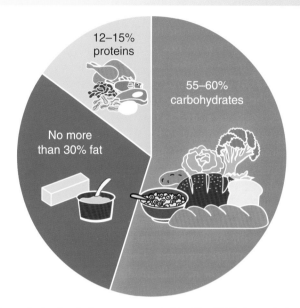

Percentage of calories recommended by the USDA for carbohydrates, proteins, and fats.

ommended percentages of calories from the three nutrients are shown in the figure.

Carbohydrates

Carbohydrates provide you with your main source of energy. The two kinds of carbohydrates are simple and complex. Most of our carbohydrate calories should be complex. Complex carbohydrates are sugars found in foods such as whole-grain breads, vegetables, and grain. Complex carbohydrates are called nutritionally dense because they contain large amounts of nutrients for the number of calories they provide. The majority of the carbohydrates in your diet should be complex in nature. Simple carbohydrates should account for 15 percent or less of the total calories in your diet. Some simple carbohydrates are better than others. For example fruit juices are simple carbohydrates that are high in simple carbohydrates but also contain vitamins. Others, such as candy, pastries, and soft drinks are considered to be empty calories because they contain many calories but contain few vitamins or minerals.

Fiber is a type of complex carbohydrate that your body cannot digest. Fiber supplies no energy. Fiber sources include the leaves, stems, roots, and seed coverings of fruits, vegetables, and grains. Examples of foods high in fiber are whole-grain breads and cereals, the skin of fresh fruits, raw vegetables, nuts, and seeds. Fiber helps you avoid intestinal problems and might reduce your chances of developing some forms of cancer.

Proteins

Proteins are the group of nutrients that builds, repairs, and maintains body cells. They are called the building blocks of your body. Animal products, such as milk, eggs, meat, and fish, contain proteins. Some plants, such as beans and grains, also contain proteins. Proteins provide energy but do not provide as many calories for energy (12 to 15 percent) as carbohydrates or fats. If more protein is consumed than needed to build body tissues, the calories will be used to produce energy for daily activities or stored as body fat.

During digestion, your body breaks down proteins into simpler substances called **amino acids,** which your small intestine can absorb. Your body can manufacture 11 of the 20 existing amino acids. You need to get the other nine amino acids—known as the essential amino acids—from food.

Foods with all nine essential amino acids are said to contain **complete proteins.** They come from animal sources, such as meat, milk products, and fish. Foods that contain some, but not all, essential amino acids are said to contain **incomplete proteins.** Beans, nuts, rice, and certain other plants contain incomplete proteins. A daily diet that includes foods with both complete and incomplete proteins usually provides ample essential amino acids. People who do not eat meat need to eat a variety of incomplete proteins that together provide all the essential amino acids.

Fats

Fats are in animal products and in some plant products, such as nuts and vegetable oils. Fats are necessary for the growth and repair of cells. Fats dissolve certain vitamins and carry them to body cells. In addition, they enhance the flavor and texture of foods.

Fats are classified as saturated or unsaturated. In general, **saturated fats** are solid at room temperature, and **unsaturated fats** are liquid at room temperature. Saturated fats come mostly from animal products such as lard, butter, milk, and meat fats. Unsaturated fats come mostly from plants such as sunflowers, corn, soybeans, olives, almonds, and peanuts. Also, fish produce unsaturated fats in their cells.

According to the USDA, less than 30 percent of the total calories you consume should be from fat. It is recommended that no more than 10 percent of your total calories come from saturated fat or **transfatty acids.** Transfatty acids are made from unsaturated fats such as vegetable oils using a process that makes them solid at room temperature. Solid margarine is an example of

a transfatty acid. Transfatty acids have been found to be similar to saturated fats in their effect on the body. For years food labels have informed you of how much saturated fat is in food, but only recently have labels included information on transfatty acids (transfats).

Cholesterol is a waxy, fatlike substance found in the saturated fats of animal cells, including those of humans. You consume cholesterol in foods high in saturated fat such as meat. Because you are an animal, you produce your own cholesterol. People who consume high amounts of saturated fat and transfatty acids produce more cholesterol than those who limit the amounts of these fats in the diet. High levels of cholesterol in your blood can contribute to atherosclerosis and other heart diseases. Medical experts recommend eating foods low in cholesterol, low in saturated fat, and low in transfatty acids.

Nutrients That Do Not Provide Energy

Minerals, vitamins, and water have no calories and provide no energy, but they all play a vital role in staying fit and healthy. Minerals and vitamins are sometimes called **micronutrients** because the body needs them in relatively small amounts compared to carbohydrates, proteins, and fats.

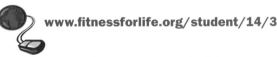

www.fitnessforlife.org/student/14/3

The Food and Nutrition Board of the Institute of Medicine provides standards for the amounts of micronutrients called Dietary Reference Intakes **(DRI).** The three types of DRIs are used to help you know how much of each vitamin and mineral you should consume. The first is called the Recommended Dietary Allowance **(RDA).** RDA refers to the minimum amount of a nutrient necessary to meet the health needs of most people. The second, Adequate Intake **(AI),** is used when there is not sufficient evidence to establish an RDA. Tolerable Upper Limit **(UL)** describes the maximum amount of a vitamin or mineral that can be consumed without posing a health risk. For more information concerning all of the DRIs consult the Web site on the previous page.

Minerals

Minerals are essential nutrients that help regulate the activities of cells. Minerals come from elements in the earth's crust. They are present in all plants and animals. You need 25 different minerals in varying amounts. Table 14.1 shows some major functions of the most important minerals as well as some food sources for them.

If you eat a balanced diet, you will most likely be getting the proper amounts of minerals. Nutrition experts still recommend that the best way to get adequate minerals and vitamins is with a balanced diet. Recently the American Medical Association recommended that most Americans take a vitamin and mineral supplement because many do not eat regular meals and for this reason do not get the vitamins and minerals they need. If you take a vitamin and mineral supplement, it should contain only the RDA or AI value for each mineral and vitamin. Supplements should not provide more than the UL for any vitamin or mineral. An excessive amount could lead to health problems. For example, too much calcium can interfere with other medications you may take. Too much magnesium can deplete the body of calcium and phosphorus. Too much zinc can deplete the body of copper.

Some minerals are especially important for young people. Calcium is one of them. Eating calcium-rich foods is important for health. An important function of calcium is building and maintaining bones, and the body needs calcium to build bones during the teen years. At about age 20, your bones become less efficient in getting calcium out of the food you eat and your bones begin to lose calcium. Because of a change in hormones when women reach about age 55, they

have much more bone loss than men. A large percentage of older women develop osteoporosis, a condition in which the bones become porous and break easily. Men can have this disease, but they get it less often and much later in life. Getting enough calcium and doing weight-bearing exercises (such as walking and jogging) and resistance exercises all of your life help reduce the risk of osteoporosis.

Iron is a mineral needed for proper formation and functioning of your red blood cells. The red blood cells carry oxygen to your muscles and other body tissues. Iron deficiencies are especially common among girls and women. When you have insufficient iron in your body, you have iron deficiency anemia. This condition causes you to feel tired all the time.

The best sources of iron are meat (especially red meat), poultry, and fish. Iron from these foods is more easily absorbed than iron from other foods. An adequate amount of vitamin C also helps your body absorb iron. Eating a variety of foods that contain iron is the best way to get an adequate amount.

Sodium is a mineral that helps your body cells function properly. Sodium is present in many foods. It is especially high in certain foods, such as snack foods, processed foods, fast foods, and cured meats such as ham. For many people, sodium in the diet comes primarily from table salt (sodium chloride).

Most people eat more sodium than they need. It is wise to limit the amount of sodium in your diet. People with high blood pressure, or hypertension, need to be especially careful to limit sodium. It can cause their bodies to retain water, helping keep their blood pressure high.

Vitamins

Vitamins are needed for growth and repair of body cells. Vitamin C and the B vitamins are water soluble,

Table 14.1

Functions and Sources of Minerals

Mineral	Function in the body	Food sources
Calcium	Builds and maintains teeth and bones; helps blood clot; helps nerves and muscles function	Cheese; milk; dark green vegetables; sardines; legumes
Phosphorus	Builds and maintains teeth and bones; helps release energy from nutrients	Meat; poultry; fish; eggs; legumes; milk products
Magnesium	Aids breakdown of glucose and proteins; regulates body fluids	Green vegetables; grains; nuts; beans; yeast
Sodium	Regulates internal water balance; helps nerves function	Most foods; table salt
Potassium	Regulates fluid balance in cells; helps nerves function	Oranges; bananas; meats; bran; potatoes; dried beans
Iron	Helps transfer oxygen in red blood cells and in other cells	Liver; red meats; dark green vegetables; shellfish; whole-grain cereals
Zinc	Aids in transport of carbon dioxide; aids in healing wounds	Meats; shellfish; whole grains; milk; legumes

so they dissolve in blood and are carried to cells throughout your body. Your body cannot store excess B and C vitamins. You need to eat foods containing these vitamins every day. Vitamins A, D, E, and K dissolve in fat. Excess amounts of these vitamins are stored in fat cells in your liver and other body parts. Table 14.2 gives you more information about specific vitamins.

Folacin, or folic acid, is one vitamin that is especially important to girls and young women. Research has shown that children born to women low in folacin are at risk of birth defects.

Water

Dietitians usually say that water is the single most important nutrient. It carries the other nutrients to your cells, carries away waste, and helps regulate body temperature. Most foods contain water. In fact, your own body weight is 50 to 60 percent water.

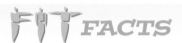

The term *nutritionist* is frequently used for an expert on nutrition. In fact, a dietitian is more likely to be a true expert than those who call themselves nutritionist. In many states anyone can use the title nutritionist. The term *dietitian* is reserved for those with a degree in nutrition and who are registered (registered dietitian).

Your body loses two to three quarts of water a day through breathing, perspiring, and eliminating waste from the bowels and bladder. In very hot weather, or when you exercise vigorously, you lose even more water than usual. Then you need to drink plenty of extra fluids. The best beverages for this purpose are water, fruit juice, and milk. Soft drinks that contain caffeine are not as effective as water. Also, sports drinks sold commercially usually contain sodium and other ingredients that you do not need unless you exercise for several hours in high temperatures.

Planning a Balanced Diet

As you have learned, you need to eat foods containing all six nutrients in order to get a healthy, balanced diet. In addition, other guidelines have been developed to help you choose healthy foods.

Health Goals in America

America has national goals, called Healthy People 2010 goals, to promote health and prevent disease. These goals are the Healthy People 2010 goals related to nutrition:

▶ Reduce dietary fat, especially saturated fat.

▶ Increase complex carbohydrates in the diet.

▶ Increase the amount of calcium in the diet.

▶ Decrease the amount of salt and sodium in the diet.

▶ Reduce the incidence of iron deficiency.

Table 14.2

Functions and Sources of Vitamins

Vitamin	Function in the body	Food sources
B_1 (thiamin)	Helps release energy from carbohydrates	Pork; organ meats; legumes; greens
B_2 (riboflavin)	Helps break down carbohydrates and proteins	Meat; milk products; eggs; green and yellow vegetables
B_6 (pyridoxine)	Helps break down protein and glucose	Yeast; nuts; beans; liver; fish; rice
B_{12} (cobalamin)	Aids nucleic acid and amino acid formation	Meat; milk products; eggs; fish
Folacin	Helps build DNA and proteins	Yeast; wheat germ; liver; greens
Pantothenic acid	Involved in reactions with carbohydrates and proteins	Most unprocessed foods
Niacin	Helps release energy from carbohydrates and proteins	Milk; meats; whole-grain or enriched cereals; legumes
Biotin	Aids formation of amino, nucleic, and fatty acids and glycogen	Eggs; liver; yeast
C (ascorbic acid)	Aids formation of hormones, bone tissue, and collagen	Fruits; tomatoes; potatoes; green, leafy vegetables
A (retinol)	Helps produce normal mucus; part of chemical necessary for vision	Butter; margarine; liver; eggs; green or yellow vegetables
D	Aids absorption of calcium and phosphorous	Liver; fortified milk; fatty fish
E (tocopherol)	Prevents damage to cell membranes and vitamin A	Vegetable oils
K	Aids blood clotting	Leafy vegetables

MyPyramid

Our national health goals are based on dietary guidelines developed by the United States Department of Agriculture (USDA). MyPyramid, an outcome of the dietary guidelines, was designed to help you make smart choices from every food group, to help you get the most nutrition from the calories you consume, and to help you find a balance between food and physical activity. The new pyramid contains multicolored bands representing six food groups. Also new is a stairway, to the left of the pyramid, designed to represent your need for regular physical activity. In this book, each step in the stairway is labeled with a type of physical activity to illustrate the variety of activities included in this book. The combination of the pyramid and the stairway emphasizes the importance of the balance between food and physical activity in maintaining a healthy weight.

A higher proportion of your total calories should come from food groups with wide colored bands than from food groups with narrower colored bands. The orange band represents grains. It is wide because grains should make up a large part of a healthy diet. At least half of your grain choices should be whole grain. Look for the whole grain label on bread, cereal, and other grain products.

The green band represents vegetables, and the red band represents fruits. The bands for vegetables and fruits are wide because both foods should constitute relatively larges proportions of your total diet. There

are five vegetable groups: dark green, orange, dry peas and beans, starchy, and other. The guidelines emphasize getting most of your vegetable servings from the dark green and orange vegetables. Fruits can be fresh, canned, frozen, or dried. Fruit juices (100% juice) are a source of fruit consumption, but the guidelines suggest that you not consume them too much because of their high content of simple sugar.

The other relatively wide colored band in MyPyramid is blue. It represents dairy products, including milk, cheese, milk-based desserts, and yogurt. It is recommended that you consider low-fat and fat-free products when making choices from this food group.

The purple band represents meats and beans. The foods in this group are important because of their protein content. You do not need to eat as much of these foods as you do of other foods, but they are essential to good health. Included in this group are red meats (such as beef and pork), poultry (including eggs), fish, dry beans, nuts, and seeds. Dry beans, nuts, and seeds are important sources of protein and are included in the vegetable group as well. Consuming fish and lean cuts of meat is recommended.

Oils are represented by the yellow band. Oils are types of fat, so they should be used sparingly. Monounsaturated oils (such as canola oil) are a healthy choice. Polyunsaturated oils (such as corn oil) are preferred over saturated fats such as butter, lard, and trans fats (oils with hydrogen added, such as margarine). Saturated fats (including

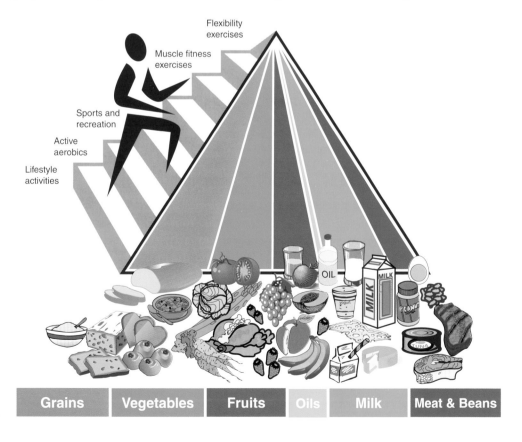

MyPyramid.

Table 14.3

Recommended Number and Size of Servings

FOOD GROUP	CALORIE RANGE			EXAMPLES OF SERVING SIZES
	1,600	2,200	2,800	
Grains	6 servings	9 servings	11 servings	1 slice bread; 1/2 cup cooked cereal, rice, or pasta; 1 cup cold cereal; 1/4 cup wheat germ; 1 6-inch tortilla
Vegetables	3 servings	4 servings	5 servings	1 cup raw leafy vegetables; 1/2 cup other vegetables (chopped or cooked); 3/4 cup vegetable juice; 1/2 cup cooked vegetables
Fruit	2 servings	3 servings	4 servings	1 orange; 3/4 cup fruit juice; 1 cup cooked fruit
Milk	2-3 servings	2-3 servings	2-3 servings	1 cup milk or yogurt; 1/2 cup cottage cheese; 1-1/2 oz cheese
Meat and beans	2 servings	2-3 servings	3 servings	1 serving = 2-3 oz of any cooked meat, poultry, or fish; Equivalent = either 1/2 cup of cooked dried beans, 2 tablespoons peanut butter, or 1 whole egg; Quantity and type of fat vary in each protein source

animal fats and some vegetable oils) are solid at room temperature but are still considered oils in MyPyramid. Fish oils, especially those high in omega 3, are a healthy addition to the diet when not consumed in excess.

Although not represented by a colored band, a category called "discretionary calories" is described in MyPyramid. Included are sources of calories such as condiments (such as ketchup and mayonnaise) and simple sugars (such as soft drinks and candy). These sources of calories can be part of a healthy, well-planned diet when priority is given to choosing adequate foods from the principal groups and when consumed in small proportions.

The new dietary guidelines emphasize that no single diet is best for all people. The exact amount of food that should be consumed from each food group depends on factors such as age, gender, and activity level. Find out more about MyPyramid and learn about alternative pyramids developed by certain groups (for example, the American Heart Association developed a pyramid for people with heart problems) at the Web site. Ethnic food pyramids are also available.

 www.fitnessforlife.org/student/14/4

Recommended Servings
How much do you need to eat? It depends on your caloric needs. The total calories you need each day is listed next.

▶ 1,600 calories: primarily sedentary women

▶ 2,200 calories: most children, teenage girls, active women, and sedentary men

▶ 2,800 calories: usually teenage boys, active men, and very active women

Most experts agree that one of the main reasons why so many Americans are overfat is because of an increase in food portion size. Some of the current portions are two or three

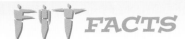

One reason for the increase in portion sizes in recent years is the marketing of larger sized meals sometimes referred to as super size. For example, the original size of most French fries had 450 calories. The size of a large order currently promoted by many fast food places has over 600 calories. Another example is buffets that offer all you can eat for a specific price. People often take large portions because they want to get their money's worth.

times as large as portions served in the past. What you are served may really be several servings, not just one. Table 14.3 lists the recommended servings from each food group.

Balancing Calories
You learned in chapter 12 that many factors, including metabolism, heredity, maturation, and physical activity, influence body fatness. These factors also influence the number of calories you need to eat. You need to balance the number of calories you consume with the number of calories you expend in order to maintain a healthy weight. Your body burns calories for energy. The more vigorous activity you do, the more energy your body uses and the more calories you need.

Lesson Review
1. How much dietary carbohydrate, protein, and fat are desirable for good health?
2. Why are vitamins and minerals necessary for good health?
3. What is MyPyramid? How can it help you plan for healthy eating?

Self-Assessment

Body Measurements

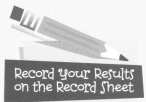

Record Your Results on the Record Sheet

In earlier chapters you learned how to assess all of the parts of health-related physical fitness because good levels of health-related fitness are related to good health and wellness. The two assessments that you will do in this chapter do not measure physical fitness, but the factors that you will assess are very much related to health and wellness.

You will use a tape measure to do both assessments. As you do the assessments, follow these guidelines:

▶ Use a non-elastic tape to make the measures.

▶ Pull the tape snugly against your skin but not so tight as to cause an indentation in your skin.

▶ Be sure that the tape is horizontal when measures are made. If the tape sags, measurements will be larger than they should be.

Body weight (lb)	% Fat	Waist (in.)
		45
120	40	40
140	30	
160	25	
180	20	35
200	15	
220	10	
240	5	30
260		
		25

Body measurement for males.

PART 1: Estimating Body Fat From Body Weight and Body Girths

You already know that having too much body fat can cause health problems. You can use body measurements to estimate your percentage of body fat. Males use weight and waist measurements, and females use height and hip measurements. Work with a partner to take the measurements.

Males: Waist and Weight

1. Measure your waist even with your navel.
2. Weigh yourself while fully clothed, but without shoes. Find your weight to the nearest pound.
3. Use the body measurement figure to estimate your percentage of body fat. To do so, place a ruler so that it cuts across the left vertical line at the mark for your weight and across the right vertical line at the mark for your waist measurement. Your estimated percentage of body fat is the number where the ruler intersects the center vertical line. Write this information on your record sheet.
4. Find your rating in the rating chart for body fatness on page 227. Record your rating.

249

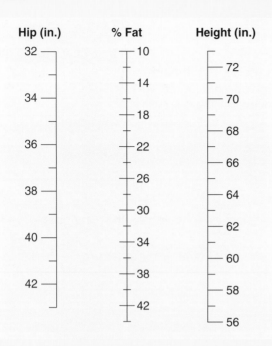

Body measurement for females.

Females: Hip and Height

1. With clothes on, measure your hips at the widest point. Measure to the nearest half inch.
2. Remove your shoes and measure your height to the nearest half inch.
3. Use the body measurement figure to estimate your percentage of body fat. To do so, place a ruler so that it cuts across the left vertical line at the mark for your hip measurement and across the right vertical line at the mark for your height. Your estimated percentage of body fat is the number where the ruler intersects the center line. Record this information.
4. Find your rating in the rating chart for body fatness on page 227. Record your rating.

PART 2: Waist-to-Hip Ratio

Scientists now know that people who have more weight in the middle of the body have a higher risk of disease than people who have more weight in the lower body (legs and hips). Those who have too much weight in their mid-section are said to have an apple body type, while those who have more weight in their hips are said to have a pear body type. Overfat people who have a pear body type have less risk for disease than overfat people with an apple body type. In general, women are more likely to be a pear type, and men are more likely to be an apple type. This fact may in part explain why women have less risk of heart disease than men. The waist-to-hip ratio is a simple method of assessing the risk associated with your body type.

1. Measure your hips at the largest point (largest circumference of the buttocks). Make sure that measurements are made while standing with your feet together. Record your measurement.
2. Measure your waist at the smallest circumference (called the natural waist). If there is no natural waist, measure at the level of the umbilicus. Measure at the end of a normal inspiration (just after a normal breath). Do not suck in to make your waist smaller. Record your measurement.
3. Calculate your waist-to-hip ratio using the formula on your record sheet.
4. Find your ratio in table 14.4. Record your rating.

Table 14.4

Rating Chart: Waist-to-Hip Ratio

	Males	Females
Good health zone	<.90	<.80
Borderline risk	.91-1.0	.80-.85
Higher risk	>1.0	>.85

Making Food Choices

Lesson Objectives

After reading this lesson, you should be able to

1. Explain how to use the FIT formula to meet your nutritional needs.

2. Explain how reading food labels can help you make healthy food choices.

3. Recognize some common myths about nutrition and explain why they are not factual.

Lesson Vocabulary

food label (p. 251), food supplement (p. 254), junk food (p. 251)

 www.fitnessforlife.org/student/14/5

You have learned how to use recent nutritional guidelines and MyPyramid to choose foods for a nutritious diet. You also learned how following the dietary guidelines can help you attain and maintain good health. In this lesson, you will learn more about choosing healthy foods for a balanced diet.

The FIT Formula and Nutrition

Table 14.5 shows how you can use the FIT formula as a guideline for nutritional fitness. Note that the FIT formula recommends that you use the MyPyramid to help you choose foods.

Keep in mind that to have a healthy diet, you need to eat foods with the proper amounts of all the nutri-

Table 14.5

Fitness Target Zones and Nutrition

Frequency	Eat three meals a day. An occasional snack is fine.
Intensity	The number of calories you consume each day should fall within the range recommended for your sex and age group unless you are extremely sedentary or very active.
Time	Eat meals at regular intervals, such as morning, noon, and evening.

Consume the recommended number of servings from the food groups shown in the MyPyramid.

ents. Remember that a steady diet of **junk food,** fad diets, fast foods, and incorrect use of vitamin and mineral supplements can all be harmful to your health. Also remember that eating properly and doing regular physical activity are important for maintaining a proper level of body fatness. Be aware of the signs of eating disorders that you learned in chapter 13.

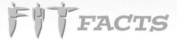

The National Dietary Guidelines suggest that we should follow the ABCs for Good Health: A = aim for fitness, B = build a healthy base, and C = choose sensibly. To **A**im for fitness, aim for a healthy weight and be active each day; to **B**uild a healthy base, choose foods from the base of the pyramid; and to **C**hoose sensibly, choose many servings of fruits and vegetables daily.

When selecting foods, you need to determine your own nutritional requirements. As you learned, a person's nutrient needs vary according to age, sex, height, and weight. Young people who are going through puberty and those who are still growing have special nutritional needs. They need to eat foods high in potassium, calcium, and iron. These minerals aid in the development of bones and blood. By eating the correct number of servings from each of the food groups, you probably are consuming a diet that will meet your nutritional needs.

Food Choices

Many teenagers do not plan meals, shop for groceries, or cook for a family. However, maybe you do help with these activities. Most likely, you do sometimes purchase snacks for yourself. How do you know whether the food you are purchasing is nutritious? Reading food labels can help you determine how nutritious a food is. In fact, according to law, manufacturers must now use a standard format for food labels.

Food Labels

You probably have noticed that most foods have a nutrition label and an ingredient list. Look at the **food label** shown on the next page. First, notice the number of servings in the container. Four servings are listed on the label for the food. Next, notice the calories per serving. For the food with this label each serving contains 90 calories. The total calorie content of the food package is 360 ($90 \times 4 = 360$). Some people think that the calories listed (90) is the amount in the total package.

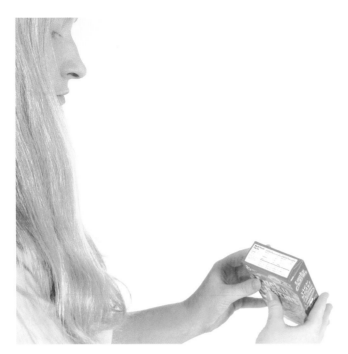

Reading food labels will help you select healthy foods.

This is not true. Keep in mind that if you double the serving size listed, you need to double the nutrient and caloric values. On the other hand, if you eat only half the serving size, you need to cut the nutrient and caloric values in half. This information can help you keep track of how many calories and nutrients you consume.

FIT FACTS

Most soft drinks contain approximately 150 calories for each 12-ounce can. Many teens drink several cans a day. Three cans a day equals 450 calories. A 60-ounce drink, such as those sold at many fast food and convenience stores, has 900 calories. Studies show that excessive consumption of soft drinks may be one of the reasons for the high incidence of overweight in our society. Water quenches your thirst and has zero calories. If all other aspects of your diets stayed the same, adding one soft drink a day would result in 15 pounds of fat gain in a year.

Listed beside each nutrient is the percentage of the daily requirement contained in one serving. Total fat, saturated fat, and trans fat should be limited to no more than 100% of the daily value. Sodium is a mineral that also should be limited in the diet.

Carbohydrate is a major source of calories in your diet. Dietary fiber, one type of carbohydrate, is encouraged in your diet. Simple sugars should be limited. Adequate protein in the diet is essential. However, certain types of protein can cause allergic reactions, so the food label must indicate that these types of protein are contained in a food. The foods are milk, eggs, fish, crustacean shellfish, tree nuts, peanuts, wheat, and soybeans. Food labels also list several key vitamins and minerals.

Nutrition Facts

Serving Size 1 cup (228g)
Servings Per Container 2

Amount Per Serving		
Calories 250	Calories from Fat 110	
		% Daily Value*
Total Fat 12g		**18%**
Saturated Fat 3g		**15%**
Trans Fat 3g		
Cholesterol 30mg		**10%**
Sodium 470mg		**20%**
Potassium 700mg		**20%**
Total Carbohydrate 31g		**10%**
Dietary Fiber 0g		**0%**
Sugars 5g		
Protein 5g		

Vitamin A 4%	•	Vitamin C 2%	
Calcium 20%	•	Iron 4%	

*Percent Daily Values are based on a 2000 calorie diet. Your daily values may be higher or lower depending on your calorie needs:

		Calories	2000	2500
Total Fat	Less than		65g	80g
Sat. Fat	Less than		20g	25g
Cholesterol	Less than		300mg	300mg
Sodium	Less than		2400mg	2400mg
Total Carbohydrate			300g	375g
Dietary Fiber			25g	30g

Calories per gram:
Fat 9 • Carbohydrate 4 • Protein 4

Food label.

FITNESS Technology

The development of the Internet has made it possible to easily find sources that allow you to determine the contents of various foods. It is now easy to determine the amount of each nutrient in food. To do this, you should keep a daily log of everything you eat. Write down the name of the food and the size of the serving. Then log on to the Web site listed below. You can use the information at this Web site to determine the contents of the foods you eat. Ask your teacher about a log sheet that you can use to keep track of the foods that you eat each day. You can also use a computer program called Nutrigram to calculate the content of the foods you eat. Ask your teacher whether Nutrigram is available in your school.

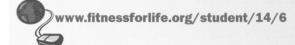 **www.fitnessforlife.org/student/14/6**

Look at the column on the food label that lists percent daily values. This information tells you what percent of your daily requirements for a nutrient are met by this food. For fat, saturated fat, cholesterol, and sodium, choose foods with a low percent daily value. For total carbohydrate, dietary fiber, vitamins, and minerals, your goal is to reach 100 percent of your daily value.

Claims on Food Labels

You might have noticed terms such as those shown in table 14.6 on many food containers. These terms relate to fat in food and can be displayed on food containers only if the food meets legal standards set by the government. The terms were developed to prevent false advertising. Even with the standardized terms shown in the table, you can still be fooled concerning advertisements relating to fat in foods. Some foods such as milk and packaged meats advertise that they are 2 percent fat or 98 percent fat free. This is true if measured by weight of the product, but not true when measured by the total number of calories in the product. For example, 2 percent of the weight of a glass of 2-percent milk is fat, but over 30 percent of the calories in a glass of 2-percent milk is fat.

You can calculate the true percentage of fat calories in food. Simply divide the calories per serving into the calories from fat. For the food label shown on page 252, the calories per serving is 90 and the calories of fat per serving is 30, so the percentage of calories in this food is 33 percent (30 ∏ 90 = 0.33).

You also might see health claims such as "good for heart health" on some food labels. Manufacturers must comply with government regulations regarding such labeling. For example, if a product advertises that its fat content is good for the heart, the product must be low in fat, saturated fat, and cholesterol. Fruits, vegetables, and grain products that make such claims must not only be low in fat, saturated fat, and cholesterol, but

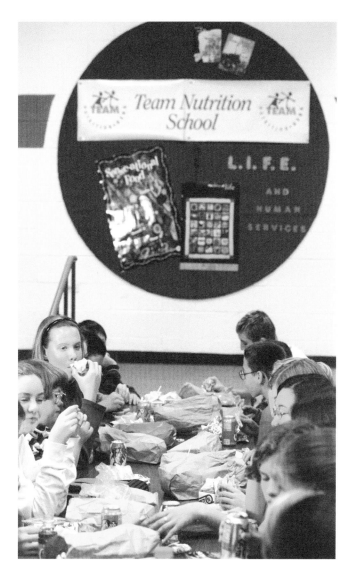

When you eat properly, you are more likely to be fit, look better, feel better, and have fewer health problems than people who are overfat and unfit.

also contain at least the minimum amount of fiber for each serving. Foods that display health claims related to blood pressure must be low in sodium. Some food labels now contain information about transfatty acids.

Table 14.6

Key Words on Food Labels and What They Mean

Key words	What they mean
Fat free	Less than 0.5 gram of fat
Low fat	3 or less grams of fat per serving
Lean	Less than 10 grams of fat, 4 grams of saturated fat, and 95 milligrams of cholesterol
Light (lite)	1/3 fewer calories or no more than 1/2 the fat of the higher-calorie, higher-fat version; or no more than 1/2 the sodium of the higher-sodium version
Cholesterol free	Less than 2 milligrams of cholesterol and 2 or less grams of saturated fat per serving

Common Food Myths

You may have heard a number of incorrect or misleading statements about nutrition. Some common nutrition myths are listed here.

▶ **Myth:** Skipping meals is a good way to lose weight.

▶ **Fact:** Studies show that people who skip meals typically eat more than those who eat regular meals. Skipping meals stimulates the appetite, so having fewer meals can lead to eating more food at each meal, while

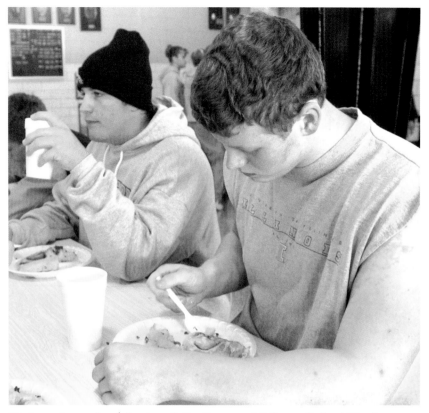

Most people can do moderate activity after a meal if they wait about 30 minutes to an hour. However, if you have problems doing activity after eating, you may need to modify what you eat.

having more meals usually means having less food at each meal. Skipping breakfast or lunch is common but is ineffective in weight loss and results in lower work and school performance.

▶ **Myth:** A **food supplement** is tested for safety and to insure that it meets claims advertised by the seller.

▶ **Fact:** Since 1994 food supplements have been unregulated. This means that they are not tested by the government either for safety or to insure that they meet the claims made for them. Beware of food supplements that make claims that are too good to be true.

▶ **Myth:** High protein diets are best for losing weight and maintaining good health.

▶ **Fact:** A review of a large number of studies shows that a balanced diet based on the Food Guide Pyramid and the percentages of nutrients listed in the first lesson of this chapter is most effective in fat loss and for weight maintenance. The popular high protein diets cause quick loss of body water but are only effective in fat loss if they result in consuming fewer calories. Because these diets are high in fat, experts fear that they can result in increased health problems if used for a long time.

▶ **Myth:** If you limit the amount of fat in foods, you do not need to be concerned with how many calories a food contains.

▶ **Fact:** It is the total number of calories you consume that makes a difference in weight maintenance. Fats do contain more calories per gram than carbohydrates and proteins, but many foods advertised as low in fat actually contain more calories than foods higher in fat. For good health it is wise to limit fat intake, but for weight maintenance total calorie intake is what is important.

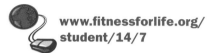
www.fitnessforlife.org/ student/14/7

Because health and nutrition quackery is so commonplace, many other myths also exist. When making choices about nutrition, be sure to follow the dietary guidelines and the guidelines presented in the MyPyramid. Use information that comes from reliable sources. Some of these sources include: the Food and Drug Administration (FDA), the United States Department of Agriculture (USDA), the American Dietetic Association (ADA), the American Medical Association (AMA), the American Heart Association, and the American Cancer Society.

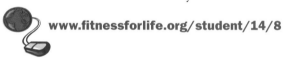
www.fitnessforlife.org/student/14/8

Eating Before Physical Activity

Most people can do moderate activity after a meal if they wait about 30 minutes to an hour. People who have problems doing activity after eating may have to wait longer or modify what they eat. If you plan to do vigorous physical activity or participate in a highly competitive athletic event, you may have to modify your eating patterns. Here are some guidelines for eating before physical activity:

▶ **Special diets are typically not necessary before athletic competitions.** Some athletes think they need a steak or a food supplement before they compete. Steak is high in protein and fat, both of which are digested slowly. Steak eaten within two hours of the event might interfere with a person's performance. In general, you can eat what you like as long as it does not disagree with you.

▶ **Allow extra time between eating and activity before vigorous competitive events.** Eat one to three hours before competing. Allow more time if the foods you have eaten are difficult to digest.

Taking Charge: Saying "No"

Sometimes the single act of saying "no" is the best way to avoid a situation that is potentially harmful. While it may seem easy to say this simple word, the action may actually be very difficult to carry out successfully.

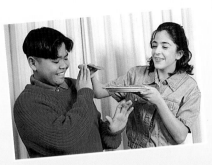

Manny was invited to spend the holiday with his girlfriend's family. Plans were made to spend the afternoon water-skiing at a nearby lake and then have a big party. His girlfriend, Rita, warned Manny that her mother always prepared huge amounts of food for the party. It was her family's tradition to stuff themselves until they couldn't move. She told him to make sure he came with a big appetite. Unfortunately, Manny's doctor had just instructed him to restrict the amount of fats and calories he consumed.

Manny arrived at the party just as Rita's mother was setting out the food. The table was loaded with tortilla chips, guacamole, beef and bean burritos, chiles rellenos, and fresh corn, as well as cakes, pies, and cookies. Manny knew that he faced a difficult situation as

Rita came forward with a plate piled with cookies. "Manny, you're just in time. The food is great!"

Manny replied, "Everything looks good, but I have to watch my diet."

Rita offered him a cookie, knowing they were Manny's favorite. "But you've got to try my mother's cookies. Everyone says they're the best. You'll hurt my mother's feelings if you don't eat one."

For Discussion

In what way does the party put Manny in a difficult situation? How can Manny say "no" to Rita without embarrassing her or hurting her feelings? What can he do so that his refusal won't hurt Rita's mother? What could he have done before actually going to the party to prepare for this situation? In what other situations would saying "no" be the best response? Fill out the questionnaire provided by your teacher to find out whether you are more likely to say "no" and mean it or give in under pressure. Consider the guidelines on page 256.

▶ **Before competition, reduce the size of your meal.** Small meals are easier to digest than large ones. If you get very nervous or often have an upset stomach before competition, try a liquid meal of about 900 calories in 16 ounces of liquid. In general, liquid meals are not recommended.

▶ **Drink fluids before, during, and after activity.** Whether you are competing or not, it is important to drink water. Added salt or sugar are not typically needed, except for especially long events or events in high heat and humidity. Using drinks with too much sugar can actually detract from performance.

Lesson Review

1. How can the FIT formula help you determine how often to eat?
2. What are three examples of information you can find on a food label?
3. What are two common food myths? How are they incorrect or misleading?

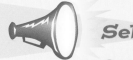

Self-Management Skill

Saying "No"

Most of us try to eat well, do regular physical activity, and practice healthy lifestyles. Sometimes the situation we are in or the people we are around make it difficult to keep doing healthy behaviors. We are tempted to do things that we would not normally do. You can take steps to make it easier to say "no" when you are in situations that encourage you to do behaviors you know are not best for you. The following guidelines are designed to help you say "no" to eating food that you do not want or need. You may be able to use these strategies to help you say "no" in other situations related to health behaviors.

▶ **Say "no" to food offered on special occasions.** Eat a light meal before a holiday event so that you are not hungry. Practice ways to refuse food so that you do not hurt the feelings of the host or hostess. Avoid standing near food. When you feel the need to eat, talk to someone or find something else to do.

▶ **Say "no" to extra food when eating out.** Plan in advance what you will eat. Resist ordering foods that are advertised or that others eat. Choose small servings—avoid big orders such as large burgers and large fries. Say "no" to special deals that include foods you do not want—order single items you want instead. Say "no" to extra sauces, toppings, and condiments such as mayonnaise.

▶ **Shop with a strategy.** Preparing a list ahead of time and sticking with it helps you say "no" to foods high in empty calories. Use food labels and avoid those foods high in calories per serving. Look for better choices. Eat before you shop so that you are not hungry.

▶ **Consume healthy snacks.** Eating snacks of vegetables and fruits can help you say "no" to snacks that are high in empty calories such as potato chips, cookies, and candy. Avoid sugared soft drinks. Carry a water bottle. Drink water rather than high-calorie drinks such as soft drinks or sport drinks when you are thirsty.

▶ **Eat healthy foods at school.** Prepare your own lunch or snacks for school to help you say "no" to food in snack machines. If you have free time, find a way to be active to avoid thinking about eating things you do not really want or need. If you eat school food, ask for small servings to avoid eating too much. If you have free time with friends, ask them not to bring high-calorie foods.

▶ **Say "no" to large servings and seconds.** Reject large or second servings. Tell family members and friends not to offer seconds. Limit servings of desserts.

▶ **Eat slowly and avoid eating while studying or watching television.** Some experts recommend that you limit your eating to the kitchen or dining room to help you say "no" to unwanted food.

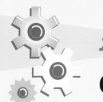

Activity 2

Cooperative Aerobics

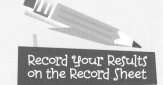

Record Your Results on the Record Sheet

Previously you learned about aerobic dance and step aerobics. Both are good forms of active aerobics and are good for expending calories. In this activity you will work with others to develop an aerobic exercise routine. You will also learn about calories expended by performing this activity.

▶ **Step 1.** Your class will be divided into several groups of 3 to 4 people. Each person in the group will make up an arm and leg pattern to teach to the other group members. Listen to the music your instructor plays as you invent your combinations. Arrange the patterns created by each group member into a routine for the group. Look at the arm movements and leg movements that are listed. You can use these movements in any combination to create a dance step. On the other hand, you may prefer to use your imagination and make up your own movements.

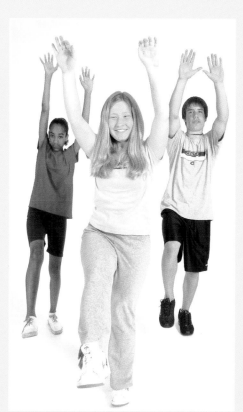

▶ **Step 2.** Perform the routine created by your group to music. Determine the total number of minutes in the routine. Multiply the number of minutes in the routine by the number of calories (per minute) expended in the routine. Use table 14.7 to determine calories per minute.

▶ **Step 3.** One chocolate-covered peanut candy contains 9 calories. How many minutes of cooperative aerobics would you have to perform to expend the calories in one chocolate-covered peanut candy? How many minutes would of cooperative aerobics would you have to perform to expend the calories in one serving (20 in a serving)? Record your results on the worksheet supplied by your teacher.

Table 14.7

Calories Expended Per Minute During an Aerobic Routine

Your weight (lbs)	90	100	110	120	130	140	150	160	170	180	190+
Calories/min	4.5	5.0	5.5	6.0	6.5	7.0	7.5	8.0	8.5	9.0	9.5

Leg Movements to Choose From

Note that R stands for right, and L stands for left.

1. Step-Heel
   - Step R, touch L heel to floor.
   - Repeat with L step and R heel.
2. Step, Close-Step, Heel
   - Step R, slide L foot to R.
   - Step R, point L heel forward.
3. Step, Close-Step, Kick
   - Follow directions for step, close-step, heel, except kick instead of pointing heel forward.
4. Step-Close
   - Step R, slide L foot to R.
   - Repeat with step L, close R.
5. Stair-Step
   - Walk forward—R, L.
   - Walk backward—R, L.
6. Step-Kick
   - Step R, kick L.
   - Step L, kick R.
7. Step Knee-Lift
   - Step R, lift L knee.
   - Step L, lift R knee.
8. Grapevine
   - Step R.
   - Cross L behind R, and step.
   - Step R.
   - Cross L in front of R, and step.

9. Box Step
   - Step forward R.
   - Cross L over R, and step.
   - Step back R.
   - Step back L.
10. Pony (similar to dance called Cha-Cha)
    - Step R, slow.
    - Step L, quick.
    - Step R, slow.
    - Repeat, starting L.
11. Rocker
    - Step R, point L heel forward, lean back.
    - Step L, point R heel backward, lean forward.
12. Hustle Forward and Backward
    - Step forward, R, L, R.
    - Hop R, lift L knee.
    - Step backward, L, R, L.
    - Hop L, lift R knee.
13. Elbow to Knee
    - Step R, lift L knee to R elbow.
    - Step L, lift R knee to L elbow.
14. Charleston
    - Point L toe forward, step back L, toe then heel.
    - Point R toe back, step forward R, toe then heel.
    - Repeat.
15. Mambo
    - Step forward R, back L.
    - Step R, L, R, in place.

Arm Movements to Choose From

1. Arm Press
   - Push arms down and up from chest to waist.
2. Biceps Curl
   - Move as though weightlifting.
3. Triceps (French) Curl
   - Move arms overhead as in weightlifting.
4. Front Scissors
   - Swing arms across each other in front of chest then out to sides.
5. Back Scissors
   - Scissor arms behind back.
6. Double-Arm Swing
   - Swing arms together across front of chest.
7. Arm Circles
   - Alternate circling R arm clockwise and L arm counterclockwise.
8. Chicken Wings
   - Bend elbows and flap them up and down at your sides.

9. Windshield Wipers
   - Bend elbows and move hands in front of face like windshield wipers.
10. Rowing
    - Move arms as though rowing a boat.
11. Cheerleader
    - Pump arms up and down alternately overhead.
12. Hustle Arms
    - Swing both arms backward, then forward, with a clap on the hop.
13. Elbow-to-Knee Arms
    - Twist and touch R elbow to L knee.
    - Twist and touch L elbow to R knee.
14. Drive a Big Truck
    - Move both arms as if turning a very large steering wheel.
15. Picking Cherries
    - Reach up with both arms as if to get a cherry and put it in your pocket.

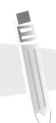

14 Chapter Review

Reviewing Concepts and Vocabulary

Number your paper from 1 to 6. Next to each number, write the word (or words) that correctly completes the sentence.

1. Your body breaks down proteins into simpler substances called _____.
2. Your body can use _____ for energy with little or no change during digestion.
3. You need to limit your intake of _____, a fatlike substance found in animal cells.
4. _____ contain more nutrients than do simple carbohydrates.
5. _____ are food substances required for the growth and maintenance of your cells.
6. A food that is _____ contains a large amount of nutrients for the number of calories it provides.

Number your paper from 7 to 11. Next to each number, choose the letter of the best answer.

Column I	Column II
7. carbohydrate	a. contains some, not all, essential amino acids
8. proteins	b. cannot be digested by the body
9. fiber	c. provides you with energy
10. complete protein	d. contains all nine essential amino acids
11. incomplete protein	e. building blocks of your body

Number your paper from 12 to 15. On your paper, write a short answer for each statement or question.

12. Describe and refute a myth some athletes have about eating before physical activity.
13. Explain how complete proteins are important for your health.
14. Explain how calcium is important for your health, and tell what you can do to help keep your bones strong.
15. Why is water considered an important nutrient, and why might a person who is exercising need extra amounts of it?

Thinking Critically

Write a paragraph to answer the following question.

Your friend asks your advice about her diet. She wonders whether the food choices she makes are important or whether she only needs to count calories. She has started to increase her physical activity and wonders how that will affect her caloric and nutritional needs. What advice would you give your friend?

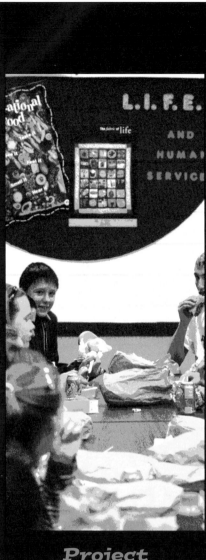

Project

Because people eat out often, it is important to make good food choices when you do. Make the assumption that you are going on a one-day trip. Your only food choices are fast foods. List what you would typically order for breakfast, lunch, and dinner for the day of your trip. Write down the name and amount of each food on your list. Use the Web site shown below to look up the calories in each food on your list. On a separate sheet of paper, list more healthy choices you could have made from the fast food menu. Calculate the calories in your healthy choice list. Make a comparison of the calories in each diet.

15

Making Consumer Choices

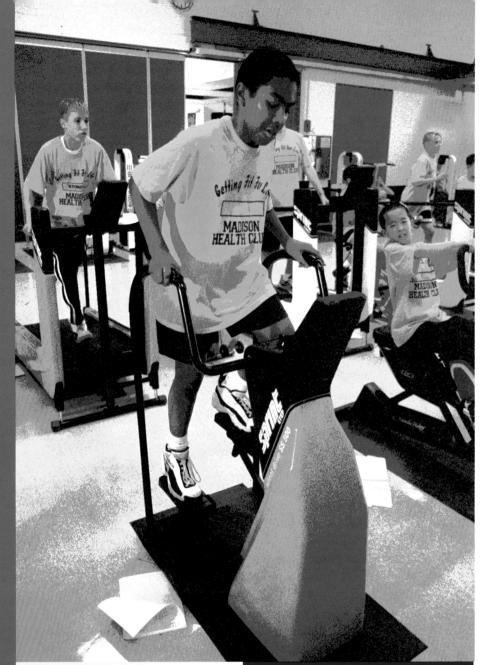

In this chapter...

Activity 1
Continuous Rhythmical Exercise

Lesson 15.1
Health and Fitness Quackery

Self-Assessment
Reassessing Body Composition, Flexibility, and Strength

Lesson 15.2
Evaluating Health Clubs, Equipment, Media, and Internet Materials

Taking Charge
Learning to Think Critically

Self-Management Skill
Learning to Think Critically

Activity 2
Active Learning: Isometric Exercise Circuit

Activity 1

CONTINUOUS RHYTHMICAL EXERCISE

Continuous Rhythmical Exercise (CRE) was invented by Dr. Thomas Cureton at the University of Illinois. He wanted to develop an exercise program that would build many parts of health-related fitness, including cardiovascular fitness, flexibility, and muscular fitness, as well as to help control body fatness. CRE involves doing flexibility and muscle fitness exercises with continuous motion (for cardiovascular fitness) between exercises. You will try a sample program that lasts about 10 minutes. You can repeat this program or develop one of your own.

Health and Fitness Quackery

Lesson Objectives
After reading this lesson, you should be able to
1. Explain the importance of being an informed health consumer.
2. Name reliable sources of health-related and fitness-related information.
3. Name and describe examples of health and fitness misconceptions and quackery.

Lesson Vocabulary
con (p. 261), fraud (p. 261), passive exercise (p. 263), quack (p. 261), quackery (p. 261)

 www.ffitnessforlife.org/student/15/1

You probably have seen and heard newspaper, magazine, radio, and television advertisements for health and fitness products and services. Is a product or service effective simply because it is advertised? In this lesson, you will learn how to become a wise consumer, or purchaser, of health and fitness products.

What Is Quackery?

Some people are in a hurry to lose body fat or gain muscle strength. Often, people who want quick results are persuaded to purchase useless health and fitness products and services. They may become victims of quackery. **Quackery** is a method of advertising or selling that uses false claims to lure people into buying products that are worthless or even harmful. Some people who practice quackery actually believe that the products that they are selling do work. They may have good intentions but still do harm. A person who practices quackery is sometimes referred to as a **quack.**

Some people who practice quackery are guilty of **fraud.** People who practice fraud try to deceive you and get you to buy products or services that they know are ineffective or harmful. A person who practices fraud is called a **con.** Cons try to convince you of something that is untrue. Because what they do is often illegal, they may be convicted of a crime.

Detecting Quackery and Fraud

People who commit quackery and fraud use a variety of deceptive practices to get you to buy their products or services or use products they endorse. Separating fact from fiction can be difficult. Use the guidelines in the following section to help you spot health and fitness quackery and fraud.

Check Credentials
Be sure that the person you think is an expert really is an expert. A con might claim to be a doctor or to have a college or university degree. However, the degree might be in a subject unrelated to health and physical fitness. It might come from a nonaccredited school, or it might be falsified. You can verify credentials by checking with your local or state health authorities or professional organizations.

If you have questions about health or fitness, be sure to ask an expert's advice. For medical advice, talk to a physician (MD or DO) or a registered nurse (RN). For questions about general health, ask a certified health education teacher. A physical educator, a person with at least a bachelor's degree in exercise science or kinesiology, or a registered physical therapist (RPT) is qualified to advise you about exercise and fitness. These experts have college degrees and training in their area of specialization.

A registered dietitian (RD) is best qualified to advise you about diet, food, and nutrition. Keep in mind that a person who uses the title nutritionist is not necessarily an expert. Similarly, staff members in health clubs are often not required to have college degrees. Those members with certifications from a well-respected organization are more qualified than those without certifications, but certification without a degree is not adequate to be considered an expert. Neither nutritionists nor health club employees are considered reliable sources of health or fitness information unless they have the credentials just described.

Be Wary of Advisors Who Sell Products
People who sell products make money by selling them. Salespeople often have little training in health, fitness, and wellness. For example, people who sell exercise equipment or food supplements may know less about their products than their customers. Salespeople are often willing to stretch the truth to make a sale. It is best to consult a true expert before you make purchases.

Check the Organizations of the Experts You Consult
Many well-known and reputable associations for qualified doctors, fitness experts, and nutrition experts exist.

Examples of well-established and legitimate organizations are the American Medical Association (AMA), the United States Department of Agriculture (USDA), the Food and Drug Administration (FDA), the Centers for Disease Control and Prevention (CDC), the American Alliance for Health, Physical Education, Recreation and Dance (AAHPERD), and the American College of Sports Medicine (ACSM). These organizations are either government groups charged with protecting your health (USDA, FDA, and CDC) or private organizations of experts including teachers and coaches, medical doctors, college professors, and researchers with advanced degrees (AAHPERD, AMA, and ACSM). Quacks and cons sometimes try to get you to believe that they know more than the experts from these organizations. Be wary of people who claim they know more than well-known experts and who try to discredit the organizations just listed.

Sometimes quacks and cons use names and initials of phony organizations with important sounding names similar to well-known organizations. Anyone can form an organization and use it to try to impress you. Check the background of anyone who claims to be a member of an organization whose name you have never heard.

Be Wary of Those Who Promise Immediate Results

Be suspicious if a salesperson promises immediate, effortless, or guaranteed results.

Be Suspicious of Sales Pitches That Promise Results Too Good to Be True

Look for words and phrases such as *miracle*, *secret remedy*, *scientific breakthrough*, and *endorsed by movie stars*. A quack or con is likely to use these and similar terms in a sales pitch for an item that is useless.

Be Cautious About Mail-Order and Internet Sales

Be cautious of mail-order and Internet sales offers. You cannot examine mail-order and Internet products before buying them. Money-back guarantees may seem to protect you, but a guarantee is only as good as the company that backs it. Do business only with reputable firms.

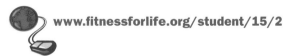
www.fitnessforlife.org/student/15/2

Be Wary of Product Claims

A favorite trick of some cons is to claim that a product is "brand-new" or is just now being offered for the first time. Others may claim to be "available in the United States for the first time." They try to make you think that you are getting something special. Claims made by cons are typically false.

Be Wary of Untested Products

Quacks do not subject their products to thorough scientific testing. The product is rushed on the market in order to make money as quickly as possible. Also, quacks and cons try to get you to believe their product is popular in Europe, Asia, or some other location. This technique is usually used to impress you. One way to tell whether a product or service is a good one is when it is supported by good research. Good research is published in respected journals and conducted by qualified experts. Using untested products can pose significant risks for a consumer. Journals of the organizations described earlier are good sources of scientific research.

Health Quackery

Many people are willing to try new health products. In fact, the market is flooded with health products, many of which are useless. Although some of these products may not be harmful, false advertising claims give people unrealistic expectations about the benefits these products can provide. Be aware that many advertisers promote myths about health and fitness. You can recognize health quackery when advertisers make unrealistic claims about a product. Examples include claims that a product will promote hair growth, cure acne, make wrinkles disappear, or remove cellulite (fat tissue).

Food Supplements

A food supplement is a product that is not a part of the typical diet but is added to the regular diet. Supplements often are produced as syrups, powders, or tablets. Generally, they are sold in health food stores or through the mail. Common supplements are protein (amino acids), vitamins, minerals, and herbs. Packaged

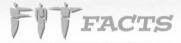

Cellulite is a term that is often used for fat that causes the skin to look rippled or bumpy. Cons would have you believe that cellulite is a special kind of fat that can be eliminated with creams or other special products. In fact, cellulite occurs when fat cells become enlarged. It is best reduced by expending more calories than you consume.

foods such as canned goods (e.g., canned vegetables and fruits), boxed goods (e.g., cereal, cake mix), and frozen foods (e.g., ice cream, frozen dinners) must have a food label that informs you of the product's ingredients (see chapter 14). Such labels are not required of food supplements.

Most Americans believe that food supplements are regulated by the government in the same way as drugs and foods. This is not true. A law passed in 1994 changed the regulation of supplements from government control to manufacturer control. Manufacturers do not have to prove that a supplement works before they sell it, and the law does not regulate the contents of a supplement. For this reason, you cannot be sure that you are buying what you think you are buying when you purchase a supplement. More than a few people have died from taking supplements that were contaminated or contained ingredients that were not supposed to be in the supplement. Also many illnesses and even deaths have occurred when people have taken supplements claiming to result in fat loss or performance enhancement. An example is the herb ephedra that has been implicated in several deaths. It is now banned by the FDA.

Some supplements are not harmful but simply do not provide the benefits promised by those who sell them. Since the regulation of supplements was changed in 1994, the sales of supplements have more than doubled. Many people are wasting money on products that do not work.

Some supplements can be beneficial when recommended by a physician. For example, the AMA suggests that taking a daily multivitamin can be beneficial if it includes no more than the RDA for each vitamin. But even vitamins can be dangerous if taken in amounts that are too large. Vitamins and minerals that are not harmful typically provide no benefits when taken in larger than recommended amounts. It is especially important to consult with your parent or guardian as well as your family physician before taking supplements. You can find more information about supplements at the Web site below.

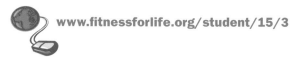

www.fitnessforlife.org/student/15/3

Sport Supplements

A current fad is the use of sport supplements or sport vitamins—products sold to enhance athletic performance. As described in chapter 12, these supplements are also called ergogenic aids. Many supplements sold as ergogenic aids

are actually quack products. Many supplements can be harmful to health.

Fad Diets

"Lose pounds a day on the ice-cream diet!" "Rice diet works wonders!" "Fruit diet dissolves fat!" How many similar weight-loss claims have you heard? Each claim is false and an example of a fad diet. Although fad diets are popular because they usually promise fast results, nearly all fad diets are nutritionally unbalanced. They often restrict eating to only one or two food groups, or even one specific food. As you have learned, a combination of physical activity and eating fewer calories is the only safe, effective way to reduce body fatness and lose weight. Eating healthy, low-calorie foods such as those being eaten by the teens in the picture can help you control your calorie intake.

Fitness Quackery

Many useless products are being sold to promote fitness. For example, you may have seen advertisements for thigh creams to reduce fat in the thighs. Such claims are a myth. These creams do not reduce body fat. Also be alert for the following worthless fitness devices and methods.

Exercise Programs

Programs that use **passive exercise** are ineffective because, instead of using your own muscles, they use machines or other outside forces to move your body.

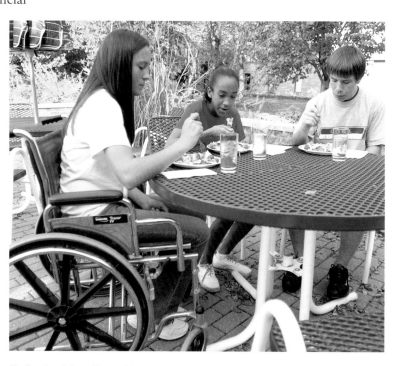

Eating healthy will provide you with the proper nutrients.

A variety of devices provide passive exercises. For example, rollers are machines that roll along your hips or legs. Vibrating machines shake body areas and are said to break up fat cells. Motorized belts, cycles, tables, and rowing machines are advertised for fat reduction and weight loss. These claims are false.

Figure Wrapping

Wearing nonporous garments and soaking in baths are often advertised for weight loss. These practices can cause overheating and dehydration and can be extremely dangerous to your health.

Spot Reducing

An unqualified fitness instructor might recommend spot exercises. Spot exercising refers to doing an exercise to remove fat in a specific location. Research shows that no type of exercise will cause fat loss at one specific location. You can do spot exercises to strengthen muscles in a certain part of the body, but they do not remove fat at that location. Physical activity does help reduce fat all over the body.

Reaching Goals Safely

Attaining health and fitness goals takes planning and time. No diet, product, or exercise program can work magic. Recognizing myths and misconceptions, such as those described here, can help you save your money and your health. Education is the best safeguard against quackery. In the next chapter you will learn how to set goals and plan your personal physical activity program.

FITNESS Technology

You learned in previous chapters about many technological innovations that make our lives better. Some help us to assess fitness and health accurately (e.g., DEXA) as well as help us exercise (e.g., isokinetic exercise machines). However, not all technological devices are safe and effective. Some unscrupulous people sell devices that are not only ineffective but also can be quite dangerous. One example is a device with electrodes that are placed on your abdominal muscles. Electrical current is sent through the electrodes, causing the muscles to be stimulated. People who advertise these devices claim that they build strong abdominal muscles without doing any regular abdominal exercises such as crunches or curl-ups. Studies show that these devices do not work to build fitness, and the current from the electrodes can cause the heart to beat irregularly. Be wary of devices that promise fitness without exercise.

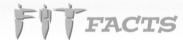

FIT FACTS

It is possible to lose a lot of weight in a short period of time as a result of dehydration. If you do not drink enough fluid or you lose excessive water through sweating, you will become dehydrated and lose water weight. Some people think this loss in weight is permanent. It is not. Losing water weight can be dangerous (see discussion of heat-related illness in chapter 2). Products that cause water loss do not help you lose body fat and can be dangerous to your health.

Lesson Review

1. Why is learning to recognize quackery and fraud important?
2. To whom should you direct questions about health and fitness?
3. What are two examples of health-related or fitness-related quackery?

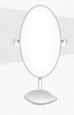

Self-Assessment

Reassessing Body Composition, Flexibility, and Strength

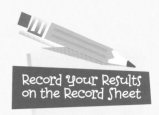

Record Your Results on the Record Sheet

You can determine your present state of fitness by reassessing the five health-related components. Reassessing your fitness is important for several reasons. First, practicing self-assessments will help you know how to do self-assessments properly throughout your life. Second, you can select the self-assessments that you think you will most likely use when you are doing them independently. Finally, these reassessments will allow you to see whether your fitness in any category has changed since the assessments you did earlier in the class. If you do not see changes, keep in mind that it normally takes about six weeks for any significant improvement to occur in physical fitness. You can do periodic reassessments of fitness throughout your life to determine your personal fitness progress.

In this self-assessment, you will reassess your body composition, flexibility, and strength. Choose assessment items that you think are best for you personally. Refer to the page number following each self-assessment for instructions and ratings. If time allows, perform more than the designated number of self-assessments. When you are finished with your reassessment items, record your results and ratings on your record sheet. Also, indicate the reasons for performing the assessment items that you chose. *Note:* Assessments with an asterisk (*) are *FITNESSGRAM* tests.

Body Composition

Choose at least two of the following methods to reassess your body composition.

1. Skinfolds* (chapter 13, pages 226-227)
   ▶ Triceps
   ▶ Calf

2. Body mass index* (chapter 5, pages 81-82)
   ▶ Height
   ▶ Weight

3. Height–weight chart (chapter 13, page 228)
4. Body measurements (body fat levels) (chapter 14, pages 249-250)
5. Waist-to-hip ratio (chapter 14, page 250)

Flexibility

Choose at least one assessment from each category to reassess your flexibility.

1. Upper body
   ▶ Arm lift (chapter 10, page 159)
   ▶ Zipper* (chapter 10, page 159)
   ▶ Wrap around (chapter 10, page 160)

2. Lower body
   ▶ Knee to chest (chapter 10, page 161)
   ▶ Back-saver sit and reach* (chapter 5, page 82)
3. Trunk
   ▶ Trunk rotation (chapter 10, page 160)
4. Ankle
   ▶ Ankle flex* (chapter 10, page 161)

Strength

Perform the 1RM assessments for the arms and legs. You may also choose to do the additional 1RM and/or the isometric assessment.

1. Isotonic assessments: If resistance machines are available, perform the 1RM self-assessments that follow. If only free weights are available, you can use the bench press to assess arm strength.

   ▶ Arm press using a resistance machine (chapter 11, page 183) or bench press using free weights (page 193).
   ▶ Leg press using resistance machine (chapter 11, page 183).
2. Additional 1RM Assessments
   ▶ 1RM for other basic 10 exercises (chapter 11, pages 193-198)
3. Isometric Assessment
   ▶ Isometric grip strength (chapter 11, page 184)

265

Evaluating Health Clubs, Equipment, Media, and Internet Materials

Lesson Objectives

After reading this lesson, you should be able to

1. Evaluate health-related and fitness-related facilities.
2. Describe the proper clothing and equipment that you need for physical activity.
3. Evaluate printed material, videos, and Internet resources related to health and fitness.

Lesson Vocabulary

spa (p. 266)

www.fitnessforlife.org/student/15/4

People are more interested in health and fitness now than at any other time in our history. More people belong to health and fitness clubs than ever before. Exercise equipment sales are setting records. Many magazines totally dedicated to health and fitness are being published. The development of the Internet has created another source of health and fitness information. In fact, the Internet has become the leading source of health information throughout the world. In this lesson, you will learn about health and fitness clubs as well as exercise clothing and equipment. You also will learn how to evaluate literature and Internet resources. Finally, you will read about reliable consumer organizations.

Health Clubs

You do not need to join a health club, **spa,** or gym to attain or maintain fitness. Health clubs have special equipment and personnel for the benefit of members. Modern spas have saunas, whirlpool baths, and provide other services such as hair/skin care and massage. Some people find that joining a club helps motivate them to exercise and remain physically active. But these services are expensive. Well-educated people can save money and still get the benefits of regular exercise by designing their own fitness and activity programs without the need for a special facility or equipment.

Many low-cost programs are offered through community centers, universities, churches, and other groups. Your school may be one of the many that have

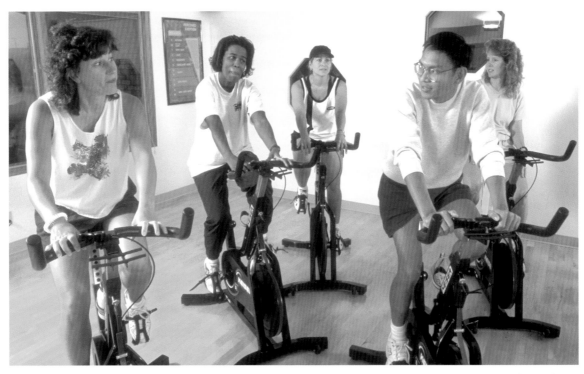

When choosing a health club, be sure to pick a well-established club that includes activities that you enjoy such as a spinning class.

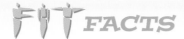

FIT FACTS

Be wary of advertisements that promise to build muscle tone. *Tone* is a word created by advertisers. Health-related physical fitness can be measured using the self-assessments in this book. Tone cannot be easily and accurately measured. For this reason, it is easy to claim that a lotion or a cream improves muscle tone, but it is very hard to prove. Also, be wary of fitness leaders who claim to build muscle tone. Place your trust in experts who help you build sound exercises programs that produce gains in fitness using sound tests of fitness.

built fitness centers. These programs can provide the same benefits and motivation as more expensive clubs. Still if you feel that it would help you say active, you may be interested in joining a commercial club, spa, or gym at some point. Some schools have made cooperative arrangement with fitness clubs that allow students to work out at special rates or that allow school classes to use club facilities. Follow these guidelines when making decisions about joining a group.

▶ **Join on a pay-as-you-go basis, if possible.** If you do sign a contract, make it a short-term one. Read the fine print carefully. Do not sign a contract right away. Too often people pay a lot for a long-term contract and then stop using the facility. It is best to pay for a short membership until you are sure that you will stick with it. The fine print may contain special clauses that will cost you money. For example, do you still have to pay if you move? Also there is often high pressure to sign a contract on a first visit—it is best to think about it for a while before signing.

▶ **Choose a well-established club.** Such a club is less likely to go out of business. Make sure the facility has qualified fitness experts such as those described earlier in the chapter. Be alert for signs of fitness quackery. If you notice signs of quackery, quit the club.

▶ **Make a trial visit to the club.** Visit at a time when you would normally use the club. Make sure you feel comfortable with the employees and other patrons. Also, make sure the equipment and facilities are available for your use.

▶ **Choose a club that meets your personal needs.** For example, a person who has joint pain may prefer to avoid activities such as jogging, choosing

instead to swim for cardiovascular fitness. In such a case, a facility that includes a swimming pool would be necessary.

▶ **Consider special medical needs.** If weight loss is your primary goal, consider joining a program recommended by your physician or sponsored by a hospital, rather than joining a health club. If you have a special medical need, you may need the help of a physical therapist.

Special Clothing and Equipment

A good fitness program requires a minimum of clothing and equipment. The following section provides guidelines for choosing proper clothing and equipment for exercise.

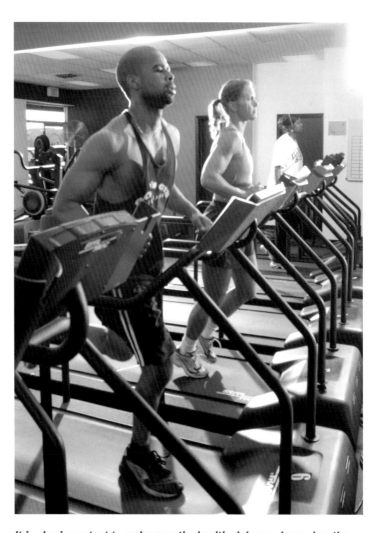

It is also important to make sure the health club you choose has the equipment you are interested in using and has a sufficient number so that you don't have to wait to use it.

Clothing and Footwear

Fashionable exercise clothing and footwear are popular, but not necessary. You need only wear what is comfortable and safe. Review what you learned in chapter 2 about proper clothing and footwear for safe physical activity.

Exercise Equipment

Some people choose not to join a club, choosing instead to buy home exercise equipment. If you are considering home exercise equipment, follow these guidelines:

▶ **Consider inexpensive home equipment.** You can use homemade weights, inner tubes, or rubber or latex bands for resistance exercises. You can use jump ropes, stepping benches, or stairs to build cardiovascular fitness. If you are interested in fitness for health and wellness, this equipment may be all you need.

▶ **Consider your personal needs before buying equipment.** If you are interested in higher levels of fitness for sports or high-performance jobs, you may choose to purchase machines or other equipment for use at home. Free weights or home exercise machines are available for building muscle fitness. For cardiovascular fitness, home exercise machines such as treadmills, bicycles, or stair steppers are available. A regular bicycle is also a good choice if you have a safe place to ride. Exercise equipment is often quite expensive, so making a good choice is important. Rather than depending on the advice of a salesperson, consult an expert, the Web site of the ACSM, or the *Consumer Reports* magazine. Buy from a well-established company that will honor the warranty, service the product, and have replacement parts available.

▶ **Be sure before you buy.** Avoid investing money in exercise equipment until you are sure you will use it. Many people buy equipment but do not use it after the first few months. You can see evidence of this behavior in the many ads for slightly-used equipment found in the classified sections of newspapers. Some of the high-tech equipment described in this book can be useful, such as pedometers and heart rate watches. However, some equipment can be quite expensive, and you may find that you will not use it regularly. You should see whether you can try equipment owned by a friend or by the school before making the decision to buy the product. Some high-tech products do not justify the cost. For example, expensive electrical devices for measuring body fatness are not worth the personal investment when an inexpensive caliper can give accurate fat measurements. Follow the advice in the previous section before buying equipment so that you can be confident that it will benefit you.

▶ **Make sure you have the space to put the equipment.** One of the main reasons people do not use the exercise equipment they buy is that they do not have a good place to keep it. If you have to get the equipment out each time you use it or move it from place to place, you are less likely to use it than if you have a room or a place where you can set it up permanently.

Evaluating Books and Articles

A growing emphasis on health and fitness has led to the publication of many books and articles on weight control and exercise. Much of the information presented through the media is misleading or incorrect. How can you evaluate information about health and fitness that you read, see, and hear? Follow these guidelines to help you decide which ones are worthwhile:

▶ **Consider the credentials of the author.** The author(s) or consultant(s) should be a registered dietitian, should have completed advanced study in nutrition, or should have advanced degrees in an exercise-related field such as exercise science, kinesiology, or physical education.

▶ **Check for sound information.** The book or article should provide information about a balanced diet and physical activity that is consistent with the information presented in this book. Books that promise quick and easy fitness or fat loss are not good sources. The information in the book or article should not use techniques used by quacks and cons described in lesson 15.1. Exercise discussions should include the principles of overload, progression, and specificity, in addition to the FIT formula for each type of physical fitness.

▶ **The recommended exercises should be safe and effective.** The exercises should require the use of your own muscles and should not recommend effortless devices.

Evaluating Exercise Videos

You probably have noticed many exercise videos for sale. Follow these guidelines to help you evaluate an exercise video:

▶ **Apply the same guidelines as recommended for books and articles.**

▶ **Choose a video that includes appropriate warm-up and cool-down exercises (cardiovascular and flexibility).**

▶ **Make sure the video contains only safe exercises.** Safe exercises, as well as dangerous exercises to avoid, are identified in chapter 2.

▶ **Choose a video that rotates the use of muscle groups and all parts of fitness.** For example, use arms, then legs, then back, then abdominal muscles, and so on. If the video claims to be a total fitness program, make sure it includes activities for all parts of fitness. Exercises for the different parts of fitness should be rotated.

▶ **Choose a video that is appropriate for all ability levels.** Make sure that the activities on the video are appropriate for you. Is it says for beginners, is it really appropriate? Is it appropriate for intermediate or advanced levels, as labeled?

▶ **Make sure the exercises start gradually and progress in intensity.**

▶ **Choose a video with a fun and interesting routine.**

▶ **If the video does not meet all of these guidelines, modify it.** For example, change the order of the routine to make it better.

Evaluating Internet Resources

As mentioned earlier, more and more adults are depending on the Internet for health and fitness information. Research has unfortunately shown that more than half of all Internet sources provide incorrect information. Ask yourself these questions when using the Internet to locate information concerning health, fitness, and wellness:

▶ **Who developed the Web site?** Web sites with the best information are developed by government agencies or professional organizations. Governmental health agencies have .gov at the end of the Web address, and professional organizations have .org at the end of theirs. Choose Web sites of well-known agencies and organizations such as those listed in the following section. Choosing sites with .gov or .org at the end will often lead you to more reliable sources than those that end in .com or .net. Remember, however, that any organization can obtain a .org Web address, so it does not insure that the information on the Web site will be sound. Conversely, some Web sites with .com and .net provide good information. Consult the Web site at the end of the list for information about good Web sites for health and fitness.

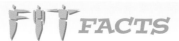

Advertisers often photograph models who are underweight to sell women's clothing. This practice promotes an unrealistic weight standard. Very few people can be, or should be, as thin as these models.

▶ **Does the Web site sell products?** Web sites that sell products are more likely to provide false information than those that do not.

▶ **Do you recognize any suspicious techniques?** Be wary of Web sites that use the techniques of quacks and cons described in lesson 15.1.

▶ **Do experts find the Web site credible?** The Web site should be recommended or highly regarded by health and fitness experts.

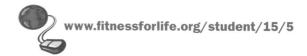

www.fitnessforlife.org/student/15/5

Reliable Consumer Agencies and Organizations

Many organizations work to protect consumers from misleading advertising and quackery. Some of the governmental agencies include the CDC, Consumer Product Safety Commission (CPSC), the Federal Trade Commission (FTC), the FDA, the USDA, and the United States Postal Service. Some reputable private organizations include AAHPERD, ACSM, AMA, American Dental Association, Better Business Bureau, Consumers Union, Cooper Institute, Mayo Clinic, and National Council Against Health Fraud. Some Web sites of highly respected individuals such as former Surgeon General C. Everett Koop are not sites of professional organizations but are considered by experts to present sound and factual information.

As a consumer, you need to be informed about the products and services you use. Do not assume that every advertised product is safe and effective. While agencies such as the ones just named can provide information, you make the final decision about buying a product or service.

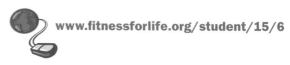

www.fitnessforlife.org/student/15/6

Taking Charge: Learning to Think Critically

A misconception is a belief based on incorrect or misunderstood information or lack of facts. The best way to counter a misconception is to increase knowledge so that you can interpret facts correctly.

Mary Lou had tried several exercise programs but did not find one she felt would meet her goal of attaining strength and muscle fitness. She never even considered weight training because she believed she would develop big, bulky muscles.

One day Mary Lou's physical education teacher took her class to the weight room. There, she explained how to use the free weights and machines for the best benefit. Over the next several weeks, the class practiced the correct use of the weight training equipment. As a class assignment, Mary Lou's physical education teacher had each member of the class find one newspaper or magazine article on weight training and write a report on it. Mary Lou learned that muscles will not become bulky if weight training is done properly.

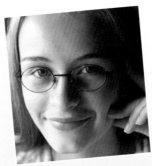

Mary Lou realized that the correct weight training program would give her exactly what she was looking for. Now she works out with weights three days each week. The knowledge Mary Lou gained about weight training has dispelled her original misconceptions.

Now Mary Lou is trying to help others change their irrational beliefs about weight training. When friends ask her why she is trying to build big muscles, she tells them, "If strength and muscle fitness are what you're after, you should give weight training a try."

For Discussion

What misconception did Mary Lou have? How was she able to build knowledge to dispel her misconception? What are some other misconceptions people have about physical activity? Fill out the questionnaire provided by your teacher to find out about your knowledge regarding physical activity and how you use it to make decisions about being active. Consider the guidelines on page 271.

Lesson Review

1. What are some guidelines to consider regarding the joining of a health or fitness club?
2. What should you consider before buying exercise equipment?
3. What are the guidelines for evaluating exercise videos, books, or articles?
4. What are the guidelines for choosing a Web site for health and fitness information?

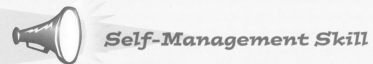

Self-Management Skill

Learning to Think Critically

Thinking critically means that you follow a problem-solving or decision-making process before making important decisions. You can follow several steps to solve problems or make good choices. These steps are listed next with an example for selecting exercise equipment. You can use the same steps to solve other problems or to make decisions about other important topics.

▶ **Step 1: Identify the problem to be solved or clarify the decision that must be made.** If you know that you want to improve your muscle fitness but are not sure how, you have to define the problem more clearly. Do you want to do your exercises at school, join a health and fitness club, buy exercise equipment, or use inexpensive equipment? You will also need to clarify your reasons for wanting to build muscle fitness. Do you want to improve your health or improve your appearance, or do you want to get fit for sports performance? In this case, let us assume that you want to make a decision about what equipment you want to use to build muscle fitness for health. The problem has been defined.

▶ **Step 2: Collect information and investigate.** Performing self-assessments for muscle fitness is one way to collect information. Knowing your current strength and muscular endurance levels will help you. You can also consult with experts, reliable Web sites such as that of the ACSM (www.acsm.org), or books such as this textbook. You might want to check *Consumer Reports Magazine* or the *Consumer Reports Year Book* for more information. In this case, you would also want to try out several options. You could try using the school exercise room. You could visit health and fitness clubs in your area. You could go to the sporting goods store and try some of the machines that are for sale. You could try several of the inexpensive equipment options your learned in this book. Focus on finding information that will help you solve the specific problem you identified in step 1.

▶ **Step 3: Develop a plan of action.** Use the information from your investigation to formulate a plan. The results of step 2 may have indicated that the school exercise room was not open when you had free time to use it. Health and fitness clubs were too far from your home and cost too much. Some of the exercise equipment available in stores was quite expensive. After trying all options, you decide to use rubber band exercises. The equipment is inexpensive and you can do all the exercises necessary to meet your goal. You decide to choose several of the exercises described in this book. You make a written plan that includes the days of the week you will do each exercise and how many reps and sets you will do each day.

▶ **Step 4. Put your plan in action.** For a plan to be effective, you must use it. The sooner you begin to act after preparing your plan, the more likely you are to change your behavior. In this example, you would use the plan developed in step 3 to get going.

▶ **Step 5. Evaluate the effectiveness of your plan.** Use self-monitoring to keep records and use self-assessments (reassessments) such as those in this chapter and chapter 16 to chart your progress.

You can use the same five steps to help you think critically to solve various problems and make important decisions about health, fitness, and wellness. When you create your personal fitness and activity plan in chapter 18, you will use many of these steps.

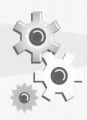

Activity 2

Active Learning: Isometric Exercise Circuit

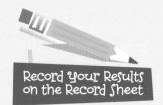

Record your Results on the Record Sheet

You already know that isometric exercises help develop muscle fitness. Isometric exercises can be done with little or no equipment. You can use your own body, a wall, or a towel as immovable resistance when performing isometric exercises. This activity includes examples of isometric exercises good for strengthening muscles that can be done at home at little or no cost. Write your results on your record sheet.

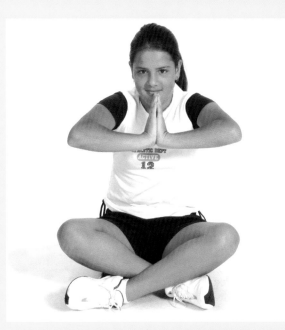

This exercise uses the arms and shoulder muscles.

Hand Push

1. Sit on the floor with your back straight. You may cross your legs if you prefer. Place the palms of your hands together.
2. Raise your hands and elbows to shoulder height. Push your hands against each other as hard as you can. Hold the position for 7 seconds; rest for 30 seconds.
3. Repeat the exercise 2 or 3 times as time allows.

Back Flattener

1. Lie on your back with your knees bent.
2. Pull in your abdomen by contracting your abdominal muscles as tightly as possible. Flatten your lower back against the floor. Hold the position for 7 seconds; rest for 30 seconds.
3. Repeat the exercise 2 or 3 times as time allows.

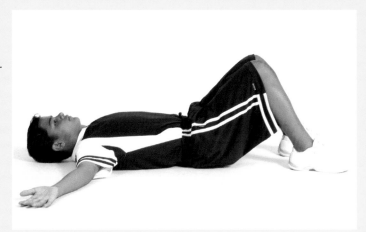

This exercise uses the abdominal muscles.

Knee Extender

1. Hold onto something for support and stand on your left foot. Lift your right foot behind you, bending the knee to a 90-degree angle.
2. Loop a towel under your right ankle; hold the ends of the towel in your right hand.
3. Push downward with your foot, trying to straighten your leg against the resistance of the towel.
4. Repeat the exercise 2 or 3 times with each leg as time allows.

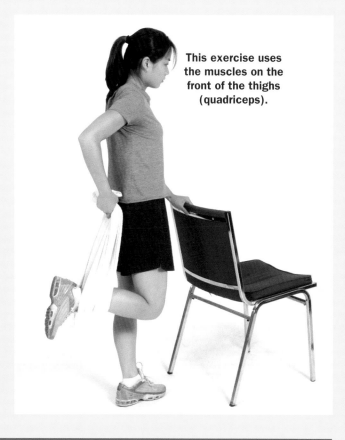

This exercise uses the muscles on the front of the thighs (quadriceps).

Wall Push

1. Stand with your back against a wall.
2. Move your feet out as you lower yourself into a half squat. Keep your thighs parallel to the floor.
3. Push your back against the wall by pushing with your legs as hard as you can. Hold the position for 7 seconds; rest for 30 seconds.
4. Repeat the exercise 2 or 3 times as time allows.

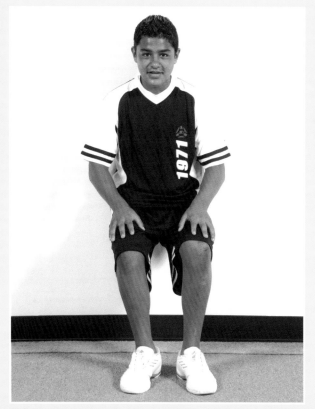

This exercise uses the muscles of the legs and abdomen.

Biceps Curl With Towel

1. Stand with your back straight and your knees slightly bent.
2. Loop a towel under the back of your thighs.
3. Grasp the towel ends with your palms up. Keep your elbows against your sides.
4. Pull up on the towel as hard as possible. Hold the position for 7 seconds; rest for 30 seconds.
5. Repeat the exercise 2 or 3 times as time allows.

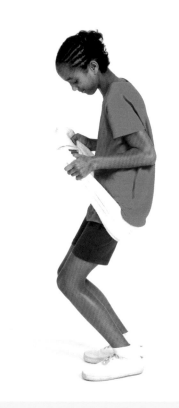

This exercise uses the muscles of the front of the arm (biceps).

Toe Push

1. Sit on the floor using good posture.
2. Hold the end of a jump rope or towel in each hand. Loop it over the balls of your feet so that it is tight against the soles.
3. Push with the balls of your feet as you pull on the rope or towel. Keep your back straight. Hold the position for 7 seconds; rest for 30 seconds.
4. Repeat the exercise two or three times as time allows.

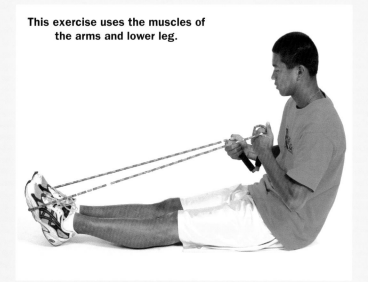

This exercise uses the muscles of the arms and lower leg.

Leg Curl

1. Stand on your left leg. Hold onto a chair or wall for balance.
2. Loop a towel behind your right ankle and stand on the ends of the towel with your left foot.
3. Keeping your posture erect and your back straight, try to bend your knee against the resistance of the towel. Hold the position for 7 seconds; rest for 30 seconds.
4. Repeat the exercise 2 or 3 times with each leg as time allows.

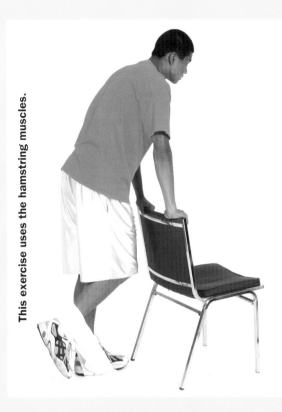

This exercise uses the hamstring muscles.

Bow Exercise

1. Stand in a position that an archer would take when shooting a bow.
2. Hold a towel with your right arm as if you were holding a bow.
3. Hold the other end of the towel with your left hand near the chin as if holding the string of a bow.
4. Push with your right hand and pull with your left hand. Hold the position for 7 seconds; rest for 30 seconds.
5. Repeat the exercise 2 to 3 times with each arm forward as time allows.

Safety Tip: Breathe normally while doing these exercises. Do not hold your breath. Holding your breath can cause dizziness and possibly a blackout.

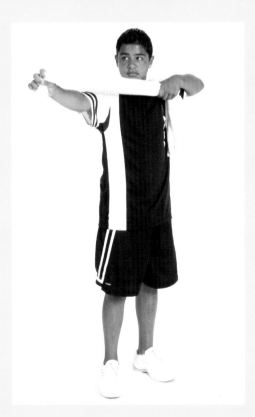

This exercise uses the muscles of the arms and shoulders.

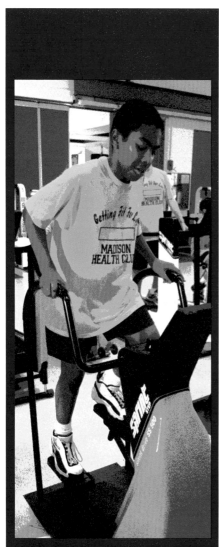

15 Chapter Review

Reviewing Concepts and Vocabulary

Number your paper from 1 to 5. Next to each number, write the word (or words) that correctly completes the sentence.

1. Many products sold as _____, or ergogenic aids, are quack products.
2. A _____ exercise uses machines or outside forces to move your muscles.
3. A method of advertising or selling that uses false claims is called _____.
4. A food _____ is a product intended to add to a person's nutritional intake.
5. A _____ diet often promises quick results but is usually nutritionally unbalanced.

Number your paper from 6 to 10. Next to each number, choose the letter of the best answer.

Column I	Column II
6. medical doctor	a. may not be an expert
7. certified health education teacher	b. provides medical advice
8. registered physical therapist	c. offers advice about diet and nutrition
9. dietitian	d. has information about fitness
10. nutritionist	e. answers concerns about general health

Number your paper from 11 to 12. On your paper, write a short answer for each statement or question.

11. Describe three ways you can recognize quackery.
12. Explain the effect of spot exercises on levels of body fat.

Thinking Critically

Write a paragraph to answer the following question.

Your friend Lee visited a health food store and got interested in taking a supplement. He says that he can make his own decision because the products must be safe and must work or they would not be on the shelves of the store. What advice would you give your friend? Explain your reasons.

Unit Review on the Web

 www.fitnessforlife.org/student/15/7

Unit V review materials are available on the Web at the address listed above.

Project

Choose one of the following projects. You may use a worksheet provided by your teacher as part of the project report.

1. Visit a local health club. Use the guidelines in this chapter to write a brief report on the club.

2. Choose an article on exercise from a popular magazine. Use the guidelines in this chapter to write a report on the contents of the article.

3. View an exercise video. Use the guidelines in this chapter to write a brief report on the quality of the video.

4. Select a Web site related to health or physical fitness. Use the guidelines in this chapter to write a brief report on the quality of the Web site and the information included.

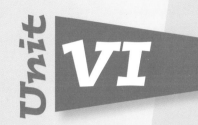

Unit VI

Wellness and Personal Program Planning

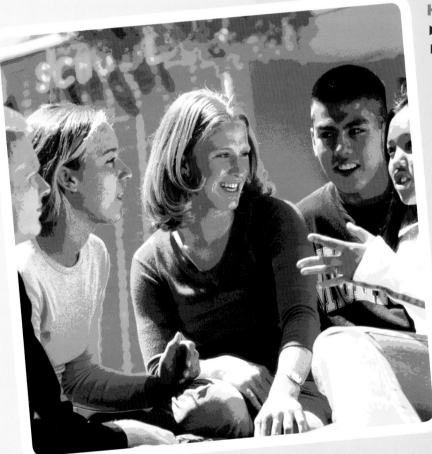

Healthy People 2010 Goals

▶ Improve mental health.
▶ Ensure access to mental health services.
▶ Decrease suicide and suicide attempts among teens.
▶ Increase availability of stress reduction programs.
▶ Increase availability of treatment for depression.
▶ Increase availability of treatment for anxiety disorders.

Unit Activities

▶ Cooper's Aerobics
▶ Your Health and Fitness Club
▶ Frisbee Golf
▶ Relaxation Exercises for Stress Management
▶ Exercising at Home
▶ Performing Your Plan

16

A Wellness Perspective

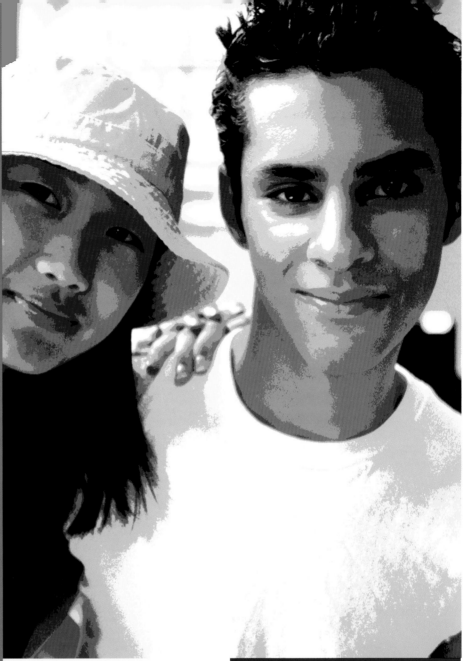

In this chapter...

Activity 1
Cooper's Aerobics

Lesson 16.1
All About Health and Wellness

Self-Assessment
Reassessing Cardiovascular Fitness and Muscular Endurance

Self-Assessment
Wellness

Lesson 16.2
Healthy Lifestyles and Environments

Taking Charge
Thinking Success

Self-Management Skill
Thinking Success

Activity 2
Your Health and Fitness Club

Activity 1

COOPER'S AEROBICS

Aerobics is a physical activity program that was originally developed by Dr. Kenneth Cooper for use by the U.S. Air Force. Now the program is widely used by people of all ages and includes many kinds of activities. In Cooper's Aerobics, you earn points for various activities. Your teacher will provide information on how to plan Cooper's Aerobics workouts. You may find out the point values of different activities at the Web site listed below.

 www.fitnessforlife.org/student/16/1

All About Health and Wellness

Lesson Objectives

After reading this lesson, you should be able to

1. Explain how wellness relates to good health.
2. Identify the components of good health and describe the positive and negative aspects of each.
3. Explain how the positive aspect of each component can contribute to good health.

Lesson Vocabulary

wellness (p. 279)

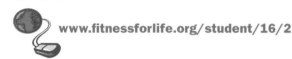

www.fitnessforlife.org/student/16/2

What would you wish for if you could only have one wish? Some people would say $1,000,000. Some would wish for other material things, such as a new car or a new house. But after thinking about it, many people indicate that they would wish for good health for themselves and their family. If you possess health and wellness, you can enjoy life to its fullest. Without health, no amount of money will allow you to do all the things you would like to do. In this lesson you will learn about the components of good health and the relationship of wellness to good health.

Good Health Includes Wellness

The World Health Organization (WHO) issued a statement in 1947 indicating that health was more than disease or illness. This recognition led to the development of a more comprehensive definition of health, which now includes wellness. According to the WHO statement, you are not well just because you are not sick. **Wellness** is the positive component of health that includes having a good quality of life and a good sense of well-being as exhibited by having a positive outlook on life and being happy and fulfilled. The illustration at the top of the page shows that a healthy person is not ill (blue outer circle) but also has a strong wellness component (green inner circle).

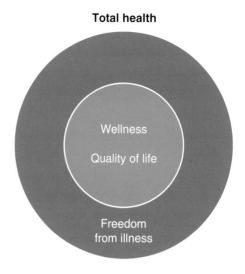

Being healthy means having wellness as well as not being ill.

Components of Good Health

In chapter 3 you learned about many of the health and wellness benefits of physical activity. Most of these benefits were physical, which might lead you to conclude that good health and wellness are only physical concerns. It is true that good physical fitness is important to overall health and wellness, but you now know that health and wellness have many components. A chain is often used to show the different components of health and wellness. The chain in the figure represents different components of health and wellness. For a chain to be strong, each link must be strong. Because health and wellness have many components, it is important not to focus on just one. The physical component is one that has been emphasized in this book because physical activity is so important to health and wellness. But other components are also important.

The goal for good health and wellness is to promote the positive while avoiding the negative in each component. Look at the positive and negative aspects of each component shown in table 16.1.

If you achieve the positives of each component, you will be well on your way to the quality of life and sense of well-being that the Healthy People 2010 goals

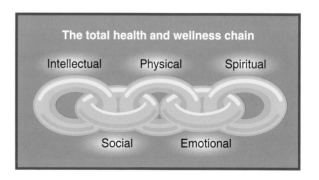

Table 16.1

Components of Health and Wellness

Negative aspect (avoid)	Component	Positive aspect (goal)
Depressed	Emotional	Happy
Ignorant	Intellectual	Informed
Lonely	Social	Involved
Unfit	Physical	Fit
Unfulfilled	Spiritual	Fulfilled
Illness	Health	Wellness

Adapted, by permission, from C. Corbin et al., 2004, *Concepts of fitness and wellness*, 5th ed. (St. Louis, MO: McGraw-Hill).

suggest are important. If you are happy, informed, involved, fit, and fulfilled, you have incorporated the positive aspects of the health components into your life. You will possess wellness, and your risk of illness will be decreased.

Moving From Illness Treatment to Health and Wellness Promotion

Did you know that a person born in 1900 had a life expectancy of only 47 years? But a person born today could expect to have a lifespan of approximately 77 years. What is the reason for such an increase in life expectancy? One major factor is the advances in medical science. Prior to 1900, killer diseases such as pneumonia, small-pox, and polio killed thousands, resulting in a relatively short life for the average person. During that same time, treatment of illness was a major concern because cures such as the antibiotics and vaccines we have today were not available. But as medical science conquered many diseases, research began to focus more on how lifestyles affected disease. The focus shifted from treatment to the prevention of illness and the promotion of wellness.

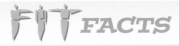

The leading causes of death in North American and other automated countries are chronic lifestyle diseases such as heart disease, cancer, stroke, and diabetes. These conditions also can influence well-ness by limiting your ability to function effectively in daily living and limiting your ability to enjoy your leisure time.

With this expanded definition of health in mind, the U.S. Department of Health and Human Services has set forth health goals called Healthy People 2010. These goals focus on developing health for all. These national objectives were described at the beginning of each unit of this book. While some of the goals are designed to ensure that all people get treatment for illness, many of the goals emphasize disease prevention and wellness promotion. As shown in the picture on page 281, all three phases (treating illness, preventing illness, and promoting health and wellness) are important. But a principal goal for the year 2010 is to help all people to be not only free from illness but also to live healthy, happy, and productive lives.

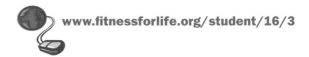

www.fitnessforlife.org/student/16/3

Wellness for All

Because wellness often is considered the opposite of illness, people sometimes think wellness is impossible for a person with a disease or medical problem. Most experts now agree that anyone can have wellness, even if he or she has a disease that is being treated. For example, a person who has had diabetes since birth has a disease. However, with treatment, the person can live a relatively normal life. By practicing healthy lifestyles a diabetic can develop good health and wellness. This, in turn, will enable the person to reach his or her fullest potential.

Most of us have health problems at some point in our lives. These problems may be short- or long-term conditions. However, even with problems, you can develop and practice healthy living to enhance your

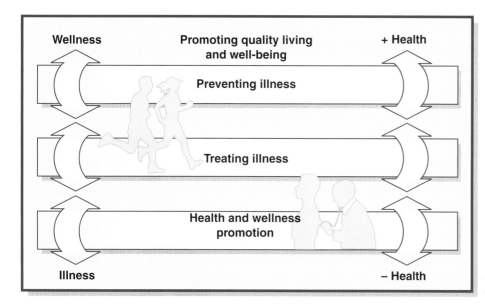

| Wellness | Promoting quality living and well-being | + Health |
| Preventing illness |
| Treating illness |
| Health and wellness promotion |
| Illness | | – Health |

Good health includes the promotion of wellness.

sense of well-being and your quality of life. For example, maintaining a positive attitude can help you overcome physical problems that are beyond your control.

One way to gain the information and support you need is to join a health club. Throughout this chapter your class will work together to create a health club. Your teacher will provide you with the information you need to begin.

Lesson Review

1. How does wellness relate to good health?
2. What are five components of health and wellness? Describe the positive and negative aspects of each.
3. How can the positive aspect of each component contribute to good health?

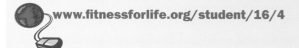
FITNESS Technology

Scientists have developed many products that help prevent diseases. For example, special high-tech machines can test to see whether you have fats and other substances in your blood that can lead to heart disease. X-ray and MRI machines can be used to detect cancers. These devices are important, but we also know that some very simple self-exams can help you prevent illnesses. For example, you can check your skin for moles that change in color or shape. Check the Web site listed above for more information on self-exams.

www.fitnessforlife.org/student/16/4

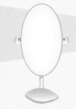

Reassessing Cardiovascular Fitness and Muscular Endurance

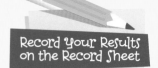

Record Your Results on the Record Sheet

In chapter 15 you had the chance to reassess your body composition, flexibility, and strength. Remember that reassessments can be good because they give you a chance to practice self-assessment procedures, they allow you to choose those fitness assessments you think meet your personal needs best, and they allow you to see whether your fitness changes over time.

In this self-assessment you will reassess your cardiovascular fitness and muscular endurance. All of the assessments are good, but you will have a choice. Choose those assessments you think are best for you. Refer to the page references following each self-assessment for instructions on doing the assessment and for determining your ratings. If time allows, perform more than the designated number of self-assessments from the lists that follow. When you are finished doing the reassessments, write your results and ratings on your record sheet. Also indicate the reasons for performing the assessments you chose.

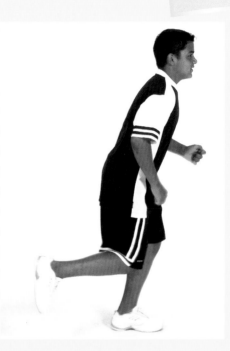

FIT FACTS

Other cardiovascular fitness tests exist, such as a treadmill test, a bicycle test, and even a swimming test. If you have performed one of these tests in addition to the one you tried in this self-assessment, you can record your results on the sheet provided by your teacher.

Cardiovascular Fitness

Choose one of the following tests to reassess your cardiovascular fitness.

1. PACER (chapter 8, page 123)
2. Step test (chapter 7, page 108)
3. One-mile run (chapter 7, page 109)
4. Walking test (chapter 6, page 94)

Muscular Endurance

Choose at least one item from each area to reassess your muscular endurance. *Note:* These items also assess strength, but because they are typically done for more than a few repetitions, they are included in the muscular endurance section of this reassessment.

1. Upper body
   ▶ Push-up (90-degree) (chapter 2, page 30)
   ▶ Bent arm hang (chapter 12, page 206)
   ▶ Side stand (chapter 12, page 204)

2. Lower body
   ▶ Leg change (chapter 12, page 206)
3. Abdominals
   ▶ Curl-up (chapter 2, page 29)
   ▶ Sitting tuck (chapter 12, page 205)
4. Back and trunk
   ▶ Trunk lift (upper back) (chapter 8, page 122)
   ▶ Trunk extension (chapter 12, page 205)

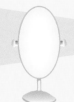

Self-Assessment

Wellness

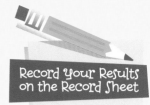

Record Your Results on the Record Sheet

In the previous lessons you learned about wellness and its several components. The following questionnaire will help you to self-assess your current wellness. This extra self-assessment is included here so that you can assess your wellness for your own personal information. Record your results on a separate sheet of paper. Follow these directions.

1. Read each statement about wellness. You can strongly agree, agree, disagree, or strongly disagree with each statement.
2. On the worksheet provided by your teacher, circle the response for each statement.
3. Write the number of your response in the box at the right of the question.
4. Calculate a score for each of the five components of wellness by adding the three questions for each component.
5. Add all five wellness scores to get an overall wellness score.
6. Use table 16.2 to get wellness ratings for each wellness part. Your teacher may provide you with a separate copy of the wellness self-assessment for use as a class assignment.

Table 16.2

Rating Chart: Wellness

Wellness rating	Three-item score	Total wellness score
Good	10-12	50+
Marginal	8-9	40-49
Low	<7	<39

283

Wellness Questionnaire

Wellness statement	Strongly agree	Agree	Disagree	Strongly disagree	Score
1. I am physically fit.	4	3	2	1	
2. I can do the physical tasks needed in my work.	4	3	2	1	
3. I have the energy to be active in my free time.	4	3	2	1	
Physical Wellness Score =					
4. I am happy most of the time.	4	3	2	1	
5. I do not get stressed often.	4	3	2	1	
6. I like myself the way I am.	4	3	2	1	
Emotional Wellness Score =					
7. I have many friends.	4	3	2	1	
8. I am confident in social situations.	4	3	2	1	
9. I am close to my family.	4	3	2	1	
Social Wellness Score =					
10. I am an informed consumer.	4	3	2	1	
11. I check facts before making health decisions.	4	3	2	1	
12. I consult experts when I am not sure of health facts.	4	3	2	1	
Intellectual Wellness Score =					
13. I feel a sense of purpose for my life.	4	3	2	1	
14. I feel fulfilled spiritually.	4	3	2	1	
15. I feel strong connections to the world around me.	4	3	2	1	
Spiritual Wellness Score =					
Total Wellness Score =					

Adapted, by permission, from C. Corbin et al., 2004, *Concepts of fitness and wellness*, 5th ed. (St. Louis, MO: McGraw-Hill).

Lesson 16.2

Healthy Lifestyles and Environments

Lesson Objectives

After reading this lesson, you should be able to

1. Explain the difference between controllable risk factors and noncontrollable risk factors.
2. Identify and describe several healthy lifestyles.
3. Identify and explain some environmental and social factors that affect health and wellness.

Lesson Vocabulary

controllable risk factors (p. 285), lifestyle (p. 285), noncontrollable risk factors (p. 285)

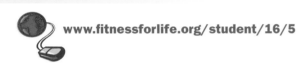

www.fitnessforlife.org/student/16/5

If you asked every person you know, you would probably find that all of them would like to have good health and wellness. But how many of them are aware of all the things they can do to achieve it? In this lesson you will learn about healthy lifestyles and how they can help you achieve good health and wellness. You will also learn about some of the environmental and social factors that can influence your health and wellness.

Healthy Lifestyles and Risk Factors

You probably know by now that lifestyle is a word that refers to the way you live. A healthy **lifestyle** is a way of living that helps you prevent illness and enhance wellness. In fact, healthy lifestyles are ways that you can reduce **controllable risk factors**—risk factors that you can act upon to change. Healthy lifestyles are in your control and, if you practice them, they reduce your risk of many of the major health problems. For example, sedentary living is a controllable risk factor, so by being active you can reduce the health risks.

As you can see in the diagram at the top of the page, four major factors contribute to early death. The largest number of early deaths result from unhealthy lifestyles. This means that these problems could be prevented if people would change the way they live. It is

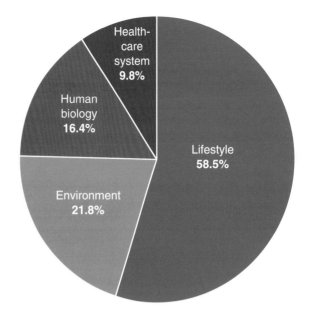

Four main factors contributing to early death.

important to know that practicing healthy lifestyles not only reduces the risk of disease and death from disease but also enhances wellness. For example, not smoking greatly reduces the risk of heart disease and cancer and also increases the quality of your life. You can breathe better, have a keener sense of smell, and spend less money on tobacco and medical care.

Some risk factors, such as age and gender, are not in your control. These factors are called **noncontrollable risk factors.** Because you cannot do anything about these risk factors, focus on those that you can control. This chapter focuses on healthful lifestyles over which you have some control.

Choosing Healthy Lifestyles

Doing regular physical activity is a healthy lifestyle that health experts feel is among the most important. Not only does it help you prevent many of the major illnesses and enhance your physical fitness and health, but also it can contribute to good health in other areas as well. Though doing physical activity is the healthy lifestyle that is emphasized in this book, others also are important. The list on the next page includes some lifestyles that you can adopt to promote good fitness, health, and wellness. These lifestyles are only of benefit if you choose to do them. The choices you make have much to do with your fitness, health, and wellness.

Be Physically Active

You have been learning throughout this book why physical activity is important to good health. The benefits to good health and wellness were outlined in

Healthy Lifestyles

▶ Be physically active.
▶ Eat properly.
▶ Manage stress.
▶ Adopt good personal health habits.
▶ Avoid destructive habits.
▶ Adopt good safety practices.
▶ Seek and follow appropriate medical advice.

detail in chapter 3. Among the health goals set forth in Healthy People 2010, being physically active is one of the most important. It was listed first among all of the goals because changing inactive people to active people (changing lifestyles) would do more for the health and wellness of people than any other change. For example, being physically active can help you manage stress, so the benefits are doubled.

Eat Properly

What kinds of food do you typically eat? Are your meals generally high in fat? Do you eat plenty of fruits and vegetables, as well as grains and meats? Many children, teens, and adults eat more fat than they should and, in general, do not eat a balanced diet. Another major health goal is to improve the nutrition of all citizens. The goals set forth in Healthy People 2010 outline ways to improve health and wellness by changing eating habits. You studied nutrition and general guidelines for eating properly in chapter 14.

Manage Stress

You probably have had periods of stress and know how it can affect you for the short term. But did you know that stress can cause health problems and detract from personal well-being and quality of life? While most people are well aware of the stress experienced by business people, elected officials, and other people in high-stress jobs, many sometimes forget that stress effects everyone—including teens. Managing stress is a healthy lifestyle that is important to good health and wellness. You will study stress in greater detail in chapter 17.

Adopt Good Personal Health Habits

In kindergarten or first grade, you most likely learned about personal health habits, such as regularly brushing and flossing your teeth, washing your hands before meals and after using the bathroom, and getting enough sleep. But how many of these habits have you adopted? Using good health habits is one way you can prevent illness and promote optimal quality of living. For example, if you have an illness that could have been prevented through proper health habits, you will feel ill and you will have at least a temporary reduction in your quality of living.

Avoid Destructive Habits

Just as adopting healthy habits contributes to good health, possessing destructive habits detracts from health and wellness. Smoking, other tobacco use, legal or illegal drug abuse, and alcohol abuse are just a few of the destructive habits that detract from total health. These destructive habits can impair your fitness, detract from your performance of physical activities, and result in various diseases, lowered feelings of well-being, and reduced quality of life.

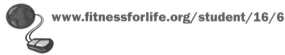

www.fitnessforlife.org/student/16/6

Adopt Good Safety Practices

News accounts of injuries or deaths caused by motor vehicle accidents fill the newspapers each day. Other common causes of death or injury include falls, poisonings, drownings, fires, bicycle accidents, and accidents in and around home. Many of these injuries or deaths could have been prevented if simple safety rules had been followed. A national health goal is to reduce the number of deaths and injuries from accidents. Things you can do to adopt healthy lifestyles include wearing

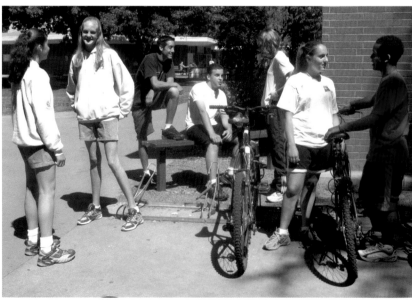

Supportive friends are important to good health and wellness.

seat belts, wearing helmets while riding bikes or inline skating, making sure that poisons are properly labeled, installing and maintaining smoke detectors, practicing water safety, and keeping your home in good repair to reduce the risks of accidents. And don't forget—being physically fit can help prevent accidents too.

Seek and Follow Appropriate Medical Advice

Even if you adopt and adhere to healthy lifestyles, you may become ill occasionally. In those cases, seeking and following appropriate medical advice is important. In fact, for best results, regular medical and dental checkups are recommended to help prevent problems before they start. Consult your own physician and dentist to determine how often you should have a checkup. Some people avoid seeking medical help because they fear they may be ill. Because early detection of health problems is important to an ultimate cure, this practice can be dangerous.

Practice Other Healthy Lifestyles

Other lifestyles that will help improve health and wellness include being an informed consumer (not buying quack products) and learning first aid (learning CPR).

www.fitnessforlife.org/ student/16/7

The Environment and Wellness

Sometimes people refer to something called environmental wellness, but environmental wellness is not a personal characteristic. Rather, an environment can be referred to as unhealthy if it causes health problems or if it detracts from the five components of personal wellness. In fact, the second most important contributor to early death (see figure on page 285) is an unhealthy environment. Especially important to your health and wellness are your physical and social environments.

Physical Environment

The physical environment refers to the air, the land, the water, the plants, and other physical things that exist around you. We know that certain physical environments can be very harmful to your health. People who live in polluted cities are at greater risk than those who live in the country where the air is cleaner. People who work in coal mines and people who work in areas that allow smoking have a higher risk of illness than those who work in less polluted areas. Your work environment is sometimes referred to as your vocational environment.

You may not be able to change some of the aspects of a physical environment, such as the place where you live. You can take action to improve your environment by not exposing yourself unnecessarily to smoke-filled places, avoiding excessive exposure to the sun, and using pollutants, such as weed killers, carefully. Exercising away from heavily traveled streets can help you avoid excessive air pollution. You can also work to protect the environment by recycling and by not polluting the air, land, or water.

Taking Charge: Thinking Success

An optimist is a person who expects a good or favorable outcome from a situation. This positive thinking is an example of thinking success. The optimist thinks that he or she can succeed at a specific activity. A person who thinks success, or has positive thoughts, will more often be successful than a person who has negative thoughts.

Aaron loves baseball. For two years he played on a team that won most of the regular season's games. The team even played in the league's championship game. During that time, Aaron played well at second base and hit a few home runs.

This year Aaron moved up to a new team. Most of the players in the new level were older, bigger, and stronger than he was. During the first game, he was hit by a pitch. He struck out each other time he was at bat. In fact, he did not even hit the ball one time. The coach noticed that Aaron no longer swung at the ball with confidence.

Luckily, the coach knew that Aaron had the physical strength and skills needed to hit the ball. He only

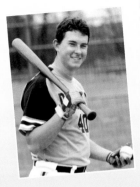

needed to change the way he was thinking. He wouldn't hit the ball until he thought he could. The coach had Aaron practice drills that he could successfully complete. He taught Aaron to mentally see himself hitting the ball and to say and believe "yes, yes, yes" as he stood waiting for the pitch. He also taught Aaron not to think obsessively about the times he struck out or failed to make a play. "After all," the coach told Aaron, "even the best professionals only get a hit about one out of three tries. The next play is the one to think about." Aaron improved his hitting as he gained confidence.

For Discussion

How did Aaron's negative feelings affect the way he played baseball with the new team? How was he able to change his attitudes to think about success? What are some other ways a person can change negative thoughts into positive ones? Fill out the questionnaire provided by your teacher to find out how negative or positive your thoughts are. Consider the guidelines on page 289.

Social Environment

Your social environment refers to your social interactions with the people around you. This environment includes interactions with friends, teachers at school, colleagues at work, and other social contacts outside of school or work and in leisure-time social situations.

Researchers have shown that teens who have friends who practice unhealthy lifestyles are likely to try risky behaviors such as abusing tobacco, drugs, or alcohol. Those who have the social support of others who have healthy lifestyles are more likely to practice healthy behaviors such as being physically active and eating well. Choosing supportive friends is important to good health and wellness. Most people are exposed to unhealthy social environments at some point in their lives, even when they would like to avoid them. If this happens to you, consider using some of the self-management skills described in this book to help you make good choices. For example, learning to think critically, learning relapse prevention, and practicing ways to say "no" can help you to stick with your healthy behaviors.

Lesson Review

1. What is the difference between controllable risk factors and noncontrollable risk factors? Give examples.
2. What are some healthy lifestyle choices? Why are they beneficial to quality of life?
3. Identify the two environmental factors that influence health and wellness and describe how they influence them.

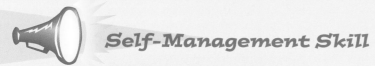

Self-Management Skill

Thinking Success

One of the main reasons some people fail to stick with a healthy lifestyle program is because they don't believe in themselves. Many people make resolutions each New Year, but not all people accomplish their goals. Follow these guidelines to help your success:

▶ **Assess your feelings about success.** Use the worksheet provided by your teachers. Use your answers to each of the questions to see where you might change to improve your chances of being successful.

▶ **Set realistic, attainable goals and use self-monitoring to reinforce your successes.**

▶ **Use self-assessments to help you set goals and evaluate your progress.**

▶ **Choose activities that you enjoy and that match your abilities.**

▶ **Practice to improve your performance skills.**

▶ **Find friends with similar interests who support you.**

▶ **Take steps to avoid relapse and to say "no" to things you do not want to do.**

▶ **Learn how to overcome barriers to success.**

▶ **Work to build your self-perceptions and self-confidence.**

▶ **Practice relaxation techniques that can help you overcome competitive stress.**

▶ **Learn the steps in planning for healthy lifestyle change.**

▶ **Become an informed consumer.**

▶ **Avoid unhealthy physical and social environments.**

▶ **Use other self-management techniques you have studied in this book.**

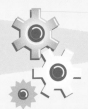

Activity 2

Your Health and Fitness Club

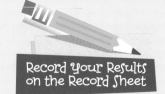

Record Your Results on the Record Sheet

Some people choose to join health and fitness clubs as a way of staying active and fit. Health and fitness clubs that are well run by educated professionals can benefit you in many ways. Unfortunately, these clubs cost money—sometimes quite a lot of money. For this reason they are not available to all people.

One way to get the benefits of health and fitness clubs is to establish one of your own. In this activity, your class will create a health and fitness club. The class will name the club, select appropriate physical activities to be offered, and prepare materials about wellness and healthy lifestyles that will be available to club members. After making these general decisions, groups will plan club activities for the club. During your activity class, you will have an opportunity to share your group's information with other classmates. You will also learn about the other groups' topics. Follow the instructions on your record sheet as you plan your health and fitness club.

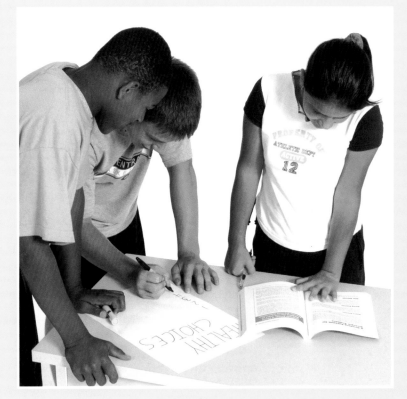

16 Chapter Review

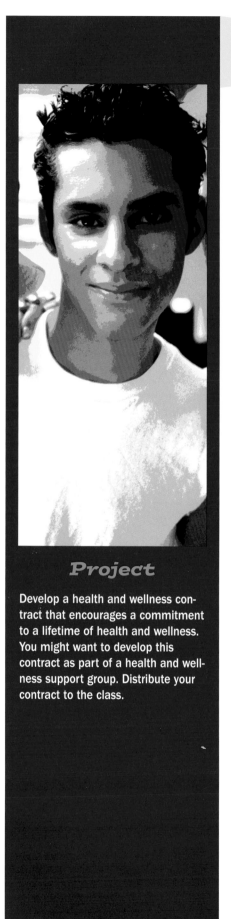

Project

Develop a health and wellness contract that encourages a commitment to a lifetime of health and wellness. You might want to develop this contract as part of a health and wellness support group. Distribute your contract to the class.

Reviewing Concepts and Vocabulary

Number your paper from 1 to 3. Next to each number, write the word (or words) that correctly completes the sentence.

1. A _____ is a way of living that helps you prevent illness and enhance wellness.
2. _____ are the largest contributors to early death.
3. _____ would do more to improve the health and wellness of American people than any other change.

Number your paper from 4 to 6. Next to each number, choose the letter of the best answer.

Column I	Column II
4. fulfilled	a. positive aspect of social component of health
5. informed	b. positive aspect of intellectual component of health
6. involved	c. positive aspect of spiritual component of health

Number your paper from 7 to 10. On your paper, write a short answer for each statement or question.

7. How has the definition of health changed during this century?
8. Explain the difference between controllable and noncontrollable risk factors. Give examples.
9. What is the focus of the national health goals as set forth in Healthy People 2010?
10. What is wellness?

Thinking Critically

Write a paragraph to answer the following questions.

What are some healthy lifestyles you now practice? How do they contribute to good health?

17

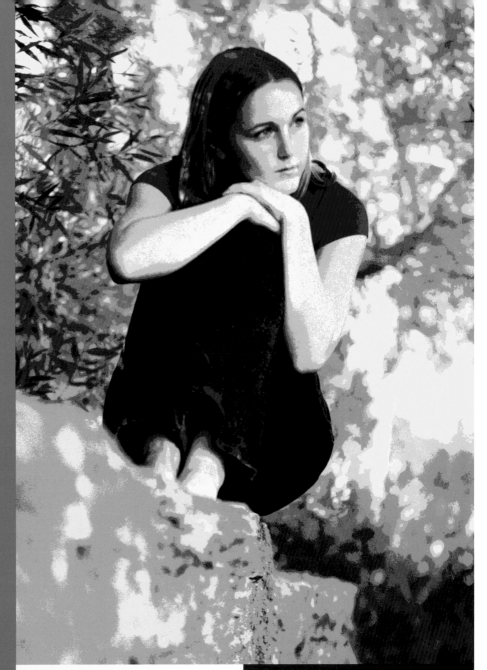

Stress Management

In this chapter...

Activity 1
Frisbee Golf

Lesson 17.1
Facts About Stress

Self-Assessment
Identifying Signs of Stress

Lesson 17.2
Managing Stress

Taking Charge
Controlling Competitive Stress

Self-Management Skill
Controlling Competitive Stress

Activity 2
Relaxation Exercises for Stress Management

Activity 1

FRISBEE GOLF

People of all ages can enjoy Frisbee golf. It is an enjoyable activity that can help you relax and reduce stress. To play the game, you try to throw the Frisbee from each "tee" into each "hole," or goal. You can design your own course using rope, baskets, plastic hoops, or chalk lines on the ground as holes.

Each hole has a "par," which is the recommended number of throws to get the Frisbee in the goal. The object is to achieve par or less for each hole. Your score is the total number of throws for 18 holes of Frisbee golf.

If you are playing for relaxation, it is best not to be too competitive. You might want to compare your score to par and try to improve rather than compare your score to someone else's.

Lesson 17.1

Facts About Stress

Lesson Objectives

After reading this lesson, you should be able to

1. Define stress and list its causes.
2. Explain the three stages in the general adaptation syndrome.
3. Explain how eustress and distress differ.
4. Discuss the effects of stress.

Lesson Vocabulary

alarm reaction (p. 293), distress (p. 294), eustress (p. 294), general adaptation syndrome (p. 293), stage of exhaustion (p. 293), stage of resistance (p. 293), stress (p. 293), stressor (p. 293)

www.fitnessforlife.org/student/17/1

How would you feel if a bear were running toward you? Most likely, you would feel frightened. Your heart rate would increase and your muscles would tense. Your body would release a chemical called adrenaline to give you energy to run away. These changes and those shown in the figure on the next page are part of the stress response, your body's way of preparing you to deal with a demanding situation. If danger presents itself, your stress response prepares your body for bursts of energy you can use to face danger or avoid it.

Encountering a bear is an unusual situation. However, you probably face stressful situations every day that affect you both physically and emotionally. In fact, two thirds of Americans report feeling stressed out at least once a week.

In this lesson, you will read more about stress. You will learn about its many causes and you will find out how it can affect you.

What Is Stress?

Stress is the body's reaction to a demanding situation. A series of physical changes takes place automatically when you are in a highly stressful situation.

A famous researcher, Hans Selye, helped us understand the effects of stress when he described the **general adaptation syndrome.** He showed that all people adapt in a general way when exposed to stressors. A **stressor** is something that causes or contributes to stress. The three phases of the general adaptation syndrome are shown in the figure below. First, the body uses its **alarm reaction** to react to a stressor. Anything that causes you to worry or get excited or anything that causes other emotional and physical changes can be a stressor and start your body's alarm reaction. For adults, stressors might include bills, vacation plans, work responsibilities, and family conflicts. Stressors for teenagers include grades and schoolwork, family arguments, and peer pressures. Other common stressors for teenagers include moving to a new home, serious illness or death in the family, poor eating habits, lack of physical activity, feelings of loneliness, a change or loss of friends, substance abuse, and trouble with school or legal authorities.

Some of the physical changes that occur when the body starts its alarm reaction to a stressor are shown in the photo on the next page. The alarm reaction may cause your heart rate to increase and other physical changes to occur. After the body has had a chance to adjust, it enters the second stage of the general adaptation syndrome. This stage is called the **stage of resistance** because in this stage the immune system starts to resist or fight the stressor. In the case of an illness, antibodies are sent out to fight. In the case of a physical stressor, such as doing heavy exercise, the heart rate goes up to supply more blood and oxygen to the body. In most cases, our resistance is enough to overcome the stressor, and we adapt by returning to our normal state of being.

In extreme cases, the body is not able to resist well enough and it enters the third stage of the syndrome, the **stage of exhaustion.** Various medical treatments may be necessary to help us resist and overcome the stressor. If the stressor is too great, as in the case of a disease that the body and medicine cannot fight, death can occur.

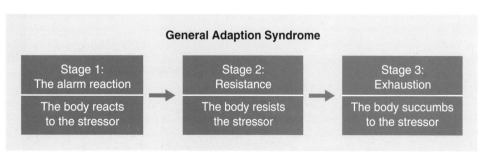

General Adaption Syndrome

Stage 1: The alarm reaction	Stage 2: Resistance	Stage 3: Exhaustion
The body reacts to the stressor	The body resists the stressor	The body succumbs to the stressor

Eustress and Distress

Not all stressful experiences are harmful. Scientists use the term **eustress** to describe positive stress. Situations that might produce eustress include riding a roller coaster, successfully competing in an activity, passing a driving test, playing in the school band, and meeting new people. Eustress helps make your life more enjoyable by helping you meet challenges and do your best.

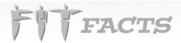

The prefix *eu* in the word eustress is taken from the word euphoria, which means a feeling of well-being.

On the other hand, unpleasant situations also cause stress. Negative stress is sometimes called **distress.** Situations that cause worry, sorrow, anger, or pain produce distress.

A situation that causes eustress for one person can cause distress for another. For example, an outgoing person might look forward to joining extracurricular activities at school or attending social events, while a shy person might dread the same situations. A similar experience can be eustressful or distressful for you at different times. For example, if you are well prepared for a test, taking that test might cause eustress. On the other hand, taking a test for which you are not prepared might cause distress.

Low levels of stress may help you prepare for more stressful situations in the future. For example, doing physical activity may be a stressor, but regular physical activity can help make you fit, healthy, and better able to handle future stressful situations. Ideally, you need to strive for the right level of stress—neither too much nor too little.

Causes of Distress

Distress can have a negative effect on your total health and fitness. To control stress in your life, you need to understand the cause of the stress you are experiencing.

Physical Stressors

Physical stressors are conditions of your body and the environment that affect your physical well-being. Examples include thirst, hunger, overexposure to heat or cold, lack of sleep, illness, pollution, noise, accidents, and catastrophes such as floods or fires. Even excessive exercise can be a stressor. Athletes who overtrain experience this kind of negative effect. However, healthy people who follow good exercise principles and achieve good fitness are better able to adapt to the changes produced by physical stressors.

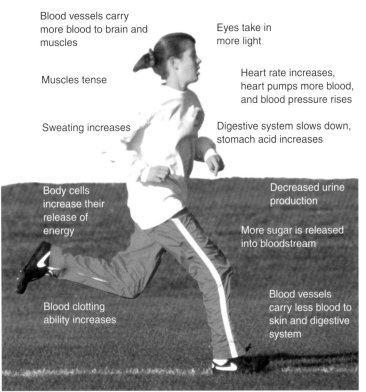

Blood vessels carry more blood to brain and muscles

Eyes take in more light

Muscles tense

Heart rate increases, heart pumps more blood, and blood pressure rises

Sweating increases

Digestive system slows down, stomach acid increases

Body cells increase their release of energy

Decreased urine production

More sugar is released into bloodstream

Blood clotting ability increases

Blood vessels carry less blood to skin and digestive system

The stress response: your body's way of preparing.

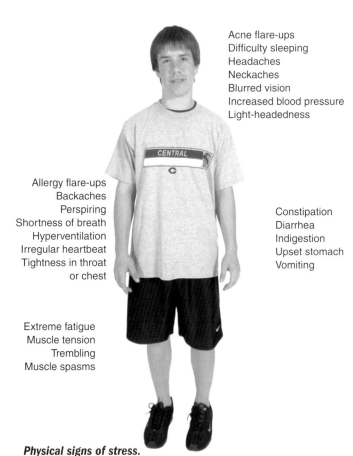

Acne flare-ups
Difficulty sleeping
Headaches
Neckaches
Blurred vision
Increased blood pressure
Light-headedness

Allergy flare-ups
Backaches
Perspiring
Shortness of breath
Hyperventilation
Irregular heartbeat
Tightness in throat or chest

Constipation
Diarrhea
Indigestion
Upset stomach
Vomiting

Extreme fatigue
Muscle tension
Trembling
Muscle spasms

Physical signs of stress.

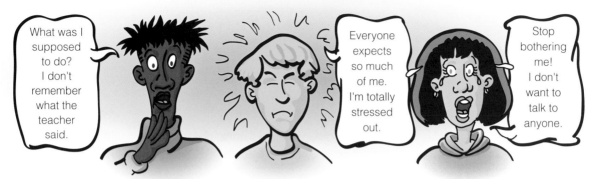

Emotional signs of stress.

Emotional Stressors

Emotions such as worry, fear, anger, grief, depression, or even falling in love are powerful stressors and can strongly affect your physical and emotional well-being.

Social Stressors

Social stressors arise from your relationships with other people. Each day, you have experiences that involve your family members, friends, teachers, employers, and others. As a teenager, you probably are exposed to many social stressors. Think about stressors in social situations in your life. Much of the stress you experience may be caused by social stressors.

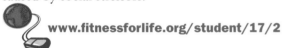 www.fitnessforlife.org/student/17/2

Effects of Stress

Stress can lead to both emotional and physical changes. Emotional effects of stress can include upset or nervous feelings; anger, anxiety, or fear; frequently criticizing others; frustration; forgetfulness; difficulty paying attention; difficulty making decisions; irritability; lack of motivation; boredom, mild depression, or withdrawal; or change in appetite. Some of these signs are illustrated in the figure above.

Have you ever experienced extreme fatigue, light-headedness, or upset stomach resulting from stress? These and other reactions shown in the figure at the left are common physical reactions to stressors. These reactions vary from one person to another. They usually last a short time, disappearing once the source of the stress is removed.

High levels of stress and prolonged periods of stress can be related to many physical conditions. For example, increased stomach acid resulting from stress can aggravate ulcers. High blood pressure can be related to stress and can lead to serious cardiovascular diseases and disorders. Prolonged stress can lower the effectiveness of the body's immune system, making a person more susceptible to certain diseases. Some doctors think that many health problems in the United States requiring medical attention are stress related. The motivation to deal effectively with stress, especially distress, is clear.

Use your self-assessment record sheet to find out how prone you are to stress. If you are prone to stress, consider using the procedures for managing stress that are described in the next lesson.

Lesson Review

1. What are some of the most common causes of stress and why do they cause stress?
2. What are the three stages of the general adaptation syndrome?
3. How do eustress and distress differ?
4. What physical and emotional effects can stress have on the body?

FITNESS Technology

Many high-tech methods exist to determine whether your body is stressed. When stressors are present, your heart rate is elevated, so the heart rate monitors you use to check your target heart rate can also be used to see whether you are stressed, especially in nonactive situations. Your body temperature is another way to determine whether you are experiencing physiological stress. Special metallic strips (stress strips) have been developed to measure your skin temperature. When you are relaxed, your skin temperature goes up; when you experience stress, it goes down. Stress strips turn red when your skin temperature goes up, indicating that your stress level is going down. They turn blue when your skin temperature goes down, indicating that your stress level is going up. You can use stress strips and heart rate to help you learn to relax.

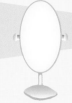

Self-Assessment

Identifying Signs of Stress

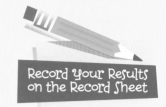

Record Your Results on the Record Sheet

All people experience some negative stress in their lives. Your body sends off certain signals when you are experiencing such distress. In this self-assessment, you will learn to identify some of the body's stress signals.

Table 17.1 lists some signs that commonly accompany stress. You may notice some of these signs when you are not under excessive stress. However, in times of great stress, these signs are often especially apparent.

One way to determine whether an activity is stressful to you is to self-assess signs and signals of stress before and after the activity. Work with a partner. Follow these steps to help each other look for signs and symptoms of stress indicated in table 17.1:

1. Lie on the floor, close your eyes, and try to relax. Have your partner count your pulse and your breathing rate. Ask your partner to observe for irregular breathing and unusual mannerisms. Then ask your partner to evaluate how tense your muscles seem. Report feeling butterflies in your stomach or other indicators of stress to your partner. Write your results on your record sheet. Have your partner lie down while you record your observations about him or her.

2. When directed by your instructor, all members of the class should write their names on a piece of paper and place the papers in a hat or a box. The teacher will draw names until only three remain in the container. The students whose names remain must give one-minute speeches about the effects of stress. Observe your partner before and during the name drawing. Look for the signs and signals of stress. Record your results on the record sheet. Also, try to remember your feelings during the drawing. Finally, observe the people who were required to make the speech. Record this information on the record sheet.

3. Finally, walk or jog for 5 minutes after your second stress assessment. Once again, work with a partner to assess your signs of stress. Write them in the third column of the record sheet. Notice that the exercise causes heart rate and breathing rate to increase. However, it may help reduce earlier signs of the emotional stress related to performing in front of the class.

Table 17.1

Signs of Stress

Heart rate	Is it higher than normal?
Muscle tension	Are the muscles tighter than usual? · arms and shoulders · legs
Mannerisms	Are unusual mannerisms present? · frowning or twitching · hands to face (nail biting)
Nervous feelings	Do you feel differently? · feeling of butterflies in stomach · tense or anxious feelings
Breathing	Have you noticed differences? · irregular · rapid or shallow

Lesson 17.2

Managing Stress

Lesson Objectives

After reading this lesson, you should be able to

1. Discuss how to manage stress in everyday life.
2. Describe health practices that can help a person deal with stress.
3. Describe competitive stress.

Lesson Vocabulary

competitive stress (p. 299), runner's high (p. 298)

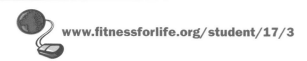

www.fitnessforlife.org/student/17/3

Perhaps you feel overwhelmed by the many causes of distress and its effects. Distress in life is unavoidable. These suggestions can help you deal effectively with it.

Effective Ways to Manage Stress

Fortunately, you can take steps to manage the stress in your life. When a situation seems distressful, follow these guidelines:

▶ **Rest in a quiet place.** Relax indoors or outdoors. The teenager in the picture is relaxing in a quiet place.

▶ **Reduce your breathing rate.** Sit or lie quietly. Take several long, slow breaths in through your nose and breathe out through your mouth.

▶ **Reduce your mental activity.** Sometimes, it is best to get rid of distressful thoughts until a later time. Try imagining a pleasant outdoor scene or listening to music.

▶ **Reduce muscle tension.** Relaxing your muscles can effectively help reduce distress. You will learn helpful relaxation techniques in the activity on pages 300 through 302.

▶ **Use exercise as a diversion.** An excellent way to relieve distress is through physical activity. Try sports or another type of physical activity you enjoy.

▶ **Identify the stressor.** Clearly identify the cause of your stress. For example, if anger is causing you stress, try to identify what is making you angry.

▶ **Tackle one thing at a time.** If several problems pile up, ask yourself, "What can I do now to change things? What can wait? What cannot be changed?"

▶ **Take action.** Rather than worrying about a problem, try to solve it. Make decisions and carry them out. When making a decision, look at several choices, consider the results of each, and choose the best one.

▶ **Manage time effectively.** Prioritize your activities so that you have time for the most important things. Learn to say "no" to new responsibilities or activities if you cannot give them the time required.

▶ **Accept what cannot be changed.** Not all problems can be solved as you would like, but you can still deal with them effectively. For example, suppose you are asked to trim the hedges. You do the job and then find that you did not do it correctly. You cannot change what you have already done, but you can deal with the stress by recognizing that all people make errors. You can learn from your mistake and get better directions the next time so that you can do a better job.

▶ **Think positively.** Positive thoughts can help reduce distress. For example, try thinking that you *will* get a hit in the softball game instead of worrying about striking out. Also, make an effort to perceive a stressor as a challenge rather than as a problem.

▶ **Do not mask your problems.** Sometimes people who are experiencing distress try to avoid the problem. Usually, masking the problem leads to more distress.

▶ **Try not to let little things bother you.** Many events in life are simply not worth stressful feelings. For example, if you are disappointed, remember that a situation might be better the next time.

▶ **Be flexible.** Learning to bend a little, or adjust to changes, can be helpful. You use this ability to help handle distress.

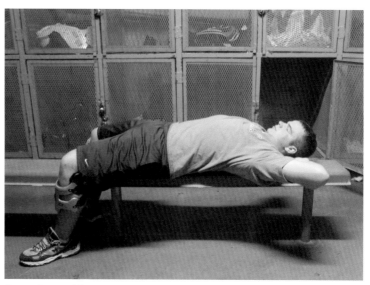

Sometimes taking a moment to rest in a quiet place can help you manage stress.

Taking Charge:
Controlling Competitive Stress

A little stress can give you more energy and help you meet a challenge. However, the effects of too much stress can interfere with your performance, especially during a competition. To do your best, you need to recognize the symptoms of stress and know ways to manage them.

Shelly watched from the bottom row of the bleachers as Willie shook his shoulders and arms. Shelly knew that swimmers did that to help them stay relaxed.

"You're the best, Willie! You're going to win." Shelly had to yell so that Willie would hear her. The crowd around them was cheering the swimmers.

Willie thought to himself, "I'm not so sure." He shook his shoulders and legs again.

"You can do it!" Shelly screamed. "You're faster than anyone. We're all behind you." She wasn't sure whether Willie heard her.

Willie had heard, and he thought, "That's the problem! The whole school is watching! My parents, too! If I don't

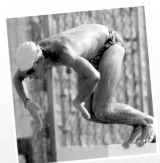

get at least second place, our team might not go on to the Regionals. The way my stomach feels, these people are more likely to see me throw up than win the 200."

Willie knew it was just stress. He had felt the same way at the last meet. Shelly had told him she felt the same kind of stress during a debate last week. The debate coach had shown her how to slow down her breathing to help her relax, and she had shown Willie.

Shelly stood up and took a deep breath. Willie saw her and did the same thing, and then he grinned to let her know he felt better. Willie was ready.

For Discussion

How were Willie's muscles affected by the stress he felt? What were his other symptoms? How was Willie's stress similar to the stress Shelly felt before her debate? Fill out the questionnaire provided by your teacher to find out how competitive stress affects you. Consider the guidelines on page 299.

Stress Management, Fitness, and Good Health

Keeping your body physically fit and in good health can help you manage stress. Follow these health practices to help you deal with stress in your life:

▶ **Eat a nutritious, well-balanced diet.** Good nutrition helps lead to good health, which can help you deal better with stress. Chapter 14 discusses the importance of good nutrition.

▶ **Avoid unnecessary, distressful situations.** If you know a situation will be stressful, you often can avoid it. For example, you can choose to avoid an event at which alcohol might be served.

▶ **Get enough sleep.** Lack of sleep can contribute to distress. In fact, lack of sleep is itself a stressor. Some problems might be easier to handle when you feel rested. Try to sleep at least 8 hours each day.

▶ **Pay attention to your body.** Pay attention to how your body reacts in different situations. If you experience physical signs of distress, use some of the stress-management techniques described in this lesson.

▶ **Have fun.** Laughter can help reduce distress. Take time to laugh and have fun. Enjoy life!

▶ **Do regular physical activity.** Doing some form of regular physical activity can help you reduce your

stress. For example, people who jog regularly report a **runner's high** that comes from their activity. As you learned in lesson 17.1, sometimes competitive activities can cause stress. Taking time out in the form of a noncompetitive activity can help you get your mind off stressful situations.

 www.fitnessforlife.org/student/17/4

Getting Help

Often people need help in managing their stress. Parents, family members, teachers, clergy members, and friends can be sources of help and support. School counselors, school nurses, physicians, and other specially trained people can provide advice about stress management. In addition, many communities have health professionals to help people manage stress. A doctor, a school counselor, or a hospital referral service can direct you to sources of help in your community.

Lesson Review

1. What are five ways to deal with a stressful situation?
2. What are some health practices that can help you deal with stress in your life?
3. What are some of the techniques you can use to cope with competitive stress?

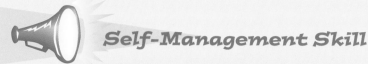

Self-Management Skill

Controlling Competitive Stress

In the next lesson, you will learn that doing regular, noncompetitive physical activity can help you reduce stress levels. However, competitive sports and other competitive activities, such as performing a music solo or giving a speech, can cause **competitive stress.** Some factors that make these activities stressful are competition, being evaluated by others, performing in front of a crowd, and feeling that the outcome is important. If you get involved in situations that cause competitive stress, follow these guidelines:

▶ **Learn to identify signs of stress.** Use the self-assessment in this chapter to help you learn to identify the signs of stress.

▶ **Avoiding competitive stress.** One way to prevent competitive stress is to avoid competitive situations or situations in which you perform for others. However, as a result, you may miss participating in activities that are fun. You also may fail to accomplish things that you are capable of doing and at which you would be successful.

▶ **Use muscle relaxation techniques.** Use the muscle relaxation techniques included in the activity for this chapter (pages 300-302).

▶ **Get experience.** Remember that most people feel stressed the first few times they compete or perform in public. With experience, competing and performing do become easier.

▶ **Practice and prepare.** Practice and preparation will help you experience eustress when competing and performing and will help you to achieve your full potential. When you practice, try to simulate the real event. Competitive practices with an audience can help you prepare.

▶ **Use mental imagery.** Some people do well in practice but not in actual competition. One method used by experienced competitors is mental imagery. During the real event, they imagine themselves as they are in practice—relaxed and confident.

▶ **Use a routine.** Golfers find that a regular routine when putting is very helpful. If you follow a routine before and during a competitive event, it can help you relax.

▶ **Take a deep breath and slow your breathing.** Taking a deep breath before a free shot or before a solo can be helpful. If you find yourself becoming tense, slow down your breathing—it can help.

▶ **Use other effective stress management procedures.** Use the effective ways of managing stress discussed earlier in this lesson.

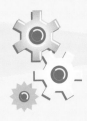

Activity 2

Relaxation Exercises for Stress Management

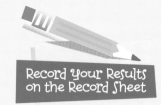

Record your Results on the Record Sheet

Did your self-assessment indicate that you have a high level of stress?
Most people need to deal with stress at one time or another. In this activity, you will get the opportunity to perform several exercises that are useful in reducing stress. You will also get the opportunity to practice a muscle relaxation procedure called contract-relax.

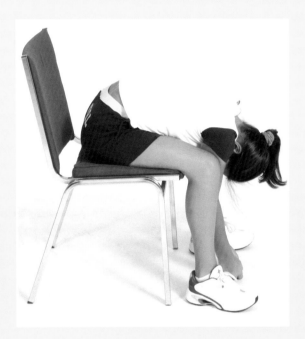

PART 1: Exercises for Muscle Relaxation

Notice that you can do some of these exercises at almost any time and almost any place. You might do them when you are sitting and studying or while you are riding or waiting for a bus. You can do most of them lying down or from a sitting position. You can even adapt some of these exercises to do them while you are standing. When you do these exercises, be sure to write your results on your record sheet.

Rag Doll

1. Sit in a chair (or stand) with your feet apart. Stretch your arms and trunk upward as you inhale.
2. Then exhale and drop your body forward. Let your trunk, head, and arms dangle between your legs. Keep your neck and trunk muscles relaxed. Remain relaxed like a rag doll for 10 to 15 seconds.
3. Slowly roll up, one vertebrae at a time. Repeat the stretch and drop.

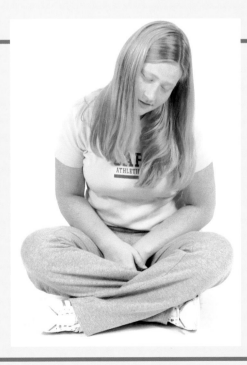

Neck Roll

1. Sit in a chair (or on the floor with your legs crossed).
2. Keeping your head and chin tucked, inhale as you slowly rotate your head to the left as far as possible. Exhale and slowly return your head to the center.
3. Repeat the movement to the right.
4. Rotate 3 times in each direction, trying to rotate farther each time, so you feel a stretch in the neck.
5. Now, drop your chin to your chest and inhale as you slowly roll your head in a half circle to the left shoulder and then exhale as you roll it back to the center. Repeat the movement to the right shoulder.

 Caution: Do not roll your head backward or in a full circle.

Body Board

1. Lie on your right side. Hold your arms over your head.
2. Inhale and stiffen your body as if you were a wooden board. Then exhale as you relax your muscles and collapse completely.
3. Let your body fall without trying to control whether it tips forward or backward.
4. Lie still as you continue letting the tension go out of your muscles for 10 seconds. Then repeat the exercise starting on your left side.

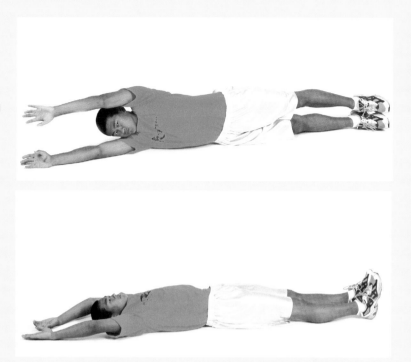

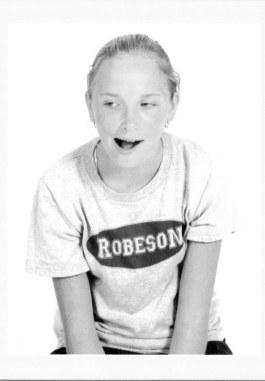

Jaw Stretch

1. Sit in a chair (or on the floor), head erect, arms and shoulders relaxed.
2. Open your mouth as wide as possible and inhale. (This may make you yawn.) Relax and exhale slowly.
3. Open your mouth and shift your jaw to the right as far as possible; hold 3 counts.
4. Repeat the movement to the left. Repeat it on both sides 10 times.

PART 2: The Contract-Relax Method of Muscle Relaxation

Lie on your back with a rolled-up towel placed under your knees. Contract your muscles in the order that they are named in the following instructions. Hold each contraction for 3 counts. Then relax the muscles and keep relaxing for 10 counts. Each time you contract, inhale. Each time you relax, exhale.

Do each exercise twice. Try this routine at home for a few weeks. With practice, you should eventually progress to a combination of muscle groups and gradually eliminate the contracting phase of the program.

1. Hand and forearm—Contract your right hand, making a fist. Relax and continue relaxing. Repeat the exercise with your left hand. Repeat it with both hands simultaneously.

2. Biceps—Bend both elbows and contract the muscles on the front of your upper arms. Relax and continue relaxing. Repeat the exercise.

3. Triceps—Bend both elbows, keeping your palms up. Straighten both elbows and contract the muscles on the back of the arm by pushing the back of your hand into the floor. Relax.

4. Hands, forearms, and upper arms—Concentrate on relaxing these body parts all together.

5. Forehead—Make a frown and wrinkle your forehead. Relax and continue relaxing. Repeat the exercise.

6. Jaws—Clench your teeth. Relax. Repeat the exercise.

7. Lips and tongue—With your teeth apart, press your lips together and press your tongue to the roof of your mouth. Relax. Repeat the exercise.

8. Neck and throat—Push your head backward while tucking your chin. Relax. Repeat the exercise.

9. Relax your forehead, jaws, lips, tongue, neck, and throat. Relax your hands, forearms, and upper arms. Keep relaxing all of these muscles.

10. Shoulders and upper back—Hunch your shoulders to your ears. Relax. Repeat the exercise.

11. Relax your lips, tongue, neck, throat, shoulders, and upper back. Keep relaxing these muscles all together.

12. Abdomen—Suck in your abdomen, flattening your lower back to the floor. Relax. Repeat the exercise.

13. Lower back—Contract and arch your lower back. Relax. Repeat the exercise.

14. Thighs and buttocks—Squeeze your buttocks together and push your heels into the floor. Relax. Repeat the exercise.

15. Relax your shoulders and upper back, abdomen, lower back, thighs, and buttocks. Keep relaxing these muscles all together.

16. Shins—Pull your toes toward your shins. Relax. Repeat the exercise.

17. Toes—Curl your toes. Relax. Repeat the exercise.

18. Relax every muscle in your body all together and keep relaxing.

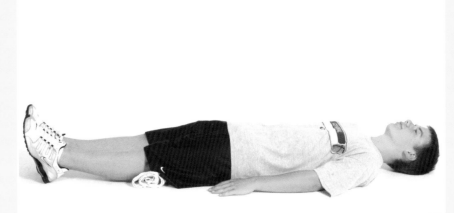

17 Chapter Review

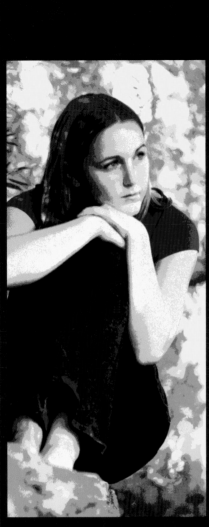

Reviewing Concepts and Vocabulary

Number your paper from 1 to 6. Next to each number, write the word (or words) that correctly completes the sentence.

1. To help reduce stress, contract and then _____ your muscles.
2. Excessive exercise, such as that done by athletes who overtrain, is a _____ stressor.
3. The _____ is your body's way of preparing you to deal with a demanding situation.
4. Worry and fear are examples of _____ stressors.
5. Stress can affect the immune system, making a person more susceptible to certain _____.
6. Getting enough _____ every night can help prevent fatigue and help you deal effectively with stress.

Number your paper from 7 to 10. Next to each number, choose the letter of the best answer.

Column I	Column II
7. stress	a. positive stress
8. eustress	b. negative stress
9. stressor	c. the body's reaction to a stressful situation
10. distress	d. causes or contributes to stress

Number your paper from 11 to 15. On your paper, write a short answer for each statement or question.

11. Describe some negative effects of competitive stress and explain how to deal with such stress in a positive manner.
12. Describe some ways of thinking that can help you deal with stress.
13. How can physical activity help you deal effectively with stress?
14. How can an activity cause both eustress and distress?
15. Name five sources of guidance and support for those who need help dealing with a stressful situation.

Thinking Critically

Write a paragraph to answer the following questions.

You have been invited to give a speech in front of your class. You are concerned that if you refuse the opportunity, you may feel disappointed in yourself. However, you are afraid that you will be too nervous to give a speech in front of a large group. What are the positive and negative consequences of each choice? What decisions would you make? How can you manage stress associated with whichever decision you make?

Project

Researchers have identified two general types of personalities—type A and type B. Research the traits of these personalities and how each personality type generally responds to stress.

18

Personal Program Planning

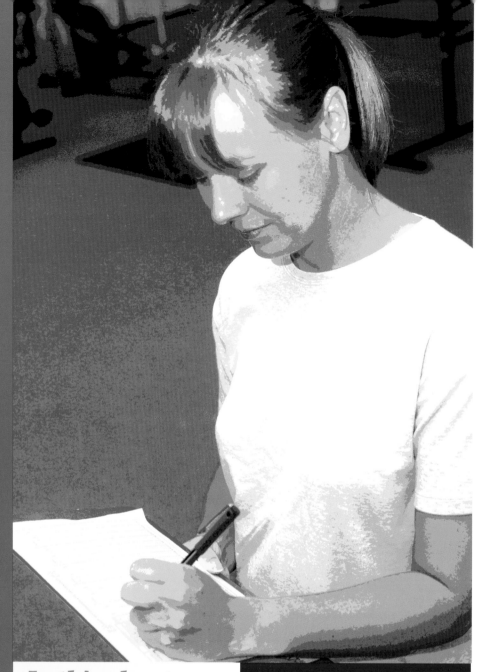

In this chapter...

Activity 1
Exercising at Home

Lesson 18.1
Program Planning

Self-Assessment
Evaluating Your Personal Program

Lesson 18.2
Staying Fit and Active

Taking Charge
Overcoming Barriers

Self-Management Skill
Overcoming Barriers

Activity 2
Performing Your Plan

Activity 1

EXERCISING AT HOME

In previous lessons you learned about many different ways to exercise to build various parts of health-related physical fitness. Many of these activities require special equipment. You can find some equipment at school, at the YMCA or YWCA, or at fitness clubs, or you can buy the equipment for use at home. But not everyone can afford to join a fitness club or to buy all the equipment they want. You can substitute common household items for more expensive exercise equipment at home. Your instruction sheet will show you how to use these household items in a variety of exercises.

Lesson 18.1

Program Planning

Lesson Objectives

After reading this lesson, you should be able to

1. Explain how to use a fitness profile to plan a personal fitness program.
2. Describe the five steps in planning a personal fitness program.

Lesson Vocabulary

fitness profile (p. 305)

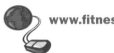 **www.fitnessforlife.org/student/18/1**

In the preceding chapters, you learned about the many activities that can be used as part of a personal activity program and about which of these types of activities is most appropriate for building each part of health-related physical fitness. In the first part of this chapter, you will have the opportunity to use this information as you go through the five steps in planning your personal physical activity program. You will notice that many of the steps in critical thinking are used in program planning. Your teacher will provide you with worksheets to help you plan.

Step 1: Collect Information

Collecting information is the first step toward making good decisions and preparing a good personal program plan. Construct a fitness profile and an activity profile to help you determine your needs and interests.

Part 1: Construct a Fitness Profile

A **fitness profile** is a brief summary of the results of your fitness self-assessments (see table 18.1). A health-related fitness profile is useful in program planning because it helps you determine the areas in which you need improvement.

To build a health-related physical fitness profile, you summarize all of your self-assessment results. A sample for Jordan, a 15-year-old, follows on page 306. You can then use the guidelines provided to determine one rating for cardiovascular fitness and body fatness. For strength, muscular endurance, and flexibility, you will determine both an upper body and a lower body rating. Write your ratings in the fitness profile on the worksheet provided by your teacher. A sample fitness profile for Jordan is shown on page 306. When preparing your fitness profile, follow these guidelines:

▶ If the ratings are different for different assessments of any fitness part, choose the rating you think is most representative of your fitness.

▶ Be sure to consider your reassessment results as well as all other self-assessment results.

▶ Use the worksheet provided by your teacher to prepare your profile or use *FITNESSGRAM* (see Web site below).

 www.fitnessforlife.org/student/18/2

Part 2: Construct a Physical Activity Profile

You can use the Physical Activity Pyramid to assess your current physical activity levels. You can determine a rating for each of the types of activity from levels 1, 2, and 3 of the pyramid. A sample of Jordan's physical activity profile is shown below. You can prepare your own profile using a similar worksheet provided by your teacher or use *ACTIVITYGRAM* (see Web site above). The four questions are the same ones used to determine the fitness of teens nationwide. Only one question exists for level 2 of the pyramid.

Table 18.1

Jordan's Fitness Profile

Rating	Cardiovascular fitness	Body composition	Muscular endurance	Strength		Flexibility
				Upper	Lower	
High performance						
Good fitness	X	X	X	X		
Marginal fitness					X	X
Low fitness						

FITNESS ASSESSMENT			FITNESS ASSESSMENT		
Cardiovascular fitness		**Rating**	**Muscular endurance**		**Rating**
PACER		Good	Curl-up		Good
Step test		Good	Push-up		High Perf
Walking test		Good	Side stand		Pass
One-mile run		Marginal	Sitting tuck		Pass
Body composition		**Rating**	Trunk extension		Pass
Body mass index		Good	Leg change		Pass
Skinfold measures		Good	Bent arm hang		Pass
Body measures (% fat)		Good			
Height/Weight		Good			
Flexibility		**Rating**	**Strength**		**Rating**
Back-saver sit and reach		Low	Arm press 1RM		Good
Trunk lift		Marginal	Leg press 1RM		Marginal
Arm lift		Pass	Arm press (per/lb/wt)		Good
Zipper		Fail	Leg press (per/lb/wt)		Marginal
Trunk rotation		Fail	Grip strength (right)		Good
Wrap around		Pass	Grip strength (left)		Good
Knee to chest		Fail			
Ankle flex		Pass			

Summary of Jordan's health-related physical fitness self-assessments.

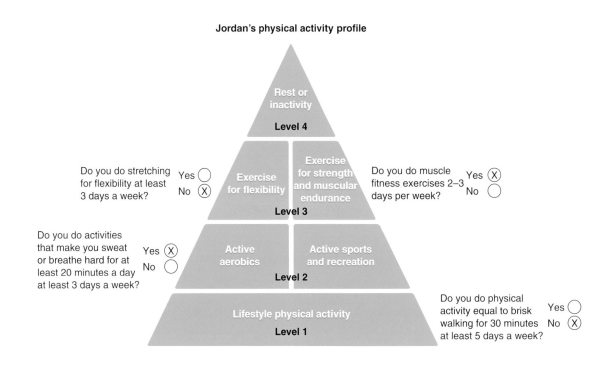

Jordan's physical activity profile

Rest or inactivity — Level 4

Exercise for flexibility / **Exercise for strength and muscular endurance** — Level 3

Do you do stretching for flexibility at least 3 days a week? Yes ◯ No (X)

Do you do muscle fitness exercises 2–3 days per week? Yes (X) No ◯

Active aerobics / **Active sports and recreation** — Level 2

Do you do activities that make you sweat or breathe hard for at least 20 minutes a day at least 3 days a week? Yes (X) No ◯

Lifestyle physical activity — Level 1

Do you do physical activity equal to brisk walking for 30 minutes at least 5 days a week? Yes ◯ No (X)

Step 2: Consider a Variety of Activities

When you plan your program you can choose from the many activities in the Physical Activity Pyramid. Consider the lifestyle activities described in chapter 6, the active aerobic and active recreational activities described in chapter 8, the active sports described in chapter 9, the flexibility exercises in chapter 10, and the muscle fitness exercises in chapter 11. Table 9.5 (page 143) will help you determine the health-related fitness benefits you will get with each activity, and table 9.2 (page 135) will help you determine the skill-related fitness benefits of different activities. Use the worksheet provided by your teacher to help you determine which activities you might want to list for your activity goals.

Jordan checked several activities on her worksheet. Volleyball and muscular endurance are activities that she is already doing. Walking, jogging, flexibility exercises, and strength exercises are new activities.

Step 3: Set Goals

Setting goals can help you build a fitness and physical activity program that will meet your personal needs. First, consider the reasons for doing your program. Are you primarily interested in fitness and physical activity for health and wellness, or are you interested in building a higher level of fitness necessary for playing a sport? Jordan is interested in health but also wants to try out for the volleyball team.

Next, consider your fitness and activity profiles. If you are low in one part of physical fitness, you may want to work on it. If you say "no" to any of the physical activity questions, you may want to do more physical activity of that type. Jordan was low in flexibility and leg strength and is not active enough to say "yes" to the lifestyle and flexibility exercise questions.

In addition to considering your reasons and your fitness and activity profiles, you should also consider the guidelines presented in chapter 5. Some of those guidelines are repeated here to help you in setting your personal goals.

▶ **Set goals for new activities established in step 2.** When setting your goals, follow these guidelines:

1. **Be realistic.** Set goals you know you can attain. People who set goals that are too hard doom themselves to failure before they begin.

2. **Be specific.** Vague or very general goals are hard to accomplish.

3. **Personalize.** A goal that is realistic for one person may be unrealistic for another. Base your goals on your own individual needs and abilities.

▶ **If you are a beginner, focus on short-term activity goals rather than fitness goals.** This approach is realistic for someone just beginning a physical activity routine, and it can help you to be successful and avoid injury.

▶ **If you are an intermediate or advanced exerciser, you can use both fitness and physical activity goals.** Consider setting short- and long-term goals for both fitness and physical activity.

You can see on page 308 that Jordan chose activities and fitness goals designed to improve weaknesses. Flexibility exercises were included to improve flexibility, and brisk walking was included because Jordan was not doing regular lifestyle physical activity. Jogging was added to improve the one-mile run score, and strength exercises were added to improve leg strength because Jordan felt that they would be helpful in performing better in volleyball. Jordan will continue to do current activities such as muscular endurance exercises and playing recreational volleyball after school. Use the worksheet provided by your teacher to prepare you program goals.

Step 4: Structure Your Program Plan and Write it Down

Use the information from steps 1, 2, and 3 to structure your program. When you established your goals, you decided how many days a week to do each type of physical activity. Now you need to decide which days you will exercise. Pick the days of the week that make exercise easiest and most convenient. Remember that exercise for some parts of fitness, such as strength, should not be done every day. Some people rotate the parts of fitness they work on each day. Review the FIT formula charts in this book before you decide on which days to exercise.

The best time of day for you to exercise is when you most enjoy exercising—a time when you are not likely to be interrupted. Keep in mind that you might complete different activities at different times.

Now you are ready to write your program. Use the worksheet provided by your teacher to prepare your written plan. List your warm-up exercises. Chapter 1 includes information about a warm-up, and chapter 10 includes stretching exercises that you might consider. Include exercises that stretch the muscles you will use while exercising. You might plan more than one warm-up to vary your program.

SHORT-TERM GOALS		
Physical activity	**Days per week**	**Weeks (up to 4)**
1. Brisk walking	5	4
2. Perform the stretching exercises on pages 167-172	3	4
3. Perform jogging	3	4
4.		
Physical fitness (not for beginners)	**Number or score**	**Completion date**
1.		
2.		
3.		
4.		
5.		
LONG-TERM GOALS		
Physical activity	**Days per week**	**Weeks (4 or more)**
1. Perform strength exercises on pages 193-198	2	8
2. Continue current muscular endurance exercises	3	8
3. Continue current active sports: volleyball	5	8
4.		
Physical fitness (not for beginners)	**Number or score**	**Completion date**
1. Improve sit and reach score	10 inches	November 15
2. Improve leg press score	1.75 lbs per lb of body weight	November 15
3. Improve mile run score	7:45 minutes	November 15
4.		
5.		

Jordan's fitness and physical activity goals.

Now list the activities you will do in each workout session. If you plan special exercises, include them in your workout. If you play sports, include practice as part of your program. Next, list your cool-down exercises. Remember to include stretching exercises for muscle cool-down and a cardiovascular cool-down.

Look at Jordan's program. It includes all of the activities listed as goals in step 3. Jordan decided to add a bicycle ride on Sunday because she enjoys biking and it provides some variety on a day that normally is an inactive one.

FITNESS Technology

A personal digital assistant (PDA) is a miniature computer. PDAs use special computer software for a variety of purposes, such as storing phone numbers and addresses, keeping personal schedules, and storing messages. Some companies have now developed physical activity program planning and self-monitoring software for the PDA. For example, you could record your self-assessment results and your program schedule and keep track of the times and dates you perform physical activity. PDAs are quite expensive and therefore may not be practical at the present time, but the cost is coming down, so they may be available to more people in the future.

Weekly Exercise Plan for <u>Oct</u> <u>20</u> **to** <u>Oct</u> <u>27</u>

Month Day   Month Day

Day	Activity	Time of Day	How Long?	
M O N	Warm up	7:30 a.m.	5	min
	Jogging	7:35 a.m.	20	min
	Special exercises for flexibility	8:00 a.m.	10	min
	Cool down	8:15 a.m.	5	min
	Warm up	3:30 p.m.	5	min
	Flexibility and muscular endurance exercises	3:35 p.m.	30	min
	Jogging	4:05 p.m.	20	min
	Cool down	4:25 p.m.	5	min
T U E	Warm up	7:30 a.m.	5	min
	Strength exercises	7:35 a.m.	30	min
	Cool down	8:05 a.m.	5	min
	Warm up	3:25 p.m.	5	min
	Volleyball club	3:30 p.m.	60	min
	Cool down	4:30 p.m.	5	min
W E D	Warm up	7:30 a.m.	5	min
	Jogging	7:35 a.m.	20	min
	Special exercises for flexibility	8:00 a.m.	10	min
	Cool down	8:15 a.m.	5	min
	Warm up	3:30 p.m.	5	min
	Flexibility and muscular endurance exercises	3:35 p.m.	30	min
	Jogging	4:05 p.m.	20	min
	Cool down	4:25 p.m.	5	min
T H U	Warm up	7:30 a.m.	5	min
	Strength exercises	7:35 a.m.	30	min
	Cool down	8:05 a.m.	5	min
	Warm up	3:25 p.m.	5	min
	Volleyball club	3:30 p.m.	60	min
	Cool down	4:30 p.m.	5	min
F R I	Warm up	7:30 a.m.	5	min
	Jogging	7:35 a.m.	20	min
	Special exercises for flexibility	8:00 a.m.	10	min
	Cool down	8:15 a.m.	5	min
	Warm up	3:30 p.m.	5	min
	Flexibility and muscular endurance exercises	3:35 p.m.	30	min
	Jogging	4:05 p.m.	20	min
	Cool down	4:25 p.m.	5	min
S A T	Warm up	10:00 a.m.	5	min
	Volleyball club	10:05 a.m.	60	min
	Cool down	11:00 a.m.	5	min
S U N	Bicycle ride	2:00 p.m.	60	min

Step 5: Evaluate Your Program After You Have Tried It

After you have tried your program for some time (depending on your goals), evaluate it. Go through the first five steps to revise your program. You can use worksheets similar to those you used in preparing your original plan to prepare your revised plan.

Lesson Review

1. How do you build a fitness and physical activity profile?
2. What are the five steps in planning a personal fitness program? Describe each step.

Self-Assessment

Evaluating Your Personal Program

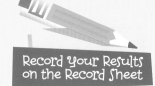
Record Your Results on the Record Sheet

In lesson 1 of this chapter, you prepared a personal physical activity plan. Select one day from your plan and perform as many of the activities as possible in class. Be sure to choose a day from your plan that has enough activities to fill a full class period. If no single day's activities last as long as one class period, supplement your program with activities from another day. If equipment is not available for the activity of your choice, select an activity that is similar in its benefits and one that you are likely to enjoy. Remember to warm up, then do your personal workout, and finish with a cool-down.

Perform other activities in your plan (those that you did not complete in class) at appropriate times of the day. On the following day, use the worksheet provided by your teacher to evaluate your plan. List the activities in your plan that you were able to complete and indicate those that you were not able to complete. If you were not able to perform some of the activities in your plan, indicate the reasons (e.g., bad weather or homework). Write a paragraph evaluating your program. Answer these questions:

1. Do you think your daily plan is one you could regularly complete?
2. Do you think you might need to make some changes in your program?
3. What changes would you make in your program and why?

It is difficult to evaluate a program after only one day, so you will need to repeat this activity after you have been performing your program for several weeks. At that time, you can evaluate the effectiveness of all days of the program using the procedures described in this self-assessment.

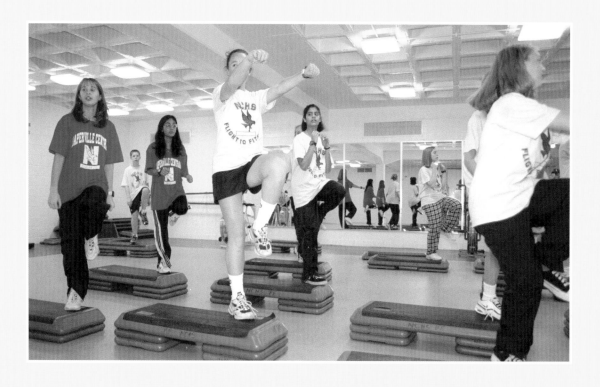

18.2

Staying Fit and Active

Lesson Objectives

After reading this lesson, you should be able to

1. Describe the five stages of physical activity.
2. Identify the strategies that help people become active and stay active at each of the stages.

Lesson Vocabulary

couch potato (p. 311), sedentary (p. 311)

 www.fitnessforlife.org/student/18/3

Think about the people you know, both young and old. Some of them are probably very active, some less active, and others not active at all. In this lesson you will learn about the activity levels of different groups of people and how to develop some characteristics that help people to stay active throughout life. You may want to use the information in this lesson to help yourself or to help a friend or family member.

Stages of Physical Activity

In chapter 5 you learned that all people are not equally active, and you learned about the five stages of physical activity. These stages are illustrated again in table 18.2. We know several things about the different stages of physical activity. People move up and down from one stage to another. For example, we know that people who were athletes in school do not necessarily

stay active throughout life. Each could even become a **couch potato**. Some people who were inactive as children become active later in life. We also know that the strategies that are useful for people at one stage are not equally useful for those at other stages.

 www.fitnessforlife.org/student/18/4

Stage 1: Couch Potato

People who do no regular physical activity from any of the first three levels of the Physical Activity Pyramid are considered to be **sedentary.** As the top level of the pyramid indicates, total inactivity or sedentary living should be avoided because it increases risk of disease. People who are sedentary are difficult to change because they are not even considering being active. However, there are some things that you can do to help them get moving. They are outlined in table 18.3.

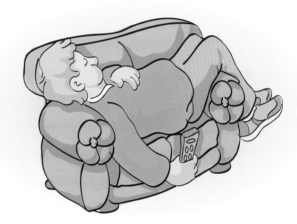

Using many of the other self-management skills described in this book can be useful in getting a couch potato going, but the three strategies in table 18.3 are often most useful.

Stage 2: Thinking About It

People who are thinking about becoming active have started thinking for a reason. Like couch potatoes, they

Table 18.2

Five Stages of Physical Activity

Stage	Stage of physical activity	Description
5	Active for life	This person is active on a regular basis. He or she can overcome obstacles that may discourage others.
4	Sometimes active	This person is active but participates inconsistently.
3	Planning to be active	This person has taken steps to get ready to be active, such as buying clothing or equipment for activity.
2	Thinking about it	This person is not active but is thinking about becoming active.
1	Couch potato	This person does no regular activity.

benefit from knowledge, beliefs, and positive attitudes. They probably have gained some knowledge and believe that becoming active will help them in some way. They may also have eliminated some of their negative attitudes and developed some positive ones. Some strategies are especially useful for people at stage 2, and they are outlined in table 18.4.

Stage 3: Planning to Be Active

People at the planning stage have taken some action. They may have made a New Year's resolution, or they may have purchased some exercise equipment or exercise clothing. They may actually have started doing some activity, but it is probably quite irregular. People

at this level can benefit from the same strategies as those for stages 1 and 2, but they are especially likely to benefit from the planning strategies outlined in the previous lesson. Other effective strategies for people at this level are listed in table 18.5.

Stage 4: Sometimes Active

People at this stage are active more frequently than those at stage 3. They may be very irregular in their activity patterns. All of the strategies for stage 3 will be useful at this level. Self-monitoring is especially important for sticking with the plan. Other strategies that are important for people at this level are listed in table 18.6.

Table 18.3

Strategies for Couch Potatoes

Knowledge	Providing information about the health benefits of physical activity may get a couch potato going. If you know someone, such as friend or relative, who is inactive, you may want to share what you have learned in this book and in this class, especially the information about risk factors (chapter 3). However, sometimes people will not be interested in knowledge from just anyone. Experts tell us that the leading reason adults start exercising is because their doctor told them to. People who wait until they have to go to the doctor are, unfortunately, already sick. If you have a friend or loved one who is inactive, you may want to encourage that person to get a check-up from a doctor. People who are active when they are young can help stay active by keeping up with the latest facts about fitness and exercise.
Beliefs	Sometimes people are aware of the latest information about physical activity but they do not believe that physical activity is that important. Believing the facts is probably as important as knowing them. A person who has had a heart attack is easier to convince than a person who seems well even if physically inactive. Sometimes people start to believe if they get encouragement from friends and loved ones as well as a doctor.
Attitudes	In chapter 6 you learned about some of the positive and negative attitudes people have about physical activity. You know you must have more positive attitudes than negative ones. You may want to review the information in lesson 2 of chapter 6 to remind you of the different types of attitudes.

Table 18.4

Strategies for Those Thinking About Starting a Physical Activity Program

Enjoyment	Some people who are not active do not enjoy activity because they have had negative experiences in the past. Finding an activity that is fun is very important. Some strategies that can be used to enhance enjoyment include trying activities that are new to you, finding friends with similar abilities, and choosing activities that are not competitive (see chapter 4).
Learning skills	An activity is much more likely to be enjoyable if you develop the skills needed for it. Consider taking lessons and consider the guidelines in chapter 9.
Self-perceptions and self-confidence	People who have good self-perceptions are happy with who they are; they like themselves. Review some of the strategies in chapter 13. They can be helpful for you or any person who is thinking about becoming active. Poor self-perceptions discourage participation. Good self-perceptions encourage participation. Self-confidence is also important. You most likely are familiar with the children's story, "The Little Engine That Could." The story's message—if you think you can, you often can—applies to becoming fit and active, especially if you do not set standards that are too high for success. Self-confidence is a very important characteristic in becoming and staying active (see chapter 2). People who think they are able to do activities usually are active. People who think they cannot, are not.

Table 18.5

Strategies for Those Planning to Become Active

Self-assessment	People at the previous two stages may not be interested in self-assessments. Those at the planning level will be ready to do self-assessments to help them set goals and plan programs.
Goal setting	People at this level can greatly benefit from setting realistic goals. Use the steps outlined in the previous lesson and in chapter 5.
Program planning	Planning a specific written personal plan is especially effective for people at this level. Follow the steps in the previous lesson.
Self-monitoring	Keeping logs to reinforce progress is very important for people at this stage and stage 4. See chapter 7 for more information.
Finding success	People at stages 1 and 2 have not done any activity. They have experienced neither success nor failure. At this level, people are trying to be active, so finding success is critical. Strategies for finding success are discussed in chapter 16.

Table 18.6

Strategies for Those Who Are Sometimes Active

Overcoming barriers	Many barriers can stop you from getting and staying active. People who are sometimes active especially need to learn how to overcome barriers. Some strategies are described later in this chapter.
Time management	The number one reason people do not exercise is because of lack of time. People at stage 5 have learned to find the time for regular activity. Following the guidelines for managing time (see chapter 12) can be especially useful to sometimes exercisers.
Social support and preventing relapse	People at all stages of activity benefit from the support of friends, relatives, teachers, and medical doctors. People at this stage get special benefits because they are starting to become active and the risk of relapse is high. Guidelines for social support and preventing relapse can be found in chapters 8 and 11. Saying "no" to those who would discourage your efforts to be active is also important for people at this level (see chapter 14).

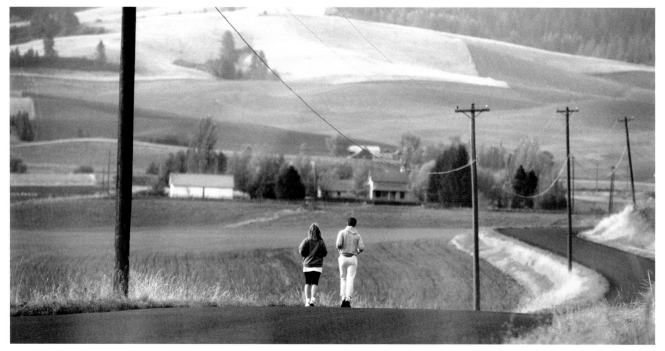

Overcoming barriers seems like taking on a long road, but the road gets easier as you continue.

Taking Charge: Overcoming Barriers

When some people face a problem beyond their control, they use it as an excuse for not being physically active. Someone might say, "I'm too short to be a basketball player, so I'm not going to try out for any sports." To be physically active, focus on what you can do—not what you can't change.

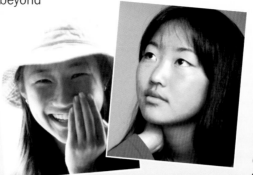

Juana stood at the window, shaking her head. "It's pouring out there! How can we go hiking today?"

Monica sighed. "I guess we're stuck spending the afternoon here, playing cards or something."

Yesterday it was too hot to go hiking; now it was too rainy. It seemed as if they were never going to have good weather. But the weather was not the only problem. The last time they tried hiking at the state park, it was sunny, but the paths were too crowded.

"I bet Miguel is at the athletic club right now," Monica said. "He can exercise no matter what the weather is. I wish we could afford memberships there!"

Juana glanced down at her sweats. "I'd need to buy more than a membership before I could go there. They wear really expensive exercise clothes at that club. I'd get laughed out of the place in these clothes."

Monica smiled. "You don't look so bad—and the rain's starting to let up now. What if we put on even older clothes, take along some rain gear, and hike around the park for a while?"

"You're right! So what if we get a little damp?"

For Discussion

What reasons do Juana and Monica give for not being active? Which of these problems can they control? They've decided not to let the weather stop them today. What other ways could they cope with the problems they've identified? Fill out the questionnaire provided by your teacher to see how well you can distinguish between controllable and noncontrollable factors. Consider the guidelines on page 315.

Stage 5: Active for Life

People who are active for life are very regular with their exercise. They can benefit from all of the strategies described for the previous four stages. They are less likely to need formal exercise plans. Many do use regular self-assessments to evaluate progress and keep activity logs. People at this stage have developed positive self-perceptions and self-confidence and have good performance skills in the activities that they perform regularly. They typically have social support, know how to find the time for exercise, and have developed self-motivation (see chapter 10).

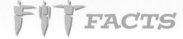

According to a report by the Surgeon General, approximately 200,000 lives could be saved each year if adults would be more physically active.

Lesson Review

1. What are the five stages of physical activity?
2. What are the strategies that help people become active and stay active at each of the stages?

Self-Management Skill

Overcoming Barriers

People face many barriers to becoming and staying active. Some are related to the environment (unsafe areas for exercise, long distance to exercise locations, bad weather, too expensive), some to personal physical characteristics (lack of physical size or skill), and some are psychological (low self-confidence, lack of time). People who are active throughout life are able to overcome barriers. Entire programs have been developed to help people overcome barriers. Follow these strategies to overcome barriers:

▶ **Find a way to exercise at home or at work.** If parks, fitness clubs, and other places for exercise are too expensive, too far away, or unsafe, find a way to exercise at home or at work. Buy some equipment that you can use at home or at work. See whether you can get the support of others at work to develop an exercise facility with equipment. If possible, exercise before or after school using school facilities. Develop a fitness club at school and ask school officials to help you find the facilities necessary for your workouts.

▶ **Develop alternate activity plans.** Consider developing multiple plans for activity. If you plan to play tennis and it rains, you can switch to your alternate plan. Your alternate plan could include performing an indoor activity. If you plan to exercise at a certain time but a meeting interferes, find an alternate time.

▶ **Get active in community or school affairs.** Many communities have developed community centers; bike, walking, and jogging trails; and other recreational facilities such as tennis courts, basketball courts, and sport fields. If these options are not available in your community, write to your city or county officials or contact school officials.

▶ **Use self-management skills to help you develop realistic plans that you will stay with for the long-haul.** Skills such as goal setting, program planning, self-monitoring, and time management can help you create a realistic plan and stick with it.

▶ **Develop a new way of thinking.** The new way of thinking involves accepting yourself as you are. Use the strategies in this book to boost your self-perceptions and self-confidence. Avoid negative self-talk.

Resolving Conflict: Sticking With a Plan

Sometimes conflict can be a barrier to participation or the reason a person does not stick to a physical activity plan. Monica and Juana (see page 314) developed a plan to walk to school five days a week for one month. Unfortunately, their friend Miguel kept offering them a ride to school. He told Monica and Juana that rejecting his offer was not very friendly. Monica and Juana wanted to please their friend, but they also wanted to stick to their plan.

Monica and Juana used their critical-thinking skills to resolve the conflict. They recognized that they did not need to exercise less or lose a friend. Instead, they modified their physical activity plan. They set a new goal of walking to school three days a week and riding with their friend two days a week. They added a 15-minute jog two days a week to make up for the missed days of walking. Juana and Monica explained their goals to Miguel and told him that it was important for them to stick to their plan. You can use the self-management skill for overcoming barriers (see previous section), for critical thinking (page 271), and for preventing relapse (page 191) to help you stick with your physical activity plan. The negotiating steps for resolving conflict on page 147 may also be useful.

315

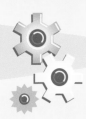

Activity 2

Performing Your Plan

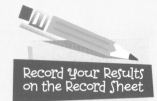

In the self-assessment activity in this chapter, you performed one day of your personal physical activity plan. You also learned how to evaluate your plan. In this activity, you may perform the same activity plan with any modifications you made as a result of your program evaluation, or you may choose to perform activities from a different day of your plan. Choose a day from your program that includes enough activities to fill a full class period. Perform the activities in class. If no single day's activities last as long as one class period, supplement your program with activities from another day. If equipment is not available for the activity of your choice, select an activity that is similar in its benefits and one that you are likely to enjoy. Remember to warm up, then do your personal workout, and finish with a cool-down. On the appropriate record sheet, write down those activities you performed in class. When you have had the opportunity to perform the activities from your plan several times, use the evaluation procedures described earlier in this chapter to revise your program.

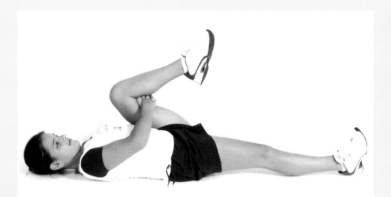

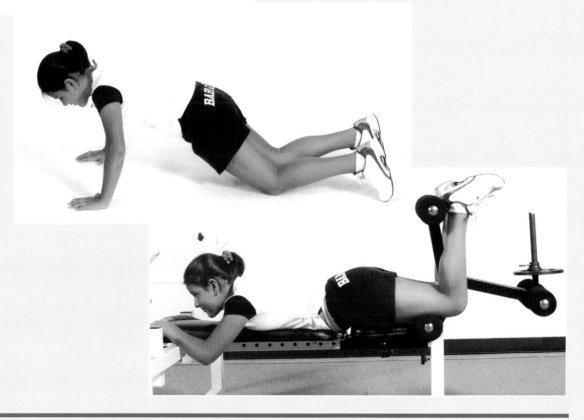

18 Chapter Review

Reviewing Concepts and Vocabulary

Number your paper from 1 to 3. Next to each number, write the word (or words) that correctly completes the sentence.

1. A _____ is a brief summary of your fitness.
2. A person who is sedentary is also called a _____.
3. You are considered to be _____ if you perform physical activity on a regular basis and have for some time.

Number your paper from 4 to 8. Next to each number, choose the letter of the best answer.

Column I	Column II
4. Step 1	**a.** Structure your program plan and write it down.
5. Step 2	**b.** Evaluate your program after you have tried it.
6. Step 3	**c.** Collect information.
7. Step 4	**d.** Set goals.
8. Step 5	**e.** Consider a variety of activities.

Number your paper from 9 to 11. On your paper, write a short answer for each statement or question.

9. Explain why constructing a fitness profile is an important part of collecting information for program planning.
10. Why is it wise to keep a fitness log?
11. Why is it necessary to periodically reevaluate your fitness program?

Thinking Critically

Write a paragraph to answer the following question.

Why is it important to develop your own fitness program and not just use one developed for someone else?

Unit Review on the Web

 www.fitnessforlife.org/student/18/5

Unit VI review materials are available on the Web at the address listed above.

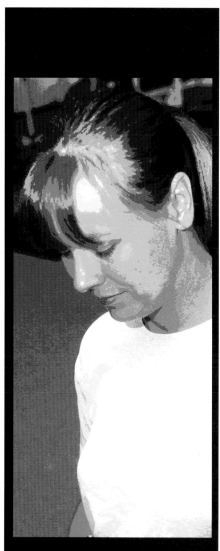

Project

FITNESSGRAM is the national youth fitness test of the American Alliance for Health, Physical Education, Recreation and Dance. It was developed at the Cooper Institute in Dallas, Texas, by an advisory board of experts. Many of the self-assessments you performed in this book are from *FITNESSGRAM*. Build a *FITNESSGRAM* profile by summarizing your results on all of the *FITNESSGRAM* self-assessments using the worksheet provided by your teacher or by entering your results on the *FITNESSGRAM* Web site. (Your school must enroll for you to use this Web site.) If you choose, you can share your fitness profile with your parents or guardians. You may want to encourage them to perform some health-related fitness assessments of their own.

glossary

A

abdominal muscles—The muscles on the front of the body between the chest and the pelvic area.

absolute strength—A term for the total amount of weight you can lift or resistance you can overcome regardless of your body weight.

Achilles tendon—The tendon on the back of the leg that connects the muscles in the calf to the bone of the heel.

active aerobic activity—Aerobic activity done at an intensity that raises the heart rate above the threshold into the target zone; many less intensive activities are aerobic (such as typing, walking, and washing the dishes) but are not considered active aerobics.

active aerobics—Aerobic physical activities (see *aerobics*) that are of enough intensity to cause improvement in cardiovascular fitness.

active recreation—Activities done during your leisure time (free time) that are of enough frequency, intensity, and time to elevate the heart rate into the target zone; examples include backpacking and skiing.

active sports—Sports that elevate the heart rate into the target zone for cardiovascular fitness.

activity neurosis—A condition that occurs when a person is overly concerned about getting enough exercise.

aerobic activity—Steady activity in which the heart can supply all the oxygen the muscles need.

aerobic dance—A combination of dance steps and calisthenics done to music.

aerobics—Physical activities for which the body can supply adequate oxygen to allow performance to continue for long periods of time.

agility—The ability to quickly change the position of the body and to control the body's movements.

AI—An abbreviation for Adequate Intake, a term that refers to the minimum amount of a nutrient a person needs for good health; it is used when there is not enough evidence to provide an RDA.

alarm reaction—The first stage of the general adaptation syndrome; occurs when you are exposed to a stressor.

amino acids—Substances that make up proteins.

anabolic steroids—Strong drugs similar to the male hormone testosterone that can make muscles bulky to enhance athletic performance but that can be extremely dangerous to health.

anaerobic activity—Physical activity done in short, fast bursts in which the heart cannot supply oxygen as fast as muscles use it.

androstenedione—A food supplement that the body converts to a substance similar to anabolic steroids and that can have harmful effects similar to those of anabolic steroids.

anorexia athletica—An eating disorder that has symptoms similar to those of anorexia nervosa in which an athlete severely restricts food intake in an attempt to be exceptionally underfat.

anorexia nervosa—An eating disorder in which a person severely restricts food intake in an attempt to be extremely low in body fat and body weight.

artery—A blood vessel that carries blood from the heart to other parts of the body.

arthritis—A disease in which the joints become inflamed.

atherosclerosis—A disease in which certain substances, including fats, build up on the inside walls of the arteries.

attitude—A person's feelings about something.

B

balance—The ability to keep an upright posture while standing still or moving.

ballistic stretching—A series of quick but gentle bouncing or bobbing motions designed to stretch muscles.

basal metabolism—The amount of energy the body uses just to keep living.

biceps—The large muscle in the front part of the upper arm.

biomechanical principles—Rules related to the study of forces that can help a person move the body efficiently and avoid injury.

blood pressure—The force of blood against the artery walls.

body composition—The makeup of the body tissues, including muscle, bone, body fat, and all other body tissues.

body fatness—The percentage of body weight that is made up of fat.

body mass index (BMI)—A method of assessing body composition.

bulimia—An eating disorder in which a person binge eats, then purges.

318

C

caliper—An instrument used to measure skinfold thickness.

calisthenics—Exercises done using all or part of the body weight as the resistance.

calorie—A heat unit referring to the energy available in food and the energy used by body activities.

cancer—A disease characterized by uncontrollable growth of abnormal cells.

carbohydrate—A nutrient in starches and sugars that provides energy.

cardiac muscle—Heart muscle.

cardiovascular fitness—Ability of the heart, lungs, and blood vessels to function efficiently when a person exercises the body.

cardiovascular system—The body system that includes the heart, blood vessels, and blood, and functions by moving oxygen and nutrients to body cells and removing cell waste.

cholesterol—A fatlike substance found in animal cells and some foods, such as meats, dairy products, and egg yolks.

circuit training—A type of physical activity program in which the person performs a group of exercises in a sequence with brief rests between exercises.

committed time—Time that is dedicated to performing job, school, and other formal daily tasks, including time spent in transit (getting to school, for example).

competitive stress—A stress condition that may be eustressful or distressful and is associated with involvement in a competitive event.

complete proteins—Proteins containing all nine essential amino acids.

complex carbohydrate—A nutrient found in starches such as breads, vegetables, and grains, that provides the body with energy; made of long chains of simple sugars.

con—Someone who practices fraud.

controllable risk factors—Risk factors a person can act upon to change.

cool-down—A series of activities to help the body recover after a workout, usually consisting of a heart cool-down and a muscle cool-down and stretch.

coordination—The ability to use the senses together with the body parts or to use two or more body parts together.

core exercises—Exercises that build the muscles of the trunk and that help the body maintain a good posture.

couch potato—A person who is sedentary or does no physical activity.

CRAC—An acronym for contract-relax-antagonist-contraction; it is one type of PNF exercise for improving flexibility.

creatine—A substance, stored in the muscles, that helps supply energy for muscle contraction and can be taken as a supplement or created by your own body.

criterion-referenced health standards—Fitness test ratings that are based on the amount of fitness necessary for good health rather than a comparison to other people.

D

dehydrated—Lacking the necessary amount of body fluid.

deltoid muscle—Muscle of the shoulder by which the arm is raised.

determinants—Factors that influence whether you will practice a healthy lifestyle such as physical activity; examples include the weather, your time schedule, and availability of facilities.

diabetes—A disease in which a person's body cannot regulate its sugar (glucose) level.

diastolic blood pressure—The force against the artery wall just before the heart beats; it is the lower of the two blood pressure numbers.

Dietary Guidelines—Recommendations developed by the U.S. Department of Agriculture for following healthful eating practices.

distress—Negative or unpleasant stress.

double progressive system—A method or system of resistance training that progressively increases (1) the amount of weight and (2) the number of repetitions used when performing an exercise.

DRI—An abbreviation for Dietary Reference Intakes, or standards for healthy eating.

E

eating disorders—Health problems that manifest themselves through starvation, eating binges followed by purging, or overeating.

electromyogram (EMG)—A test performed to determine the amount of activity in a muscle or muscle group.

ergogenic aid—A product used in an attempt to enhance performance, including some food supplements.

essential amino acid—One of the nine amino acids that the body needs to take in from food.

essential body fat—The minimum amount of body fat a person needs for good health.

eustress—Positive stress.

exercise—Physical activity done especially for the purpose of becoming physically fit.

F

fad diet—A nutritionally unbalanced diet that falsely promises quick weight loss.

fast-twitch muscle fibers—Muscle fibers that contract at a fast rate and have great strength but very little endurance.

fats—Nutrients that provide energy, help growth and repair of cells, and dissolve and carry certain vitamins to cells.

fiber—A type of indigestible carbohydrate.

fibrin—An elongated sticky cell in the blood that helps the blood clot; too much fibrin is implicated in the development of atherosclerosis.

fitness profile—A summary of the results of self-assessments of several different parts of fitness.

FITT formula—A formula in which each letter represents a factor important for determining the correct amount of physical activity: F = frequency; I = intensity; T = time; T = type.

flexibility—The ability to move the joints through a full range of motion; a part of fitness that requires long muscles.

flexor—A muscle that when contracted bends a joint in the body.

food label—The label on foods that provides information about the nutritional value of the food.

food supplement—A product intended to add to a person's nutrient consumption.

force—Energy that affects a body or causes one body to affect another (e.g., the energy of muscles results in movement of the legs and subsequent movement of the total body).

form—The placement of body parts during an exercise.

fraud—The practice of quackery with the intent of deceiving others for financial gain.

free time—Time left over when time for work, school, and other commitments has been accounted for.

frequency—How often physical activity is performed; part of the FITT formula.

frostbite—A condition that results when body tissues become frozen.

G

general adaptation syndrome—The series of phases the body goes through when it is exposed to stressors.

gluteal muscle—One of the muscles of the buttocks.

goal setting—A plan to determine ahead of time what you expect to accomplish and how you can accomplish it.

H

hamstring muscles—A muscle group located on the back of the thigh.

health—The state of optimal physical, mental, and social well-being.

health-related physical fitness—Parts of physical fitness that help a person stay healthy; includes cardiovascular fitness, flexibility, muscular endurance, strength, and body fatness.

heart attack—A sudden failure of the heart to function properly; occurs when the blood supply to the heart is decreased or blocked.

heart rate—The number of times the heart beats each minute.

heat index—A combination of temperature and humidity; a high heat index puts a person at risk of a heat-related injury.

heat exhaustion—A condition caused by excessive exposure to heat and characterized by cold, clammy skin, and symptoms of shock.

heatstroke—A condition caused by excessive exposure to heat and resulting in a high body temperature and dry skin.

heredity—Characteristics passed from parents to their offspring.

high-density lipoprotein (HDL)—A substance often referred to as good cholesterol because it carries excess cholesterol out of the bloodstream and into the liver for elimination from the body.

humidity— The amount of water vapor present in the air.

hyperkinetic conditions—Health problems caused by doing too much physical activity.

hypermobility—Range of motion that is in excess of what is considered healthy for a specific joint.

hypertension—A health problem in which blood pressure is too high for good health.

hyperthermia—Refers to an exceptionally high body temperature; may result from exercise in the heat.

hypertrophy—An increase in muscle size.

hypokinetic conditions—Health problems or illnesses that are caused partly by the lack of regular physical activity.

hypothermia—A condition often related to cold weather in which the body temperature becomes abnormally low.

I

incomplete proteins—Proteins containing some, but not all, of the essential amino acids.

intensity—How hard a person performs physical activity; part of the FITT formula.

intermediate muscle fibers—Muscle fibers having characteristics of both slow- and fast-twitch fibers.

interval training—Physical activity in which short bursts of high-intensity exercise are alternated with rest periods.

involuntary muscle—A muscle that a person cannot consciously control.

isokinetic exercise—An exercise for muscle fitness that regulates the resistance and/or speed of movement through a full range of joint movement.

isometric contraction—A muscle contraction in which no movement occurs because of an equal force in the opposite direction; the length of the muscle remains constant under tension.

isometric exercise—An exercise that involves isometric contractions in which body parts do not move.

isotonic contraction—A muscle contraction that pulls on the bones and produces movement of body parts.

isotonic exercise—An exercise that involves isotonic contractions and in which body parts move.

J

joint—A place in the body where bones come together.

joint laxity—Looseness of a joint resulting from overstretched ligaments; a condition that can lead to hypermobility and injury.

junk food—Food that is high in calories but low in nutritional value.

K

kyphosis—A posture problem characterized by rounded shoulders.

L

latissimus dorsi muscle—A large muscle attached to the back and arm.

laws of motion—Rules or principles that explain the movement of an object as a result of the application of force. They are derived primarily from Newton's three laws of motion and can be applied in a variety of physical activity and sport settings.

laxity—Looseness of the joints that allows the bones to move in ways other than intended.

leisure time—Also called discretionary time, it is time free from work and other commitments.

lifestyle—The way you live, including your typical behaviors.

lifetime sports—Sports that can be performed throughout life (as you grow older); often include individual sports such as golf and tennis.

ligament—A band of strong tissue that connects bones.

lipoproteins—Substances that carry cholesterol through the bloodstream.

long-term goals—Goals that you can expect to accomplish in several months or over the course of a year.

lordosis—A back condition characterized by too much arch in the lower back; sometimes called swayback.

low-density lipoprotein (LDL)—A substance often referred to as bad cholesterol because it carries cholesterol that is most likely to deposit in the arteries.

low-impact aerobic exercise—Exercise in which one foot contacts the floor at all times.

M

maturation—The process of becoming fully grown and developed physically.

MET—A term derived from the word *metabolism*; it is the amount of energy required to sustain life when you are resting—doing no physical activity.

micronutrients—Nutrients that are contained in foods in small amounts; vitamins and minerals.

microtrauma—An injury so small that it is often difficult to see or recognize, especially when it first occurs.

mineral—A nutrient that performs many functions in regulating the activities of cells.

moderate physical activity—Any type of exercise performed at an intensity equal to brisk walking.

motor skill—Another word for skill. "Motor" is used before the word "skill" because your "motor" nerves cause your muscles to contract when you perform a specific skill (see also **skill,** page 323).

muscle-bound—Having bulky muscles that decrease a person's flexibility.

muscle cramp—A spasm or sudden tightening of a muscle.

muscle fibers—Muscle cells, which are long, thin, and cylindrical.

muscular endurance—The ability to contract the muscles many times without tiring or to hold one contraction for a long time.

N

noncontrollable risk factors—Risk factors a person cannot change or control.

nutrient—A food substance required for the growth and maintenance of body cells.

nutrition—The study of foods and how they nourish the body.

nutritionally dense—Containing large amounts of nutrients for the number of calories provided.

O

obesity—The condition of being very overfat or having a very high percentage of body fat.

one repetition maximum (1RM)—The exertion that can be given by a muscle group when performing one repetition at a maximal level.

orienteering—A combination of walking, jogging, and map reading.

osteoporosis—A disease in which the bones deteriorate and become weak.

overfat—Having too much body fat,

overload—See *principle of overload.*

overuse injury—A body injury that occurs when a repeated movement causes wear and tear on the body.

P

PAR-Q—A questionnaire that helps you determine if you are physically and medically ready to participate in physical activity.

passive exercise—Being moved by a machine rather than using your own muscles to produce movement.

peak bone mass—A person's greatest bone mass, usually present when a person is young.

pectoral muscle—Muscle of the chest.

periodization—A method of scheduling progressive resistance exercise to provide variety and to enhance peak performance.

physical activity—Movement using the larger muscles of the body; includes sports, dance, and activities of daily life; may be done to accomplish a task, for enjoyment, or to improve physical fitness.

physical fitness—The ability of the body systems to work together efficiently.

physical skill—Specific physical task that a person performs.

plyometrics—A type of training designed to increase athletic performance using jumping and hopping and other exercises that cause lengthening of a muscle followed by a shortening contraction.

PNF stretching—A variation of static stretching that involves contracting a muscle before stretching it.

power—The ability to use strength quickly.

primary risk factor—A risk factor that is considered a major contributor to a disease.

principle of overload—A rule that states that in order to improve fitness, one needs to do more physical activity than one normally does.

principle of progression—A rule that states that the amount and intensity of physical activity needs to be increased gradually.

principle of specificity—A rule that states that specific types of exercise improve specific parts of fitness or specific muscles.

progressive resistance exercise (PRE)—The gradual increase in resistance used to improve muscle fitness.

protein—A nutrient that builds and repairs body cells.

ptosis—A posture problem characterized by a protruding abdomen.

pulse—The regular beating felt in the arteries; caused by contractions of the heart muscle.

Q

quack—Someone who practices quackery.

quackery—A method of advertising or selling that uses false claims to lure people into buying products that are worthless or even harmful.

quadriceps muscle—The muscle on the front of the thigh.

R

range of motion (ROM)—The amount of movement one can make in a joint.

range of motion (ROM) exercise—Flexibility exercise that is used to maintain the range of motion already present in the joints.

RDA—An abbreviation for Recommended Dietary Allowance, or the minimum amount of a nutrient needed for good health.

reaction time—The amount of time it takes a person to move once he or she realizes the need to act.

recreational activity—Form of exercise done during leisure time (free time) that is typically not classified as either sports or active aerobics.

registered dietitian—An expert in nutrition who is qualified to give advice about food and diet.

rehydrate—To drink liquids to replace those lost during physical activity.

relative strength—The amount of weight or resistance you can overcome for each pound of body weight (strength per pound of body weight).

repetitions—The number of consecutive times one does an exercise; usually referred to as reps.

reps—An abbreviation for repetitions; a term used to describe the number of consecutive times you perform an exercise.

resistance—A force that acts against the muscles.

resistance training—Exercises using resistance, in the form of free weights or machines, to develop muscular endurance or strength; also called weight training.

respiratory system—The body system including the lungs and air passages that functions by bringing oxygen into the bloodstream and eliminating carbon dioxide from the blood.

resting heart rate—The number of heartbeats during a period of inactivity.

RICE formula—A formula in which each letter represents a step in the treatment of a minor injury: R = rest; I = ice; C = compression; E = elevation.

risk factor—Anything that increases a person's chance of a health problem occurring.

RM—Repetition maximum; 1RM refers to the maximum amount of weight a group of muscles can lift at one time.

runner's high—The eustress people feel when they run or do exercise that they enjoy.

S

saturated fats—Fats that are solid at room temperature; found mostly in animal products.

sedentary—Being inactive or participating in very little physical activity.

self-management skills—Skills used by a person to take control of his or her lifestyle or behavior to stay physically active.

set—A group of repetitions of a specific exercise; each set of repetitions or reps is followed by a rest period before another is performed.

shinsplint—A pain in the front of the shins that is caused by overuse.

short-term goals—Goals that you can expect to accomplish in several days or weeks.

side stitch—A pain in the side of the lower abdomen that occurs as a result of vigorous activity.

simple carbohydrate—A nutrient found in sugars that can be used by the body for energy with little or no change during digestion.

skeletal muscle—Muscle that is attached to bones and makes movement possible.

skill—The capability for doing a specific task well; improves with practice.

skill-related physical fitness—Parts of fitness that help a person perform well in sports and activities requiring certain skills; includes agility, balance, coordination, power, reaction time, and speed.

skinfolds—Layers of fat under the skin that are measured to determine body fatness.

slow-twitch muscle fibers—Muscle fibers that contract at a slow rate and have great endurance.

smooth muscles—Muscles that make up the walls of internal organs such as the stomach and blood vessels.

spa—Originally a name for an establishment that had mineral baths thought to be health-enhancing. Some modern spas have saunas and whirlpool baths and provide other services, such as hair and skin care and massage.

speed—The ability to perform a movement or cover a distance in a short time.

sport skill—A specific skill necessary to succeed in sports; examples include throwing, catching, batting, kicking, and swinging a racket or club.

sport supplement—A product sold to enhance athletic performance.

sports—Activities that generally are done competitively and have well-established rules.

sprain—An injury to ligaments.

stage of exhaustion—The third stage of the general adaptation syndrome; occurs when the body is not able to resist a stressor and medical treatment is necessary.

stage of resistance—The second stage of the general adaptation syndrome; occurs when the body and its immune system start to resist or fight a stressor.

static stretching—Stretching slowly as far as possible without pain.

strain—An injury to a tendon or muscle.

strength—The amount of force a muscle can produce.

stress—The body's reaction to demanding situations.

stress response—The body's way of preparing a person to deal with demanding situations.

stressor—Something that causes or contributes to stress.

stretching exercise—Flexibility exercise that works to increase the range of motion by stretching farther than the current range of motion.

stroke—An injury to the brain that occurs when the blood supply to the brain is severely reduced or shut off, often as a result of a blood clot or other obstruction.

systolic blood pressure—The force against the artery wall just after the heart beats; it is the higher of the two blood pressure numbers.

T

target ceiling—A person's upper limit of physical activity.

target fitness zone—The correct range of physical activity to build fitness.

target weight—The weight at which a person has a healthy amount of body fat.

tendon—A band of strong tissue that connects a muscle to a bone.

threshold of training—The minimum amount of overload one needs to build physical fitness.

time—How long a person does physical activity; part of the FITT formula.

transfatty acids—Unsaturated fats that have been converted to a solid form similar to saturated fats.

triceps muscle—A muscle located on the back of the upper arm.

type— The kind of activity you do to build a specific part of fitness or to gain a specific benefit; part of the FITT formula.

U

UL—An abbreviation for Tolerable Upper Limit, or the maximum daily amount of a nutrient that can be consumed without health risk.

underfat—Having too little body fat.

underwater weighing—A technique used to assess body fat levels in which a person is immersed in water and then weighed.

unsaturated fats—Fats, such as vegetable oils, that are in liquid form at room temperature.

V

vein—A blood vessel that carries blood filled with waste products from the body cells back to the heart.

vitamin—A nutrient needed for growth and repair of body cells.

voluntary muscle—Muscle over which a person has conscious control.

W

warm-up—A series of activities, usually consisting of a heart warm-up and a muscle warm-up and stretch, that prepares the body for more vigorous exercise and helps prevent injury.

weight training—The lifting of weights to build strength; also called resistance training.

wellness—A state of being that enables a person to reach his or her highest potential; includes intellectual, social, emotional, physical, and spiritual health.

windchill factor—A combination of wind and temperature; a high windchill factor puts a person at high risk of hypothermia and frostbite.

workout—The part of the physical activity program during which a person does activities to improve fitness.

index

Note: The italicized *t* following page numbers refers to tables.

A

abdominal exercise 198. *See also* curl-ups
active aerobics 119-121, 126, 131, 142, 257*t*-258
active recreation 124-127, 231
ACTIVITYGRAM 65, 113, 305
activity logs 112, 113
activity neurosis 47
aerobic activity 63, 64, 110, 119, 231
aerobic dance 102, 119-120, 135*t*, 231*t*, 257*t*-258
age 67, 69, 221
agility 13, 19, 135*t*, 137, 141*t*
amino acids 244
anabolic steroids 33, 209
anaerobic activity 111-112
androstenedione 210
ankle flex 160
anorexia athletica 224
anorexia nervosa 223-224
appearance 5-6
arm and leg lift 57
arm curl 87
arm lift 159
arm pinch 18
arm press 88
arm pretzel 170
arm stretch 171
arteries 103, 104
atherosclerosis 43, 104
attitudes 79*t*, 95-98, 312*t*

B

back exercise circuit 55-57
back extension exercise 197, 240
back flattener 272
back problems 51
back-saver hamstring stretch 40
back-saver sit and reach 81, 82*t*, 167
Back Test, Healthy 48-50*t*
back to wall 50
backward hop 19
balance 13, 19, 135*t*, 138, 141*t*
ballistic stretching 163, 164*t*, 167
bench press 193, 236
bench step 73
bent arm hang 206
bent over dumbbell row 197
biceps curl 195, 237
biceps curl with towel 274
bicycling 120, 124, 126, 135*t*, 231*t*, 287
biomechanical principles 33-34
blood 104, 105*t*
blood pressure 44, 45
body board 301
bodybuilding 179
body composition 81-82*t*, 220-233, 241, 265, 306*t*
body dysmorphia 186-187
body fat 13, 18, 221-223, 229-233
body fat assessment 224-228*t*, 249-250*t*
body image disorder 47
body mass index 81-82*t*, 224-225
body measurements 224, 249-250*t*
bow exercise 275
bridging 215
bulimia 224

C

calcium 245*t*, 251
calf stretch 172
calories 93, 99*t*, 222, 229, 230-232, 243, 248*t*, 251-252, 253, 254, 257*t*
cancer 45
carbohydrates 243-244, 252
cardiovascular diseases 43-45, 53
cardiovascular fitness 12, 17, 103-112, 114*t*-117, 122, 123*t*, 282, 306*t*
cardiovascular fitness, self-assessment 108*t*-109*t*, 123*t*, 282
chapter reviews 21, 41, 58, 75, 89, 100, 117, 131, 150, 173, 199, 218, 241, 259, 276, 291, 303, 317
chest stretch 171
cholesterol 104, 105*t*, 244, 252, 253
circuit training 72-74*t*, 120, 135*t*, 203
clothing 24, 25-27, 34, 267-268
coin catch 20
conflict recognition and resolution, in planning 315
conflict recognition and resolution, in sport 147
conflict recognition and resolution, in the weight room 191
conflict recognition and resolution, new activities 38
conflict resolution, controlling emotions 147
conflict resolution, negotiation guidelines 147
conflict resolution, rules 191
Continuous Rhythmical Exercise (CRE) 260
cool-down 6, 11, 28
Cooper, Dr. Ken 63, 120, 278
Cooper's aerobics 278
cooperative aerobics 257*t*-258
cooperative games 42
coordination 13, 20, 135*t*, 139, 141*t*
core exercises 207-208
couch potatoes 77, 311*t*, 312*t*
creatine 210
cultural differences 95-97
Cureton, Dr. Thomas 260
curl-ups 29-30*t*, 39, 49, 55, 56, 73, 198, 240
curl-up with twist 216
Cycle of Physical Activity Benefits 5

D

dance 120-121, 135*t*, 231*t*
Delayed Onset Muscle Soreness (DOMS) 34
depression 46
diabetes 13, 45-46, 47, 221
diet 222, 229-233, 243-248, 251-256, 259, 262-263, 264, 286, 298
double-ball bounce 20
double heel click 19
double-leg lift 56
dual-energy X-ray absorptiometry (DEXA) 224

E

eating disorders 47, 223-224
elastic band exercise circuit 87-88
ephedra 210, 263
ergogenic aids 209-211, 263
ethnic groups 79, 121

exercise balls 207
exercise basics, self-assessment 7-11
exercise circuit 220. *See also* circuit training
exercise program planning 305-317
exercise videos 268-269
exercising at home 304

F

fad diets 263
family 128
    activity 128
    heredity 69
    interests 128
    risk factors 53
    tradition 265
fats 243, 244, 247-248, 252, 253
fiber 243-244
FIT formula 92*t*, 111*t*, 163, 164*t*, 188*t*, 202*t*, 230*t*, 251*t*
fitness 3-6, 12-15, 21, 67-70, 133-141*t*
fitness games 22
fitness goals 83-86, 307, 308
FITNESSGRAM 28, 29, 81-82*t*, 122-123*t*, 265, 317
fitness profile 305*t*, 306
fitness stunts 17-20, 137-141*t*
fitness trail 76
FITT formula 62
flexibility 13, 17, 63, 64, 154-165, 167-173, 232, 265, 306*t*
flexibility, self-assessment 81, 82*t*, 122*t*, 159*t*-161
flexibility exercise circuit 167-172
followers 146
food labels 251-253
food myths 253-254
food supplements 209, 210-211, 254, 262-263
force 53
Frisbee golf 292
frostbite 25, 26

G

gender 79, 121
general adaptation syndrome 293
goal setting 79*t*, 83-86, 307, 308, 313*t*
GPS (global positioning systems) technology 120
grip strength 184*t*

H

half squat 194
hamstring curl 195, 237
hand push 272
health and wellness 279-281, 283*t*-284
health clubs 266-267, 290
health-related physical fitness 12-13
Healthy Back Test 48-50
healthy lifestyles 285-288
Healthy People 2010 1, 5, 46, 59, 101, 153, 219, 246, 260, 279, 280, 286
heart 103-104, 105*t*, 106
heart attacks 43-44
heart disease 13, 43-45, 53
heart rate 9-11, 106, 111, 114*t*-116
heart warm-up 7, 27-28
heat exhaustion 24